ART THERAPY
VIEWPOINTS

ART THERAPY VIEWPOINTS

Elinor Ulman and
Claire A. Levy, Editors

Schocken Books · New York

To Bernie

First published by SCHOCKEN BOOKS 1980
10 9 8 7 6 5 4 3 2 1   80 81 82 83

Library of Congress Cataloging in Publication Data
Main entry under title:

Art therapy viewpoints.

Articles originally appeared in the American journal
of art therapy.
Bibliography: p.
Includes Index.
1. Art therapy—Addresses, essays, lectures.
I. Ulman, Elinor. II. Levy, Claire A. III. American
journal of art therapy.
RC489.A7A784   616.8'916'5   79–26087

Manufactured in the United States of America

Contents

*Numbers in parentheses following titles indicate volume and issue of the *Bulletin of Art Therapy* (Volumes 1–13) or the *American Journal of Art Therapy* (Volumes 14–18) in which the articles originally appeared.

Introduction

This collection of articles brings together in a more permanent and accessible form articles which first appeared in the *American Journal of Art Therapy*. An earlier collection, *Art Therapy in Theory and Practice*, has proved so useful that the editors undertook the present volume.

In making preliminary selections, quality of thinking and of presentation was our main criterion. After the selected articles had been sorted into appropriate groups, we were pleased but not surprised to find that, taken together, they constitute a substantial contribution to art therapy theory and to accounts of practice covering both new developments and the application of methods whose soundness has long been demonstrated. Thus this collection reflects the state of art therapy today: the field has expanded, and techniques have been introduced or modified to meet new needs; ways of working developed earlier have in some instances been refined, but they have not been superseded. We therefore have reason to believe that *Art Therapy Viewpoints* can serve as an introduction to the field for those newly interested in it and at the same time can meet the needs of students and practitioners of art therapy. The inclusion of a cross-referenced index combining content, authors, and titles makes this book readily usable as a text and as a reference work.

The book opens with a section on theory. The first article presents a symposium that seeks to broaden the conceptual basis for art therapy while setting needed limits to a field whose boundaries tend to be blurred. Also in this section, the basic ideas of earlier theoreticians such as Kramer and Ulman are further clarified, and their voices are joined by a number of new ones. For example, Brian Halsey presents a study of Freud's ideas about art (page 85), Bernard I. Levy discusses fact and fantasy concerning the bicameral mind and explains its significance for art therapy (page 32), and Laurie Wilson generalizes from careful observation of the artwork of a single mentally retarded client (page 47).

Turning from theory to practice, we outline briefly the older tradition of art therapy, sketch some newer trends, and cite articles with special relevance in these various areas. We do not, of course, mean to imply that any article is directed exclusively to one issue or another. Rather, we point to intricately interwoven threads.

In their early struggles for recognition, art therapists tended to define their field as a form of psychotherapy. Art therapy might be viewed as an independent or as an auxiliary mode of treatment, and therapy might be seen as residing primarily either in the artistic process or in verbally formulated insights based on art works. Whether people were seen individually or in groups, the focus was usually on individual psychodynamics rather than group dynamics. In *Art Therapy Viewpoints* some articles falling largely within this frame of reference are found in the section on the "Practice of Art Therapy with Adults," for example, Teller's article (page 138) and that by Lachman, Stuntz, and Jones (page 153). Meyerhoff's account of her work with two children reflects a similar approach (page 214).

When we consider recent shifts of emphasis in the art therapy field, we find that the purposeful use of art in the service of socialization has received a fresh impetus. This new development has old roots. Art therapists early recognized that art therapy groups provide special opportunities for social contact. Group members unable to approach each other directly have been seen to form relationships more readily through art works that were (because of the intrinsic nature of art) subtle, intimate self-representations. Out of such experience, in combination with recent developments in the theory of group dynamics and the practice of group therapy, *group art therapy* has developed in day hospitals and even in closed psychiatric wards. In addition, the increasing use of art therapy in a wide variety of nonpsychiatric settings—such as centers for the rehabilitation of people with substance abuse problems, residential and day-care facilities for old people and for the mentally retarded, and special schools and special education classes in regular schools—has further led art therapists to focus their skills on efforts to increase clients' awareness of one another. Zeiger's article on work with old people in a residential setting (page 187), the account by a group of students of their experience while engaged in the study of art therapy (page 121), and Geller's vivid case study (page 249) are examples suggesting the potency of art as a factor in the formation of relationships among peers.

Another aspect of art therapy receiving increased emphasis in recent years may be broadly termed educational. Cognitive skills that have never been acquired because of developmental deficiencies, or that have been lost for a variety of reasons, may be gained or recovered through specially designed procedures leading to experience of the art process. The contributions of Gitter (page 232) and Gonick-Barris (page 197) are related to this focus.

A third recent trend is the use of art experience in short-term groups of reasonably well-functioning individuals. Concepts and techniques originally developed in therapeutic work are here used as a source of inspiration and to sensitize members of the various human service professions to the potential usefulness of art to their clientele. Rhyne's contribution (page 6) to the book's first article may be looked upon as providing a theoretical basis for such applications of the art therapist's skills.

In further reviewing our selections, which include a number of articles from the *Journal*'s early years, we were gratified to find that much that has appeared in the *Journal* has stood the test of time. The oldest article, a research report by Rebecca Crane (page 358), dates back to 1962, having been published in the *Journal*'s first volume. It is a good example of the freshness and lasting value of the older material we decided to include. It describes unusually well-designed research in an area that is of vital interest to art therapists and that has been little explored even to this day.

Speaking in a more general sense, we are glad to have the chance to strike a blow against the false notion that newer is per se better in the worlds of both theory and practice. Of course there is ground for hope that *technologies* will improve, but artists—of all people—should be proof against unthinking belief in progress as a general law of life. Edith Kramer points out that art therapy "partakes in *art*, which is timeless and in *therapy*, which grows and changes." She goes on to say, "In art we strive for perfection. . . . Art does not evolve or improve over the centuries. . . . There is change, there is rise and decline, but progress there is not" (unpublished speech delivered at the Second Annual Conference of the American Art Therapy Association, Milwaukee, Wisconsin, September 16–18, 1971).

In addressing art therapists as artists, we are, perhaps, wishful; we hope that *Art Therapy Viewpoints* will help strengthen the place of *art* in art therapy. Here we touch on an issue that for more than two decades has been a source of controversy among art therapists. In speaking of the field's early history, we mentioned a division between art therapists who emphasized the healing quality of art and those who pressed for verbal interpretation as the key element in therapy. These divergent emphases need not become polarized, but they often do.

When we identify ourselves as advocates of *art*, we mean art in its most general sense, not art watered down for the disabled and certainly not art subverted for any purpose whatsoever. Thus we find it regrettable that some art therapists give up too easily the attempt to elicit from their clients genuine art expression at however humble a level, are too ready to offer easy substitutes. Others deliberately sacrifice the development of art expression for the sake of gathering endless quantities of diagnostic material, and still others actually discourage engagement in the full artistic process in order to push for verbal descriptions of feeling states and for the translation of visual statements into verbal ones.

Nevertheless it should be apparent to readers of *Art Therapy Viewpoints* that our allegiance to art does not exclude from the realm of art therapy a great deal of art work that fails to reach the full status of art. We also appreciate the great usefulness of art in personality assessment, as well as the important part that verbally expressed insights sometimes play in art therapy. But in our view *art* remains the art therapist's unique medium. It is art therapy's justification for being an independent discipline. Though such issues are not directly addressed in the pages of *Art Therapy Viewpoints*, we believe that collectively these articles by many authors support a rich synthesis that stands above partisanship, that is broadly comprehensive yet avoids the pitfalls of a shallow eclecticism.

Edith Kramer and Bernard I. Levy, Ph.D., took part in the preliminary screening of articles and made invaluable contributions to the development of ideas for this Introduction. Dr. Levy also helped with the very difficult task of deciding which articles to eliminate because of the inescapable limits of space imposed by economic considerations. The editors are grateful to these two colleagues for their help.

Elinor Ulman and Claire A. Levy

PART ONE

ART THERAPY THEORY AND PROFESSIONAL ISSUES

Symposium: Integration of Divergent Points of View in Art Therapy

Bernard I. Levy, Edith Kramer, Hanna Yaxa Kwiatkowska, Mildred Lachman, Janie Rhyne, and Elinor Ulman

Introduction

Bernard I. Levy: We are pleased to offer our thoughts on an issue close to all of us: attempting to define our discipline. To do so we will suggest what the outer limits of art therapy ought to be. We hope some of you share our ideas, but more than that we hope our ideas give rise to debate. It is not lost on us that this symposium initiates the professional-scientific segment of the Association's Fifth Annual Convention.[1] Accordingly, we hope that our ideas are provocative and the discussion lively.

Our title, "Integration of Divergent Points of View in Art Therapy," was provided us quite early in the development of the session. As we discussed our interests, it became obvious that the proffered title did not describe our task as we saw it. While divergent viewpoints can be "integrated" as a conceptual act and even rationalized with an eclectic philosophy, the rationale must not be so broad as to espouse laissez-faire. Integration of divergence need not mean that "anything goes." The best title for our symposium might be the question: "Are there limits to art therapy?" We feel there are.

What brings me together with the other participants—Edith Kramer, Hanna Yaxa Kwiatkowska, Mildred Lachman, Janie Rhyne, and Elinor Ulman—is not that I teach with four of them—Kramer, Kwiatkowska, Lachman, and Ulman—and work with Rhyne on the AATA Research Committee, but that all of us are involved in training candidates and formulating basic concepts for this new field of ours.

My task will be to set the stage for our presentation. The order of the other speakers, determined according to the logic of the content, and their topics are as follows: Ulman, "Innovation and Aberration"; Rhyne, "Divergency

1. American Art Therapy Association, New York City, October 24–27, 1974.

and Growth in Art Therapy"; Kramer, "The Unity of Process and Product"; Lachman, "A Partnership with Other Expressive Arts"; Kwiatkowska, "Technique Versus Techniques."

Sixteen years ago Kramer marshaled us against the invasion of anti-art, or crap-crafts, and it's-all-done-you-just-finish-it painting. We seem to have withstood that assault from without. Today art therapy finds itself menaced from within—menaced by ideas and practices that have little to do with art or therapy, much less with art therapy. Last year's AATA convention provided an array of alarming notions put forward to the unwary under the auspices of our national association. Reviewing papers submitted to the *American Journal of Art Therapy*, I came upon other cautionary examples.

Everybody on the platform shares a belief in the transcendent value of expressive art and its central place in art therapy. Art therapy focuses on the use of art materials to serve the patient's own expressive needs and eschews the manufacture of an arty bag of tricks. The panelists will elaborate briefly on what expressive art is and on its value to the individual and to the therapeutic process. Among major points to be emphasized will be the following:

1. Art therapy is a unique enterprise, distinct from both verbal psycho-therapy and activity group therapy. Art therapy must not be regarded as a back door into the practice of other forms of psychotherapy.

2. A corollary of the assertion that art therapy is a unique entity is that art therapy must develop its own body of knowledge expressed in its own literature if the profession is to expand and to achieve a sense of its own identity. A beginning has been made by Naumburg, by all the distinguished art therapists on the platform, by authors of recently published books (Betensky, Lyddiatt, Joseph), and many others. But this aspect of our enterprise is menaced by those who insist again and again on inventing art therapy anew, denying (rather than building upon and improving) the fairly recent but exceedingly vital beginnings of an intellectual tradition and body of practical experience.

Innovation and Aberration

Elinor Ulman: Art therapy legitimately covers a range of activities that at the peripheries verge on psychotherapy on one hand and on art education on the other. Essential to art therapy is that it partake of both art and therapy. For this purpose these terms may be briefly defined as follows: *Art* is the meeting ground of the inner and outer worlds as experienced by human individuals. *Therapy* aims at favorable change in personality or in living that endures beyond the therapeutic session itself.

These definitions exclude from art therapy recreational uses of art materials that aim at only momentary distraction at best and, at worst, at so-called success experiences intended to deceive both the executor of a prefabricated design and his audience into believing that he has created something. Also excluded is art training aimed primarily at developing the skills of people who hope to become artists—that is, who want to learn to create products that will be prized by a broad public as works of art.

These distinctions are the ones it seemed urgent to make a dozen years ago, and they are still valid and must still be borne in mind. However, today's battle to preserve both the *art* and the *therapy* in art therapy must meet new threats, some of which come from within the expanding profession of art therapy itself.

There are a number of current practices that may legitimately serve in art therapy as an entering wedge, but no more. Among these is the kind of "collage" that consists of the assemblage of ready-made pictorial matter. This can be useful so long as it is not thought of as a substitute for the actual artistic process.

Other fashionable procedures may have merit if they are presented to an individual in order to meet his needs at a given moment, but used routinely they offer less chance for real experience and personal interpretation of experience than did the traditional still life. One such procedure is the command to put into graphic form prefabricated imaginary experience. Of even more dubious merit is the occasional deliberate incitement, in the name of therapy, to acting-out with art materials. We may also ask whether art can be wedded to operant conditioning and survive. Can you work for tokens to be traded for Cokes and work to satisfy internal needs at the same time?

A popular and potentially destructive trend is the use of art materials in a variety of artificial ways to promote almost any kind of interaction among members of a group. In some instances we almost arrive at a sort of group play-therapy for grown-ups. For example, art materials may be used to turn out perfunctory symbols which are then manipulated in something like psychodrama, where homemade surrogates take the place of human beings. Too often, forced collaboration is emphasized; the aim is to promote togetherness by doing *anything* with art materials so long as it is not done alone. When this occurs, there is, at worst, a sort of grading of participants on the basis of how "cooperative" they are; at best some attention is paid to group dynamics as evidenced in an interaction that might be more appropriately carried out in a soccer match or preparing for a picnic—any activity that by its very nature demands the simultaneous participation of more than one person.

It is true that, through the manipulation of art materials with some expressive intent, people working in a group may easily be goaded into displays of competitiveness, domination, submission, passive-aggression —or even kindness, consideration, and loving helpfulness. They will demonstrate whatever is their characteristic mode of response. But this way of using art materials may be a needless, confusing, destructive prostitution of a medium that would better be reserved for what it and it alone is good for.

The social ramifications of the artistic process, among those who are trying to alleviate emotional distress as among those for whom art is a lifework, are complex and infinitely varied. But these valuable and subtle exchanges between persons presuppose the act of creation itself, and that is a *solitary* act. Even for those miracles of communication that span generations or centuries, the first audience is an audience of one—the artist himself.

Wherever he places himself between the poles of art education and psychotherapy, the art therapist's basic task is at the same time both utterly simple and infinitely complex: that is, to help people bring out from within themselves a source of motivation—the wish to organize their experience of their inner and outer worlds into a coherent form. Too many art therapists lack the faith that most people have the power to carry out this wish or perhaps some art therapists fail to recognize the many levels at which the wish for formed expression may be carried out.

Perhaps the quality most needed by the art therapist is courage. The frantic effort to plan elaborate art therapy procedures reflects the therapist's timidity, his need to attempt the impossible—that is, to chart in advance a voyage of discovery.

Divergency and Growth in Art Therapy

Janie Rhyne: When we speak of integrating divergent viewpoints in art therapy, we must each have some idea of what we consider to be the boundaries of art and what sort of activity we would label as therapy. Probably our views diverge quite a bit even in the definition of the terms *art* and *therapy*. This is not at all surprising; coming from many different backgrounds it is natural that we would view the scene of art therapy with selected perceptions consistent with our experiences, education, and personal attitudes. We have entered the relatively new profession of art therapy through many doors. Now that we are inside, how are we to arrange ourselves to use our space most constructively? There are people outside who'd like to come in; there are even some people inside whom some other people would like out.

I don't know any way to get us all to agree on a definition of what art therapy is or should be; I don't think that's even desirable. I do know, though, that integration in an organization is like integration in a personality: the more we understand the divergences that take us in different directions, the better we are able to choose what courses are wise and what are foolish.

Since integration of divergent points of view in art therapy implies understanding, I'll speak from here on about the kind of therapeutic approach I know best.

I presume that all art therapists, in addition to their artistry, function with some sort of theoretical psychological orientation to guide them. Of the three main schools of psychology—the psychoanalytic, the behavioristic, and the humanistic—I know most about the humanistic. Of course, all psychology is humanistic—or certainly should be—but psychologists and therapists who stress the humanistic orientation are more interested in exploring human potentials than they are in establishing institutions to explain and systematize the limits of human performance.

The big umbrella of this human-potentials movement—the third force in psychology—shelters a lot of diversity: existentialists, phenomenologists, mystics, Eastern philosophers—many views of the human venture. Among these is a gestalt philosophy and mode of therapy. Gestalt at its best fosters creative change and especially clear awareness of responsibilities. At its worst gestalt therapy is used as a catchall for a mishmash of "if-it-feels-good-do-it" messing around. This kind of sensation-seeking therapy is often presumed to be the norm in California.

I come from California. The encounter and personal growth movement also is considered to have traveled from California. Sometimes I feel really loaded down, being asked to justify all the kooky things people do when they get together in groups and throw paint around in the West, the East, and in the Midwest. I can't and won't even attempt to defend some of the silly, irresponsible, and sometimes dangerous things some people do in the name of art experience. I can and do say that working within the personal growth movement are many responsible people who have high regard for both art and therapy and practice conscientiously according to their belief systems of how art, in its many manifestations, can be an agent for beneficial change. Abraham Maslow, one of the humanistic movement's most honored fathers, was dedicated to an optimistic view of man's potential. His belief, based on many years of experience as a psychotherapist, was that we seek self-actualization and that the human self is by nature endowed with a patterning that guides toward healthy growth. Just as an acorn has within it the imprint of the oak tree, so the person is born with a pattern of potentials that *can* be grown into. But again, just as most acorns don't find a good place to grow and can't make it, most people don't find the best kind of conditions in this world either. Growing into one's full potential is not easy and probably none of us ever makes it. But the best of the personal growth movement hopes to provide experiences that will add some new possibilities of healthy growth.

Neither art nor therapy has provided us humans with enough nourishment to keep us from often being stunted and warped, but they are—separate and together—one of the many ways humankind has discovered to encourage a bit of leafing out. Both art and therapy are humanly created approaches to help us on our way to becoming the best that we can be. Both are subject to the needs of human development. As these needs evolve and change, art and therapy must recognize the changes and meet them.

Art therapy can meet many needs in many ways, depending upon the clients, the therapists, and the viewpoints of both of them. Neither the kind of art nor the kind of therapy is nearly as important as the kind of human qualities that are encouraged and sustained. In California the encounter-with-art is now directed more toward meditation than toward orgy. Jungian art therapists are active and respected; psychosynthesis uses art for centering; Tibetan Buddhists use it as a discipline. Gestalt art therapists focus on increasing awareness of individuals in a here/now environment. All of these aim toward creative therapy.

Art therapy, no matter how divergent may be its philosophies, has something rather special to offer. If I didn't believe that, I would never have gone into this business.

The Unity of Process and Product

Edith Kramer: Oversimplification and imprecision in our thinking that may seem negligible in themselves are apt to have far-reaching consequences. Half-truths entering our vocabulary and thereby our thinking ultimately influence the practice of art therapy and lead us astray.

I want to address myself to one such oversimplification and its consequences: the dictum "Art *teaching* is concerned with products, but in art *therapy* we are interested in processes." This implies a dichotomy of product and process. But in art, product and process are one. Whenever we judge that a product which serves no practical use but which constitutes an equivalent for experience has the quality of art, we imply that it has evocative power and inner consistency; that the medium has been used with skill and economy; that form and content are one, and conscious and unconscious meaning complement one another; the work lacks nothing and contains nothing superfluous. Either taking away or adding would diminish its quality.

Work of such profound inner unity cannot be planned, plotted, or faked. It can come about only through complex processes which engage the creator's manual, intellectual, imaginative, and emotional faculties in a supreme effort of integration. Surely all persons engaged in art in any capacity, be it as artists, art teachers, or art therapists, hope for this miracle, which we cannot force but for which we can prepare the way and set the stage.

What then are the reasons for stressing processes and denying interest in products? In part we may be reacting against the rampant malpractice of plotting for products, using methods that circumvent the creative process and replace it with prescribed procedures which, if followed obediently, will result in pseudo-products that can create the illusion of art. Much of art education and most of art in recreation subsists on such practices.

Students and patients who have been subjected to this kind of instruction need to be exhorted to forget about manufacturing products. To prevent their futile striving for a kind of preconceived perfection that is both guaranteed impersonal and guaranteed bad art, we assure them that we do not care what their work looks like. We implore them to put their ideas down any old way, to have courage to be *spontaneous*. Further, as art therapists we accept the fragmented, the chaotic, the abortive, the incomplete. We expect to assist in many processes that fail to culminate in art. Our interest in understanding such processes and working with them is indeed more keen than is the art teacher's interest in his student's incomplete efforts. It is also common knowledge that adults, whether or not their ideas about art are valid, must often be urged temporarily to suspend critical judgment, for excessive preoccupation with the final goal of artwork actually stands in the way of its achievement.

We are in trouble when we are taken in by our own propaganda and end up believing that we *really* do not care what the patient's work looks like; when, devising exercises to counteract rigidity and alleviate anxiety, we end up plotting activities that are so contrived that it would be *impossible* to achieve any finished product; when, having lost confidence in the art material's power to stimulate the desire to give form, we invent games and gambits that encroach on the patient's autonomy and smother his initiative as effectively as any stereotyped arts and crafts project; when, in order to induce "spontaneity," we encourage chaotic manipulation of art materials.

This leads me to another widespread error in thinking, an error which is twofold. First, there is the inclination to confound undisciplined, aimless manipulation of art materials with spontaneity. Actually, spontaneous art expression requires that one imagine and depict what is uppermost in one's mind, and this demands both the suspension of habitual defense and a high degree of moral courage and self-discipline. Untrammeled scribbling and messing are as unlike spontaneous, expressive use of art materials (and as unlikely to lead to it) as aimless chatter is unlike free association in psychoanalytic treatment.

Second, there is the erroneous belief that art therapy is concerned almost exclusively with spontaneous art expression—that is, with the use of art media that evokes the raw material of art but inevitably stops short of art as I have defined it. Such spontaneous production is invaluable in gaining access to the patient's inner life and therefore is a legitimate part of art therapy, but it is by no means the whole of it. Art therapy includes, as well, the task of integration. At best, this is a labor of love, but all the same it is arduous, not spontaneous.

This brings us back to the false dichotomy of process and product. When concentration on process results in systematic neglect of or disrespect for its natural culmination—the product—the patient is deprived both of his goal and of the reward for his labors. The processes that are fostered in such incomplete endeavors must remain primitive and abortive and thus they cannot serve as models of healthy functioning.

A Partnership with Other Expressive Arts

Mildred Lachman: My work has involved me very much with groups and group techniques. I've used art therapy along with other expressive media, such as movement; and I work as part of an interdisciplinary team. It has become very important for me to think through with clarity and conviction how to define what I do. Otherwise there may be a muddle; something may get lost, and it might just be my own sense of myself as an art therapist.

Take group art therapy. We are working here with two powerful therapeutic elements: group dynamics and creative graphic expression. You can structure your activity so that one element serves the other primarily. If your therapeutic focus is primarily on the group, art will tend to be used as a pictograph, a means of symbolic communication between group members. In that event, group members are likely not to be encouraged to spend the time and effort to make the best product they can. Many kinds of art-connected activities can be pursued with the clear purpose of fostering group interaction and study. I have worked this way, and with considerable success, too. But then I have to know that I am functioning primarily as a group therapist and secondarily as an art therapist.

Done the other way around, with the focus on the making of an art product, the structure of the group is quite different. Group members inevitably interact. One can focus on the interaction more or less—as when it prevents an individual member's achievement or when it enhances it. The result is something in the nature of a teaching and learning atmosphere, where creating something highly meaningful and personal is encouraged and the experience is shared. But concentration on personal interaction is avoided. Good art classes can be like this.

Somewhere in between it is possible to fuse the two—to lead an art therapy group where art is fostered and group dynamics are attended to. It is important, though, to be clear about the two elements, to know when you are making one element serve the other, and most important, whether you are using yourself as an art therapist or as a therapist who uses art tricks.

This brings me to activity groups. They are fine, especially for children. Here the participants busy themselves productively, often with materials which include art equipment; and the way they go about using the materials and relating to group members and to therapists is where the focus is. Is this art therapy? Not necessarily. For what is intrinsic to art therapy groups with children is the seriousness of intent and respect for the personal quality of the production. You let the group member know (perhaps in individual interviews beforehand) that what he makes will be—let us say—framed, that you will look at it in a special way as something coming from deep within his inner world. You expect him to take it seriously too. Activities primarily aimed at keeping the participant busy, fostering interaction, or revealing transference are not what you are after, and you can communicate this immediately if you are sure of where *you* stand.

This often means using a minimum of basic art materials rather than diffusing creative expression in exploration of various media.

Now what about using other expressive modalities along with art? I have presented workshops and written about the use of movement in art therapy and have thought through for myself some of the issues. I believe that one modality should be subordinated to another. We can use movement, say, to facilitate and further the artwork. Our own expertise is in visual imagery. Movement is a powerful means of communication, more primitive and regressive than visual imagery. It can be used carefully in your work as an art therapist. But I have too much respect for the complexity and power of movement (having been a dancer myself) to think that untrained people can presume to make full use of movement therapeutically. So, if your patient responds better to movement than to graphic art, consider sending him to a movement therapist.

The developing child goes through a progression of means of representation—kinesthetics, imagery, and finally language. It helps us to know this and to lead our patients into a flexible use of all three. But it is specifically with visual imagery that we can work with confidence. We'd best know our limitations, value what we do best, and enlist the other therapeutic modalities to serve us. Otherwise we might get into some washed-out, touchy-feeling thing or a romantic muddle.

In working with therapists from other disciplines, the same issues of professional identity and conviction arise. It is essential to communicate to your co-worker what you are doing and a sense of its meaning and value. If you don't, you run the risk of having your program watered down or downright sabotaged. To begin with, it's almost indispensable that your co-worker really get into it and work with the art materials himself. But most important, you must have arrived at a clear idea of your own function and limits and have a deep respect for this identity. Having done so, you will have gone a long way toward settling some of the issues that can be troublesome when therapists from several disciplines work together.

Technique Versus Techniques

Hanna Yaxa Kwiatkowska: I shall begin by relating to you my several-years-long fight about the letter *S*. I see astonishment on your faces, so let me explain. My fight is with The George Washington University academic editor responsible for the catalogue announcing our courses.

One of the courses I teach is consistently listed as "Technique*s* of Art Therapy," whereas I insist on its being "Technique of Art Therapy." The editor refuses to understand.

My strong conviction is that *the only technique of art therapy is the technique of relating to a patient through art.* Let us now think of why we are faced with the explosion of such a number of technical maneuvers in art therapy.

Each of us experiences anxiety before a therapy session. Will the patient respond? Will I be able to establish contact with him? Will I understand his needs? Will I be able to bear his negativism or hostility or, even worse, his refusal to handle any of the media I have so carefully prepared and am so temptingly offering him? Even when many years of experience make us aware that we can rarely expect immediate therapeutic success or even productivity from our patients, it is difficult to accept having nothing happen in the whole session or in a number of sessions. This feeling is even more intolerable for the beginner in the art therapy field, who often is inclined to think, "If the patient does not produce, then I have failed." This feeling results in an effort to have the patient produce at any price, the search for some "project"—exercise, if you prefer—which will eliminate the unbearable possibility that the patient may not participate actively in the session.

Here the imaginative and creative skills peculiar to those who enter the art therapy field go to work to find ways to stimulate the patient to artistic production, to give him subjects, ideas, tasks which will lead him into action.

To go one step further, why should we expose ourselves to the agony of not knowing what may happen, or rather, not happen, in the session? Isn't it safer to plan ahead, to come to the art therapy room with a planned assignment? "Draw in turn on each other's pictures; draw together, separately, in silence or while talking; draw things you hate, things you like; draw how you feel now, how you felt yesterday; draw your portrait and pass it around for others to draw on," and so on and so on. The sky's the limit. Let's have an assortment of art materials: tempera paints, crayons, pastels, finger paints, colored markers, oils, watercolors, clay, Plasticine. Let us also have ready scissors and magazines, from which we will cut out things to paste in our project for next time.

The generosity, lavishness, and pseudo-freedom of choice among many art media may become as limiting as is a preplanned task for the day. Offering a multitude of materials without knowing whether the patient is able to make choices and decisions may confuse him utterly and cause him to withdraw or to act out by a destructive misuse of many art materials together. However, just as with careful selection and gradual introduction of art materials, the use of certain of the approaches I mentioned earlier can be of great value when they are the natural outgrowth of the immediate experience of the individual patient or the group. For example, if the patient complains of lonesomeness or keeps separate from the group, one could suggest doing a drawing with another person or with the whole group (joint scribble or mural, according to the size of the group). Such an action may provide the group with a magnificent opportunity to become aware of the patient's difficulty.

An approach which terrifies me by its implicit brutality and invasion of privacy is requesting patients to work in turn on the work of the person next to them—for example, to modify a self-portrait or continue a clay piece that has been begun. While participating in a workshop I myself experienced the hurt of having something that was meaningful to me brutally destroyed by the next in line. An experience of this sort may drive a patient whose ego is fragile and vulnerable away from art therapy forever.

Playing "musical chairs" with art materials invites acting-out and destructiveness. But here again, at a certain period of therapy and upon the mutual agreement of the patients, collaboration on a picture or piece of claywork may be desirable and fruitful. What I protest is the automatic use of these approaches as if programmed by computer.

In conclusion, I want to emphasize that in the practice of art therapy, although we have to be acquainted with and ready to use some stimulative procedures when indicated, the primary task of the art therapist is to be in touch with his patients' experience and needs. Not less important is to be in touch with one's own experience in response to these needs. Both together lead to the understanding of messages in the individual's or the group's art products and to the development of a therapeutic relationship.

Art Therapy and Aggression

Edith Kramer

In our work as art therapists we encounter aggression in many guises: as disruptive violence that makes work impossible; as threat that calls forth defensive counter-measures; as destructive force which, without disrupting the creative process altogether, interferes with the unity of the work of art; as emotional content that is expressed and contained. Finally, according to our theory of sublimation, we must assume that part of the constructive energy that goes into the making of art derives from neutralized aggression. Aggression seems to be both one of the most disruptive forces we have to contend with, and an indispensable source of energy for constructive work.

Regarding the nature of aggression, both the psychoanalytic investigation of man and the study of the natural history of aggression as conducted by ethologists such as Lorenz[1] and Tinbergen[2] leave no doubt that it is a primary instinctive drive. Stresses such as frustration or danger call forth unusually intense aggressive behavior but these stimuli must not be mistaken for causes. The drive is innate, not a mere response to external conditions.

There is also evidence derived from psychoanalytic study of human relationships and from the investigation of bonds among other species that positive relationships always contain aggression. Neither man nor beast seems to be capable of forming a bond without simultaneously directing aggressive affect toward the same individual.

In his book *On Aggression*, Lorenz explains why the evolution of individual bonds has been of necessity tied to intraspecific aggression. His reasoning is as follows:

The prerequisite for the development of personal relationships is the capacity for *individual recognition*. This ability did not evolve in the peaceful flock, since there is no need to distinguish among the various members. It is only when cooperation develops among members of species who are as a rule inclined to be aggressive toward one another that the ability to distinguish between friend and foe becomes essential. Therefore only among such species was there sufficient evolutionary pressure for the development of a faculty for individual recognition.

1. Konrad Lorenz, *On Aggression*, New York, Harcourt, Brace & World, Inc., 1962.
2. N. Tinbergen, *The Study of Instinct*, London, Oxford University Press, 1958.

Furthermore, cooperation develops most often between male and female in the care of the young. Since adequate space is particularly important for new life, the functions of procreation and aggressive behavior are apt to be linked, and animals are often particularly aggressive when defending territory while preparing a nesting place or when they are tending their offspring. Species which develop cooperation therefore must also evolve mechanisms which effectively control aggressive behavior between individuals who have formed bonds. The greater the individual's readiness to valiantly defend those with whom he has formed a bond, the more reliable must be the inhibitions which prevent him from also attacking them.

And so it seems as if the ambivalence which characterizes passionate human relationships is foreshadowed in the mental organization of these other species. For among them the individuals' intercourse with their chosen companions is shot through with mechanisms that divert, bind, or transform aggression against the very beings whose company is ardently desired; the time of closest cooperation often coincides with periods when both sexual excitement and readiness for aggressive behavior are at their height.

Naturally, the existence of analogous situations among other species constitutes no proof of the psychoanalytic hypothesis that aggressive and libidinal drives in man are inevitably linked. It only places it in a wider perspective, making the reasons for it more comprehensible and therefore easier to accept.

I have permitted myself this digression because I feel that it is essential to approach the problem of aggression in the belief that we are dealing with a primeval force. Only on this basis can we hope to understand aggression, or to find ways of dealing effectively with its destructive aspects. Particularly when we encounter some of its pathological manifestations, it is important to remember that aggression is a vital force, in itself neither good nor evil. All vigorous and purposeful action draws part of its impetus from the same drive which, misdirected, causes untold suffering.

Dammed-up Aggression

The layman who considers the role of art therapy in the management of aggressive children usually thinks at first of art as a harmless outlet for the expression of pent-up anger. Such direct discharge can be beneficial when the individual's basic integration is not menaced by it.

For example, a child who has been forced into extreme cleanliness too early in life may be able to enjoy constructive work with clay or paint only after a veritable orgy of simple messing with the stuff. Or a very angry child may not be able to settle down to work unless he first gives vent to his anger directly. The hallmark of such healthy explosions is the sense of relief when it is over: the atmosphere is cleared and work can proceed better than before. We conclude that the outburst freed the individual from excessive

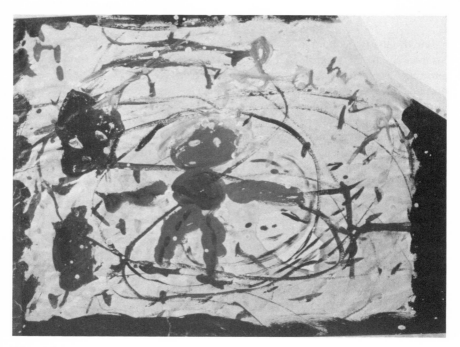

Figure 1

pressure but left essential ego structure intact. If, on the other hand, the explosion is followed by lasting disorganization or extreme distress, we must conclude that important defenses have been swept away, leaving the child more vulnerable than before.

When it frees the individual from crippling inhibitions, temporary regression to crudely aggressive art may be an emotional victory. When ten-year-old Alice, on the day of mother's expected visit, painted herself as a primitive manikin entirely scarlet with rage and surrounded by swirling streaks of paint on a paper edged in black, she bore the picture (Figure 1) in triumph to her social worker. It was the first time that she had been able to give vent to her rage at the psychotic mother who had left her in foster care, neglected her, yet pursued her with demands for filial affection.

Fifteen-year-old Philip, a very staid and stable boy whose art was usually contemplative and serene, felt great relief when he painted a crude caricature of his alcoholic father who had abandoned him and his dying mother when he was three years old.

When Mrs. Smith after a day's vacation found the cottage where she worked as a house parent in an unbelievable mess, she relieved her feelings by covering a piece of paper entirely with red paint and painting herself as a tiny brown figure, arms upraised in anger, at the bottom center of the page (Figure 2). The red background, she explained later, signified her towering rage, the primitive little figure in the middle her feeling of utter helplessness. By the time she had finished the picture, she had calmed down sufficiently to resume her duties and restore order in the cottage. The painting was more infantile than Mrs. Smith's usual work. Rage, it seems, had made her regress. It was, on the other hand, stronger than most of her more adult paintings so that we can see in it also the seeds of sublimation.

Since the two children as well as the cottage parent had sufficient ego-strength to reintegrate after their temporary regression, they experienced relief and their emotional equilibrium had not been upset.

Aggression and Control

When adequate channels for impulse discharge have failed to develop properly it is entirely different. Painful tensions are felt not only under unusual pressures; even the ordinary flow of drive energy is experienced as catastrophic and is discharged chaotically, or the ego tries to defend itself against the onslaught by unusual emergency measures that constrict or distort the child's life.

The self-representations of such children often portray this situation vividly. Like most children, seven-year-old David liked having the art therapist trace the outline of his body while he lay stretched out on a piece of brown wrapping paper, but whenever he tried to fill in the outline he soon reduced it to a seething black mess in which all body parts were lost. In his very best moments, David was able to draw a person with head, body, arms, and legs, but then it was always a robot, constructed of squares and straight lines and complete with push buttons for making it work.

Figure 2

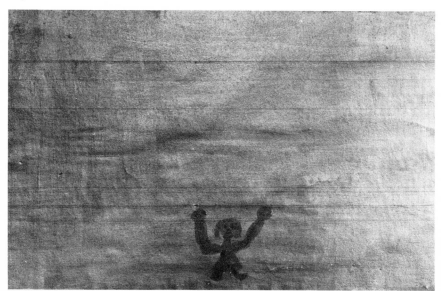

This of course does not mean that it is never advisable to offer art materials to children like David, or that aggressive manipulation of these media can never be helpful. It only means that we must not forget how easily children of this kind feel threatened by experiences that in any way tend to upset their equilibrium.

Margaret

The problem of aggression and control in the young child who is impulsive but not psychotic is exemplified admirably in Margaret's picture of a caged lion. She was a lively, emotionally deprived seven-year-old, insatiable in her demands for attention and for material goods and much given to bullying her little foster brother, Ralph. Her favorite threat, "I'll break your penis," left no doubt of her strong and open envy, but her general behavior indicated that more primitive oral aggression mingled with her overt phallic preoccupation.

One day Margaret was at a loss for subject matter. I reeled off a great many possible themes, among them a number of animals. When I pronounced the word "lion," Margaret immediately lit upon it. She produced a large, humanoid creature, which did not look particularly fierce except for a smiling but very big black mouth. Then, using the widest paintbrush, she painted strong red bars across the whole paper (Figure 3, Plate I). When I regretted that the bars had nearly obliterated her lion, she explained that this was very necessary because "the lion is dangerous and might hurt people."

Figure 3

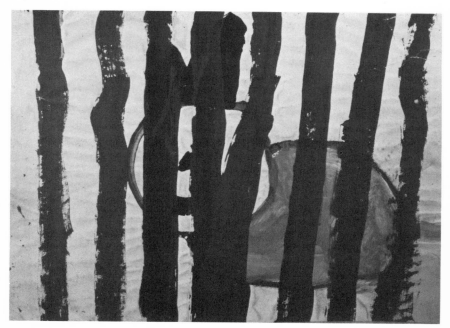

We note, however, that the lion, which officially signifies aggression, does not look very fierce. The red-hot bars, on the other hand, don't inspire confidence. We feel that they could melt any minute, join forces with the lion, and destroy us all.

I have chosen this example to present our problem in its simplest form: archaic aggression embodied in the devouring lion, crude external controls represented by the bars. Naturally the simplicity is only relative, all psychic processes being extremely complex and contradictory. We cannot just say that Margaret's aggression stands for lion, the bars for control. The lion might also stand for the controlling adult seen as aggressor; the bars, for Margaret's need to ward off external controls; or the lion might be another child (maybe Ralph) whom she wants to put behind bars. All we can be certain of is that Margaret felt both aggression and aggressive control when she painted the picture, and that both positions were internalized and sufficiently invested to produce a powerful image.

Ultimately the subject matter seems to be *"aggressive control"* per se, lion, whatever he stands for, being nearly obliterated by it. Margaret's picture draws its vitality from the state of flux which gave rise to it. Lion is obliterated by cage, but the picture began with him. When control reigns supreme, expression is apt to be lost.

In the never-ending struggle for mastery of these conflicts, we encounter Margaret at a time when she has attempted to come to terms with aggression by putting the dangerous force into a cage, which in turn constitutes an act of aggression against it. Later she may attempt to tame the lion. If she is at this time still aggressive, her ways of taming him may remain cruel and castrating.

Michael

Rather than putting them behind bars, some children are inclined to join forces with the ferocious beings they have imagined. Eight-year-old Michael was the terror of a children's psychiatric ward. Aggression permeated his life. At the time he made the father dragon and baby dragon (Figure 4), art constituted an island of relatively controlled and organized functioning in a sea of trouble. Making the sculpture extended over several art sessions. Father dragon was constructed first. He is heavily armed with spikes, is blowing fire, and is adorned with a gold crown.

The baby dragon is already able to blow fire, but he lacks the adult dragon's spikes. According to Michael these would grow as he got older. In our reproduction, baby dragon is placed for better visibility upright on the base of a clay baby carriage which Michael built for him. To it belonged an orange hood which has been removed in our picture.

Even though the sculpture looks ferocious, a great deal of Michael's play with his two dragons was tender. Talking in a soft cooing voice he would place baby dragon between father's front paws, or put him to bed in the

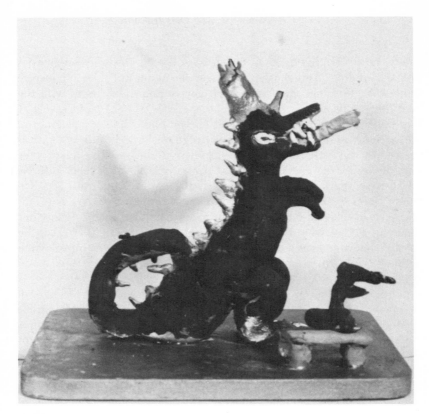

Figure 4

carriage, carefully protecting him with the hood. Whenever play was aggressive, father and son presented a united fire-spitting front against their enemies. We see that Michael plays two roles, that of the well-defended dragon king, and that of the still defenseless baby. It seems as if he tried to attain strength by identification with the aggressive male while preserving his babyhood by placing himself in father dragon's power. By playing the defenseless baby whose spikes have not yet grown, he probably also defends himself against the dragon-father's hostility. We surmise that the sculpture has grown out of a mixture of love and hate, envy and admiration, desire for independence and need for protection. There is no indication that the idea of control of hostility itself, or of good and evil, played any part in the making of the group.

We can say that Michael's pair of dragons embodies his *identification with the aggressor*. In psychoanalytic terms, this is a mechanism whereby a child defends himself against both his fear of attack and the helpless anger which such attacks arouse in him by identifying with the aggressive qualities of those persons who cause him such feelings. The most common objects of such identifications are the frustrating and controlling aspects of the parents and parent-substitutes. The process is in the main unconscious and the identifications that the child establishes constitute an amalgamation of actual experiences and the feelings and fantasies to which they give rise. What we see in images such as Michael's dragon is not the actual father, but the dragon aspect of him as it is perceived by the immature and exceedingly aggressive little son.

A child like Margaret who masters her own aggressions by aggressively controlling herself, and masters her fear of attack by controlling others, fights a battle on two fronts. She has not much energy or leeway for expressive art.

A child like Michael who attempts to master the same kind of difficulty by identifying with the power that is both admired and feared, turning all aggression against the outside, avoids inner division and preserves his narcissism. He is, at least for the time being, better able to express himself forcefully in art. Even when only the aggressive component of an authority figure has been internalized, identification has a stabilizing effect. Although father is a dragon, Michael conceives not only of his ferocity but also of his protective strength. As he forms mental representations of these qualities, his inner life is enriched.

We see that in the process of maturation both the establishment of aggressive inner controls and identification with the aggressor can be temporarily helpful. Frequently the two mechanisms complement each other. Neither position, however, is tenable for long.

Margaret's aggressively controlling personality caused her much internal suffering and brought her into unending conflict with others. It took years of struggle until Michael established reliable inner controls. At the time of the two dragons, to be alive meant being aggressive. The only time I saw him entirely well-behaved and peaceful was during an art session he spent making a sculpture of his own grave, with his mother kneeling in prayer beside his tombstone.

In Michael's case there was reason to suspect some deficiency in his psychic organization which made it difficult for him to withstand the ordinary pressures of the impulses. Although there had been stresses in his life that could have led to disturbance, there was nothing known to us which could account for his severe and intractable pathology.

Michael's story explains how it can come about that highly belligerent children become deeply and even more or less peacefully engrossed in creating pictures or sculptures.

Since the aggressive child sees enemies everywhere, and indeed makes himself enemies, he also is in constant need of protection. He is preoccupied with ideas about powerful, well-defended figures and to create their images is reassuring. For this kind of work the child is therefore ready to muster whatever controls he can. Art not being tied to any set morality, the creative process is not disturbed by the children's delinquent, often cruel imagery.

Beyond giving child and adult a moment's respite, what good can we expect of this? The process of identification is in itself beneficial. Giving form even to asocial ideas also gives substance to the aggressive child's inner life. It reduces the impact of fluctuating moods and helps to bring formerly elusive fantasies into the realm of the ego. As the child learns to love art, the activity can become a sanctuary wherein feelings and perceptions otherwise drowned in constant hostilities can be experienced for the first time. Even the most belligerent child is capable of tenderness and can enjoy some experiences that are not connected with strife. (Michael, for example, could express tenderness between father and son in his dragons.)

If all goes well, the image of aggressive authority which was the child's initial object of identification is with time transformed into a power that stands for virtue rather than mere force. The child begins to develop more benign ego-ideals.

Walter

There is, however, another possibility. Having identified with the aggressor, the child may extol delinquency rather than virtue. Even though such an ideal does not contradict his previous identification, it nevertheless makes new demands on him: Michael did not have to work on himself to live up to being a dragon or a dragon's son. For the sake of a *delinquent ego-ideal*, a child may force himself to become stronger, braver, or more cruel and ruthless. He may develop skills in handling switchblades, guns, or skeleton keys. He may build up his body or destroy it by the use of drugs. Thus even though its values are negative, the ideal exerts moral pressure. The constellation contains the seed of tragedy.

Walter painted the young man holding a switchblade (Figure 5, Plate II) when he was thirteen-and-a-half years old. It was one of a series of paintings depicting various ego-ideals. These oscillated between openly delinquent ones; exponents of lawful violence such as boxers or soldiers; and hunters, Indians, and other figures representing an adventurous but not necessarily a destructive way of life. Of these the young delinquent of Figure 5 (Plate II) a painting measuring three by four feet, was his largest as well as his most successful work of art.

The young man stands against a city street at night. His face, that of a light-skinned Negro, looks luminous against a dark building which is lit from the inside; the yellow windows contrasting with the dark walls compete for our attention, creating a feeling of restlessness. The top of the young man's head remains below the skyline so that the street envelops him completely.

Both the features and the figure as a whole show a combination of weakness and strength characteristic of the art of many delinquents. The young man's forehead and nose convey an impression of strength, but the mouth and chin are weak. The lower body seems flat and insubstantial compared with the heavy bulk of chest and arms. The hand holding the

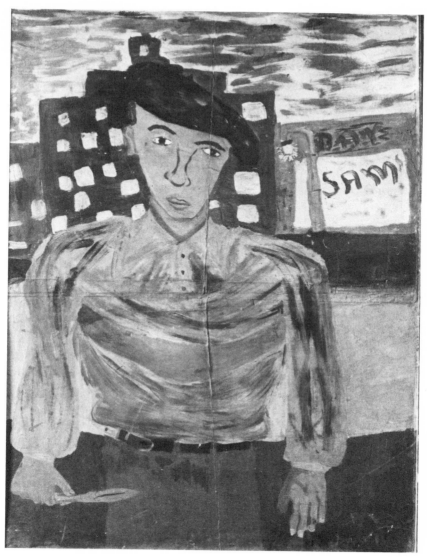

Figure 5

switchblade is turned toward the youth's own body and is painted with meticulous care. The whole is a moving image of the young delinquent, dominating the scene in narcissistic pride, yet shut in by the city, weak in spite of his overgrown muscles, but dangerous to himself and to others.

Walter was a boy of considerable personal charm with a capacity for warmth. He was a talented and prolific artist and a good student. His major weaknesses were an uncontrollable temper and suspiciousness verging on the paranoid. His saving grace was his willingness to try to reconstruct, after his frequent outbursts of temper, the actual events which had led to them. On such occasions he was willing to make amends for the damage he had wrought.

He was justly afraid of the irrational forces which menaced his precarious balance. Violence both attracted and frightened him. Walter's father had served a sentence. His paintings of prisoners showed his identification with the father as well as his ambivalence toward him.[3]

Of the limited number of possible ego-ideals of which Walter could conceive, only the delinquent one was realistically attainable. It is not easy to become an adventurer in our day, and he lacked the strength and self-discipline to become a sportsman.

When, after his discharge from the Wiltwyck School, Walter was picked up on a minor larceny charge he tried his best to pass as an adult so as to be sentenced to prison. Attaining the status of full-fledged delinquent had come to mean an assertion of manhood.

To fit into the mold Walter had to repress the softer side of his personality and relinquish his more civilized aspirations. His painting expresses both the power which he gained by identification with his ideal, and his tragedy. In its muted colors, in the tensions between light and dark, and in the expression of the boy's face, we sense a capacity for introspection and for inner suffering that we have not seen in paintings that express belligerence only.

Carl

Walter, born into a delinquent environment, developed delinquent ego-ideals. In him there was conflict between his unfulfilled dependency needs, his capacity for and need of warmth, and the delinquent ideal of hardness and self-sufficiency, but there was no moral conflict.

Carl,[4] who had grown up in the same kind of world, had nevertheless developed a sense of right and wrong. In his work there was, from the beginning, evidence of moral conflict. The forces of good and evil were frequently personified in his pictures. When he was twelve and thirteen their exponents were taken mostly from adventure stories. There were cowboys and Indians, masked assassins and their victims, and similar figures. As Carl approached adolescence the battle was more often expressed in religious terms. Figure 6, representing the angel of God casting Lucifer down to hell, is a good example of the spirit of tragedy which prevailed in these paintings. Carl produced the picture at the age of fourteen, shortly before his discharge from Wiltwyck School.

3. See the author's *Art Therapy in a Children's Community*, Springfield, Ill., Charles C Thomas, 1958.
4. *Ibid.*

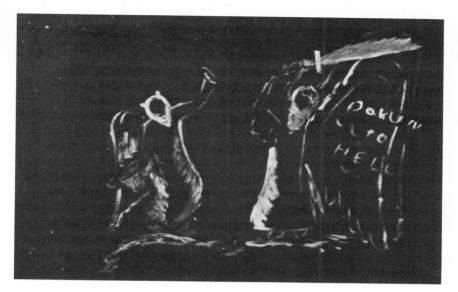

Figure 6

He had selected a large black sheet of paper on which he painted the figures in white, the angel's flaming sword being the only spot of color. Although the space is divided evenly between the two figures there is a strong feeling of motion. The angel's person completely fills his side of the surface, conveying a sense of total command and stability. By contrast Lucifer's smaller figure is set against empty black space that dramatizes his impending fall. The spectator's eye, at first attracted by the flaming sword, is led toward Lucifer's person as it is balanced before his disappearance into the pit, his arms spread in what seems to be a gesture both of warding off the blow of the sword and attempting to regain balance. It is a moment of suspense which forces upon us an intense awareness of Lucifer's doom. We cannot doubt the angel's superior power, but we are made to feel compassion for the rebel's tragedy. Thus the painting conveys to us the inner division of its creator.

Carl was talented in both music and art, and enjoyed exercising his faculties. His aspirations for a dignified life, removed from violence and delinquency and given to cultural pursuits, were genuine. Yet he felt himself menaced both from within and from the outside. He was given to rare but dangerous outbursts of violence, and he felt that being Negro and coming from a delinquent background he was doomed to failure.

Although we must not take his painting of Lucifer as an image of his total personality, the tragedy it depicts and the depressed mood which emanates from its darkness were decisive elements of Carl's character. While Margaret's conflict between aggressive impulses and need for controls resulted in aggressive controlling behavior, Carl became depressed. In him conflict had become internalized. His severe superego aggressively compelled the ego to exert controls. Since he had remained both impulsive and aggressive, the ego exhausted itself in keeping aggression within bounds and the struggle reduced his vitality. Thus the tenor of Carl's art remained muted, his joy of life subdued.

Aggression Channeled, Reduced, and Transformed

Christopher[5]

The examples so far presented have amply demonstrated the power of art to relieve pressures or to contain what is unbearable. We also have witnessed partial transformation of raw aggression into constructive energy as we saw the technical skill, the enthusiasm, and respect for art materials which many of the children developed while producing work that was loaded with aggression. We have seen art therapy contributing to temporary alleviation or partial remission of pathology.

We would like to know of examples where art therapy played a decisive role in the substantial reduction of aggression and in enduring positive changes in the child's personality. Christopher is an impressive example of such a development.

At birth he had minimal vision which then gradually diminished. At the age of seven he was totally blind but retained light perception. He was an out-of-wedlock child, who had lived in the same foster home since infancy. Because of learning difficulties and aggressive behavior he was admitted to the Guild School, a day school for disturbed blind children, when he was eleven years old. There his behavior soon became less aggressive. He began to learn and he was able to profit from psychotherapy.

I began to work with Christopher shortly after his admission. Already in the first session he told me how he loved birds, and sculptured a well-articulated pair of birds in clay. His concepts were clear and realistic. He could perceive form by touch and remember it, and he was able to shape the clay according to his ideas. Whatever Christopher's troubles were, the faculties of perception, imagination, and constructive action were intact.

Although his interest in birds was present from the beginning, Christopher spent most of his first year making images of both living and mechanical symbols of power such as cars, buses, airplanes, and ferocious animals. He always chose them for some particular capacity—the cheetah for his swiftness, the wolf for his ferocity, the bull for his horns.

Christopher's interest in wildlife was realistic, quite in keeping with his preadolescent state, yet he could not, like another child, get his ideas by looking at pictures or going to the zoo. He could form ideas about the shape of domestic animals and the tame animals at the Children's Zoo by touch. When he wanted to make sculptures of wild animals I provided the missing

5. The following case material was developed at the Guild School of the Jewish Guild for the Blind in New York City.

information by making quick clay sketches for him, being careful to shape the models so that they were comprehensible to the touch. At the same time I told him to which familiar domestic animal the wild species I had made for him was related. Christopher then formed his concepts by piecing together information from these various sources.

In the beginning Christopher had wanted to appropriate these models and use them as his own. When I objected to such cheating, he got into the habit of first feeling the model and then destroying it simply by closing his powerful hand over the soft clay figure. Often he used this very clay as raw material for his sculpture.

Three processes succeeded one another. He first took in my ideas. Then he destroyed that which was mine, not his. Some frustration about his handicap and anger against the sighted was vented in the destructive gesture. Finally my contribution was both materially and mentally incorporated, and fantasy, experience, and information were fused in a sculptural whole.

About a year later, when Christopher was twelve years old, he developed a method of making birds out of pipe cleaners, paper, and masking tape. He soon became so skillful that he was able to work at home without help. He produced innumerable birds, insects, bats, and fantastic winged creatures of his own invention, always in pairs, male and female. As his inventiveness and technical skill grew, his passion gave structure and purpose to his free time at home. His birds were much admired and made excellent gifts. Even though there was an obsessive element in his constant output, making birds gave pleasure to him and to others.

At the same time Christopher developed an obsessive preoccupation with the speed, endurance, and strength of birds. He asked endless questions. Was an eagle faster than a goose? Could a goose fly farther than a duck? If an eagle pursued a duck, would the duck escape? Could a hummingbird escape an eagle? And so on ad infinitum.

The questioning was obsessive, irrational, and joyless. It had the character of compulsive questioning which some children develop when they are preoccupied with the riddle of birth and sex. Christopher's habit of making birds always in couples points to this area as one of the motivating forces of his behavior.

It seemed, however, as if Christopher was also displacing onto birds a more general need for information. He had at this time great difficulty in admitting to any ignorance that would have put him at a disadvantage as compared with seeing people, and had developed many ingenious ways of covering up his handicap. This made it impossible for him to learn to distinguish between those things that escaped his notice because of his blindness and those that even a sighted person could not possibly know without asking.

Torturing his teachers and schoolmates with incessant questions about birds also seemed to give him considerable sadistic gratification. It looked as if the birds had come to stand not only for all that was good and desirable but also for what was unattainable and frustrating.

While Christopher was in the throes of his bird-information mania, he produced a powerful clay sculpture of a two-horned rhinoceros. It was big enough for him to sit on, and pleased him enormously. He took it home in triumph and kept it in his backyard, where it was much admired by family and friends. Inasmuch as Christopher's compulsive questioning expressed anger and the desire to be well-protected and strong, the double-horned, thick-skinned beast seemed to have been created out of a similar mood. However, in making it he was dealing with his difficulties in a constructive rather than in a neurotic way. The rhino was both culmination and end of a phase in Christopher's artistic production. From then on he no longer needed to make ferocious animals.

Meanwhile Christopher's questions were becoming more and more irritating, and answering them seemed only to perpetuate the symptom; therefore, we tried to force him to ask only sensible questions for which there were realistic answers. Thus the sadistic gratification which he had gained through his compulsive questions was no longer possible. It is likely that the frustration which this caused him helped bring about a change for the better, for somehow during a period when teachers, psychotherapist, and art therapist were making this concerted effort Christopher became more rational. His interest turned from exclusive concern with the power and speed of birds to curiosity about the lives of the local wild birds whom he could hear singing in his backyard.

He conceived a clay sculpture of a large tree with all the small domestic birds he knew sitting on its branches. The tree was to be a present to his classroom teacher. It was a major undertaking and required a wooden armature. It consisted of a roughly finished trunk from which branches, complete with large leaves, stretched in all directions. More than six bird-couples were placed in the branches and on the ground beneath the tree. While Christopher knew each bird's position and species, everything had been executed crudely and some of the birds had been mashed out of shape when he had placed them, but Christopher was in such a hurry to complete the job that he could not be bothered to repair the damage. At this point Christopher's classroom teacher visited the ceramics shop and offered to help him to perfect the work if he and I would tell her what to do.

While they were working on the tree, I suggested that he could add some nests and perhaps some eggs. Somewhat reluctantly he set out to make one. Soon there was a nest for each couple, complete with baby birds or eggs. His fervor grew and as he vividly imagined the form and position of each nest and the members of each family, the crude, somewhat disjointed structure took on a new organization. There was one couple that had eggs only, another one had both eggs and baby birds; a male woodpecker was busy making a hole in the tree trunk to accommodate his family, while another father bird was about to pull a worm out of the earth beneath the tree. Thus Christopher created for himself a representation of family life in many different constellations. It was impressive to see the sculpture become beautiful, not because Christopher was striving for esthetic perfection but because he was so totally absorbed in giving form to ideas that were alive to him.

Christopher named the sculpture (Figure 7) the *Spring Tree*. In creating it he passed from quick, prolific production toward the beginning of concern with quality in art.

The tree became possible after Christopher had relinquished some of his symptomatic behavior. This implied a certain recognition of the futility of his preoccupation with fabulous feats of strength and endurance. His new interest in real birds meant renouncing fantasies—at least up to a point.

Renunciation of sadistic gratification may have made it possible for him to move from preoccupation with the aggressive components of sexuality toward the expression of love and of Oedipal fantasies. It is not surprising that Christopher's magnificent gift of love was followed by a certain amount of negative behavior toward his teacher, whom he proceeded to tease and resist obstinately. In the space of a few weeks Christopher reexperienced, both symbolically by creating the tree and more directly in the relationship with the teacher, some of the gratifications and frustrations that belong to the Oedipal phase. Ultimately of course he, like every child, had to renounce the desire for full possession of the love-object and this could not

Figure 7

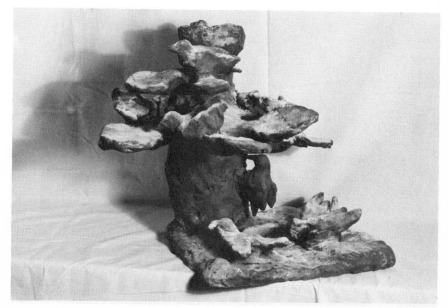

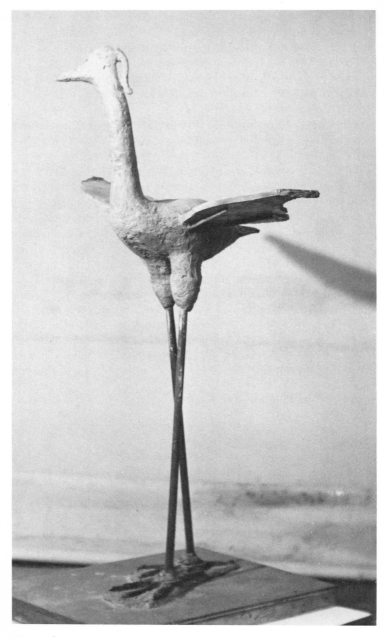

Figure 8

be achieved without a struggle. It seemed that at every juncture Christopher's emotional state was expressed in two ways, through creative work and more directly in his behavior.

Christopher's new renunciation was again followed by creative expression. After the idyllic family scene of the *Spring Tree*, Christopher established his independence by making a life-size sculpture of a blue heron (Figure 8) that was explicitly made *for himself*, not as a gift for anyone. It stood as tall as he and its wings were spread wide. The sculpture was to join the large rhinoceros at home. The difference between the crudely executed monster and the long-necked, graceful bird epitomizes the transition from defensive belligerence to a more mature and proud masculinity. It was a major undertaking and its completion took the better part of a year.

Christopher's story testifies to the necessity of teamwork. Without the sustained efforts of teachers and principal and without the help of psychotherapy Christopher's art would probably never have gone beyond the reiteration of aggressive self-assertion. His talent alone could not have given him the self-confidence he needed, nor could the discipline of creative work have instilled in him the self-discipline he lacked. But when education and psychotherapy brought about changes, art became an organizing force that helped to make each of his gains more gratifying and more secure.

Christopher's relationship to his foster family, for instance, had at the time of his admission to the Guild School reached an impasse where exasperation and despair caused all parties to show their very worst sides to one another. His destructiveness and boasting called forth punishments and derision, which in turn made him more frantically belligerent and suspicious. Consequently the first clay sculptures which he brought home were thrown away as "junk." As his behavior improved, the mother's affection for her foster son was rekindled and she was able to understand how much his sculptures meant to him. His rhinoceros was therefore given a permanent place in the garden. By the time of his discharge from the Guild School, his blue heron, adorning the front lawn, was a source of pride to the whole family. The foster mother declared that Christopher had magic in his hands and hoped that he would have the opportunity to develop his talent further.

In Christopher we can indeed observe the transformation of raw aggression into constructive energy. The change of subject matter and style is more than just an *indication* of change. Rather the creative process itself becomes a powerful force in shaping his personality and giving him the inner strength to maintain his gains in the face of continued hardship.

Review of Virshup's *Right Brain People in a Left Brain World**

Bernard I. Levy

I asked for the opportunity to review this book because I am either directing or on the committee of three doctoral dissertations dealing with the hypothesis of the bicameral mind. My students are investigating what psychological functions distinguish the cortical hemispheres in relation to race, age, handedness, site of brain damage, and field of study. The list of attributes in the preceding sentence should make it clear that our knowledge of the differential psychological functioning of the cortical hemispheres is still primitive. Research workers in this area are not yet anywhere near a Nobel award; the tentative ideas about differences between the cortical hemispheres are still controversial, not yet clearly delineated. Yet some psychologists, psychiatrists, art therapists, and popularizers have taken these conjectures and raced with them toward the goalposts. Of course as clinicians, we art therapists must try everything that might help our clients. Californian Evelyn Virshup, an energetic clinical art therapist, now has the ball and is running—I hope in the right direction.

When I think of the West Coast I think of splashes of bright color, easygoing attitudes, people focusing their energies and efforts on themselves and eschewing structure; the East Coast, on the other hand, seems full of driven people creating gray structures, organizing, rationalizing, and pushing others into the same bag: West Coast—right brain; East Coast—left brain. Virshup's book is right-brained: big, loose, splashing forms carelessly done for the sake of spontaneity, a larger-than-life format with pictures pushing to escape the confines of the book and lying uncomfortably to one side of an unconvincing assortment of words. There you have it: an East Coast left-brainer reviewing a West Coast right-brainer's book. (Of course, I don't actually know whether Evelyn Virshup is right-brained or even left-handed, the latter a good but not conclusive sign of right cortical dominance.)

First I would like to comment on the book primarily as an object. It is

*Evelyn Virshup, *Right Brain People in a Left Brain World*, Los Angeles, Guild of Tutors Press, 1978.

large, allowing ample space for reproductions of client art. Most of the reproductions are in color—intense color. The illustrations are large enough so that details are well reproduced and one can easily imagine the technique used: string dipped in black ink and allowed to fall on the paper and create random lines and shapes much like a scribble; development of a theme projected onto the random array of lines and shapes in monochrome or with colored chalks and pastels, felt pens, and blots of ink or paint. Some of Virshup's clients went quite a bit beyond the procedure itself to create highly personal and occasionally artistic works. Each illustration has a descriptive and interpretive legend near it. A flashy, mod symbolization of the bicameral mind in color, shapes, and words opens out like a double *Playboy* centerfold to reveal art by folk sculptors and well-known painters who, according to Virshup, can be taken to represent one chamber of the mind or the other.

Because of their size and color, the clients' pictures are so powerful that they clearly outweigh the text: only a quarter or so of the book is devoted to verbally expressed ideas. Evelyn Virshup selected illustrations of inherent interest because of their style, flair, and symbolism. Although she decries the focus on product, she is sometimes able to stimulate her clients to produce works that come close to personally expressive art. Thus the book seems to be primarily an exhibit of the selected work of art therapy clients rather than an exposition of the very important ideas implied by the title. (We are not even offered any evidence as to whether the clients and centerfold artists are actually dominated by their right or left cortical hemispheres.) The book also contains a Bibliography that seems more like a reference list; it makes no pretense of completeness in any of its subcategories, least of all in art therapy. Finally, on the back cover, there is a classy photograph in color of Evelyn Virshup in action, followed by two testimonials from professional workers who affirm the book's definitive representation of the drug addict's plight.

Now to concentrate on the book's content.

The title set up high expectations. I looked forward to a serious exploration of the difficulties of being right-brained in a left-brained world. Whether or not the hypothesis of the bicameral mind is valid, physically active, spatially oriented, intuitive people have serious problems in a world dominated by factual, analytic verbalists. I am particularly sensitive to this problem because of my own clinical work in psychology. I am called on to assess large numbers of adolescents and adults who have been called retarded on the basis of limitations in their verbal skills; however, when they were carefully assessed, many of them revealed not only those verbal limitations but also surprisingly high competence in nonverbal or perceptual/motor intelligence. Thus the verbal bias of our society is evident; it is even evident in the popular notion that painters are creative but not intelligent. Art is commonly viewed as intuitive; painting is a gift of the Muse, not an act of disciplined intelligence. Why? Because painting is nonverbal.

All this helps to explain the eagerness with which I opened Evelyn Virshup's book—but I was doomed to disappointment. The book has little to do with "right-brained people in a left-brained world."

True, a foreword written by Bernard B. Virshup, M.D., the author's husband, contains a pithy summary of medical thinking concerning the bicameral mind; Dr. Virshup also celebrates his wife's achievements by alluding to a breakthrough she has made in integrating both sides of the brain, although how she has done this is not made clear. In the book itself, the problem implied by the title is touched upon briefly several times but the text deals mostly with Evelyn Virshup's general ideas about art therapy.

She asserts that art is a language and that art is an extension of the self. So far, so good—she has put forward the Projective Hypothesis without crediting Lawrence K. Frank.[1] She follows Margaret Naumburg's lead when she also asserts that art can help one toward self-understanding but she does not cite Naumburg in the text (two references appear in the Bibliography). She then insists on the privacy of the creative act by arguing in several places that an external interpretation of art is unnecessary in art therapy, that the meaning resides properly in the artist.

Two problems now arise in my left cortex: first, I wonder why the discipline of art therapy is needed, since any recreation therapist, art teacher, or occupational therapist can probably encourage people to use art materials and to talk about what they've made. Why, then, does the American Art Therapy Association make such a fuss over professionalism and training for what Virshup seems to suggest is an unnecessary discipline?

The second problem is related to the first but is more complex. It has to do with the graphic language and the need for art therapists to understand it for the purpose of advancing the client's treatment. Most art therapists believe that much of the value of art comes from its capacity to symbolize (and through symbolizing, even to alleviate) inner emotional discord unconsciously—but the symbolic language of art is very difficult to understand or, if you will, to read. The original impetus for making graphic symbols lies buried in our primordial past; contemporary symbols have been influenced by cultural and personal history, further confounding their intelligibility. While in many respects personally expressive art is indubitably a representation of self, it is very difficult to assign specific meaning to it. A provocative literature of meaning exists but it is scattered, unsystematic, and of variable validity. Ideas about the meaning of art can be found in fields as widely scattered as psychology and comparative religion.

Being able to understand the graphic language is, then, the province of a few specialists. Yet many art therapists routinely urge clients to comment

---

1. Lawrence K. Frank, "Projective Methods for the Study of Personality," *Journal of Psychology*, Vol. 8, 1939, pp. 389–413.

about, react to, associate to, in effect interpret their own art. What folly! Virshup asks her clients, and urges other art therapists to ask clients, to pierce the veil of the hidden unconscious language when so few professionals can do so. The client's interpretation is likely to consist largely of secondary elaboration—which in turn will need to be interpreted. It's as though one is asked to interpret one's own Rorschach without the highly specialized training needed for the task.

What clients say about their own art is important if the process of associating to the art has therapeutic merit. On the other hand, if the client's comments delay or interfere with therapy, then the associative process should be replaced by something else. My own conviction is that clients are usually polite and cooperative enough to want to please and at times imitate the art therapist. This manifestation of transference probably does nothing worse than delay the effect of treatment. It is likely that art therapy works in spite of having the clients interpret the art.

Virshup clinches the power of the client's interpretations by implying that they are valid and the observer's or therapist's interpretations are projections! Such an idea drives the last nail into art therapy's coffin by making the art therapist nothing more than a provider of supplies and a rooter.

Of course I do not mean to brush aside the Naumburg tradition with its emphasis on the elucidation of the patient's psychological conflict and its reliance on what the patient says in association with the picture. Naumburg's term *psychoanalytically oriented art therapy* suggests her style of treatment. She devoted a great deal of time to eliciting her patients' spoken reactions to their art, sometimes encouraging them to devote their sessions with her to talking about paintings done at home. She was convinced that painting was one of the royal roads to the unconscious; to deal with such data the art had to be converted into the spoken word.

An enormous amount of material can be provoked by the artistic process and the resulting art—memories, attitudes, meanings, values, history, feelings, dreams, resistances, and on and on. Once one has been caught up in it, such a verbal outpouring could divert one's attention from the art therapy! But while the interpretation of the patient's verbal elaborations would seem to be the focus of Naumburg's treatment, she remains a true art therapist in that she brings the patient back to the art, back to the creation of art. However, pure Naumburg is clearly neither Virshup's model nor mine.

From my vantage point, the therapist's *interpretation of the art itself* is always crucial and the client's only occasionally useful. The basic process of art therapy takes place in three steps: (1) the art therapist's invitation to creative self-expression; (2) the process of creation by the client with the art therapist attentively passive; and (3) the therapist's reaction to the art. To react in a helpful way to the art just produced by the client—i.e., a way that helps the client go on to create more (and more profoundly expressive) art and thus start the basic process anew—the art therapist must have first interpreted the art. (It may or may not become useful for the client to be told about the therapist's interpretation.)

This concept of the process of art therapy demands therapists trained at a professional level. Unlike Virshup's conception, it implies the need for the discipline of art therapy.

But Virshup does not depend solely on the client's self-interpretation and the resulting self-knowledge to supply the therapy of art therapy. She asserts the importance of sublimation without citing Edith Kramer (even though one of Kramer's books is in the Bibliography) and the educational value of art without citing Rawley Silver,[2] and then, because she is humanistically oriented, she goes on to say that art therapy is also for normal people.

Finally, Virshup takes the ultimate step into the land of the Philistines by asserting that the quality of art is unimportant in art therapy: it is the *process* that carries the burden of favorable therapeutic outcome. But what constitutes the *process of making artworks?* Can a client who idly makes a few colored marks on a paper be helping himself? I agree with Kramer and Elinor Ulman that one of the secrets of art therapy is the active engagement with materials, with the struggle to formulate as complete a self-expression as possible. Engagement and struggle lead to quality, to meaning, and to knowing oneself. Insofar as Virshup's clients color scribbles or fill in shapes made by colored strings they are not engaged in the art process, and what they are doing cannot lead to art and thus to feeling better. It could abrogate art. I reiterate that any activity therapist can help people fool around with art materials if that is all that is needed. As if to make my fears come true, Virshup introduces Chapter III, "Drawing Myself Out," with these words:

> . . . I will discuss in the next chapter some exercises which are appropriate for "normal" people of any age, *by themselves,* following the simple directions, and *without the need for the art therapist's expertise.* [Emphasis supplied, p. 33]

What does Virshup mean by the "art therapist's expertise"? I hold that it must be more than having people color random shapes.

Chapter 4, "Drawing Together," deals with Virshup's conception of group art therapy. Chapter 5, "Drawing Out My Feelings," presents exercises that attempt to do just that. Chapter 6, "Drawing to a Close," attempts a summary and suggests readings.

Right Brain People in a Left Brain World is interesting but badly flawed. Its title promises more than is delivered. Despite the glowing tributes on the back cover, the text merely hints at the use of art with drug abusers. The Foreword promises that we will learn about the use of art to integrate the hypothesized bicameral mind, but this promise too remains unfulfilled.

---

2. See Rawley Silver, *Developing Cognitive and Creative Skills Through Art,* Baltimore, University Park Press, 1978, as well as many articles published earlier.

Assertions about who is and who is not dominated by the right brain fly freely, without benefit of documentation. The illustrations flow in one stream and the words in another, with only occasional points of intersection. The incomplete Bibliography betokens a lack of scholarship.

In sum, one cannot take the book seriously as a scientific or technical work. But even so, it is worth buying and studying. Its price is reasonable and much of interest is said in the illustrations and between the lines—the book dazzles the eye and the mind.

Finally, I want to thank the author for a work so provocative that it impelled me to formulate more clearly than before my own theory of art therapy.

Art Education for the Emotionally Disturbed*

Elinor Ulman

[Editor's Note: The attitude of art educators and art therapists toward each other's fields has changed noticeably in recent years. Formerly many art teachers tended to guard jealously against any ulterior demand that might distract from their concentration on the esthetic. In recent years, however, both undergraduate and graduate schools of art education have become eager to introduce art therapy offerings. At the same time, more and more art therapists have been seeking places within the educational system rather than in clinical settings.

Obvious economic motives for these shifts of attitude do not tell anything like the whole story. Sources both of conflict and of potentially fruitful exchange lie deep within the two disciplines and within their common denominator—art itself.

Interest continues to grow. The National Art Education Association has offered art therapists a place on the platform of its annual conference several times over, and the American Art Therapy Association has established a committee to study the relationship between art education and art therapy. We are reprinting the following article, first published in 1971, in the belief that it suggests a philosophical and historical basis for further dialogue.]

Children and adolescents constitute the age group within the emotionally disturbed population most likely to receive art education. Art education is often included in the programs of the treatment centers, special schools, and special classes in regular schools where these young people are segregated. Emotionally disturbed adults, if they are offered special opportunities to work with art materials, are more often engaged in recreational, occupational, or art therapy and are not likely to be participating in art education programs.

This discussion will focus on that aspect of art education which seeks to involve the student in making visual objects whose primary purpose is

---

*This essay appeared under the title "Art Education for Special Groups: The Emotionally Disturbed" in Vol. 1 (pp. 311–16) of *The Encyclopedia of Education*, Lee C. Deighton, Editor-in-Chief. Copyright © 1971 by Crowell Collier and Macmillan, Inc., New York. Reprinted by permission.

expressive rather than utilitarian. Those aspects of esthetic education which stress art history and the critical appreciation of works of art play secondary roles.

Since the usefulness of art activity to the emotionally disturbed depends in large part on values inherent in the artistic process itself, it is difficult to make a sharp distinction between art education and a certain aspect of art therapy. Looked upon by some practitioners in both fields as incompatible, in actuality they cannot always be kept apart. The arts, after all, exist to serve the psychological needs of mankind![1]

Because both art education and art therapy not only may contribute to personal well-being but also may help develop capacities for effective artistic expression, it is important to distinguish how their approaches differ from each other. A leading art educator, Viktor Lowenfeld, pointed the way toward

> a therapy specific to the means of art education [which deals with] neither the interpretation of symbols, nor a diagnosis reached by speculative inferences based on certain symbols. . . . [A] *motivation used in art education therapy only differs from any other art motivation in degree and intensity and not in kind.*[2]

Edith Kramer, the foremost exponent of art therapy with children, believes that the therapist's skills must include competence as both artist and teacher. She defines the art therapist's special function as making creative experiences available to disturbed persons in the service of emotional health; from this definition it follows that, like the art educator, the therapist must use only such methods as are compatible with the inner laws of artistic creation. The clinically trained art therapist is, however, better equipped than the art teacher to make diagnostic contributions and to establish an intimate relationship between art activity and psychotherapy.[3]

Margaret Naumburg, one of the earliest practitioners of art therapy and an outstanding writer on its theory and methods, has devoted much of her career to a form of intensive treatment which is much more closely allied to psychonalytic therapy than to Lowenfeld's art education therapy. In her teaching, however, Naumburg has demonstrated that, given additional insight into problems of personality development and the implications of graphic communication, a classroom teacher may establish by means of

---

1. Edith Kramer, "Art and Emptiness: New Problems in Art Education and Art Therapy," *Bulletin of Art Therapy*, Vol. 1, No. 1, 1961, pp. 7–16; Edith Kramer, "Amplification and Reply: Art Education and Emptiness," *Bulletin of Art Therapy*, Vol. 1, No. 3, 1962, pp. 20–24; Myer Site, "Art and the Slow Learner," *Bulletin of Art Therapy*, Vol. 4, No. 1, 1964, pp. 3–19.
2. Viktor Lowenfeld, *Creative and Mental Growth* (Third Edition), New York, Macmillan Co., 1957, p. 435.
3. Edith Kramer, *Art Therapy in a Children's Community*, Springfield, Ill., Charles C Thomas, 1958.

individual drawing sessions a highly constructive relationship with a disturbed child. This procedure can lead to substantial improvement in the child's mood and behavior. Furthermore, far from interfering with the development of creative capacity, this way of using art tends to bring about progress from the strictly esthetic point of view, adding another dimension to artistic expression.[4]

This brief sampling of opinion in the field demonstrates that although spokesmen for art education and art therapy strive to maintain the distinct identity of each discipline, the boundaries they suggest are, at best, blurred. It is interesting that the art teacher in a special school readily becomes known as an art therapist, while the mathematics teacher in the same educational setup, however benign his influence, is not likely to be mistaken for an arithmetic therapist.

Art and Maturation

The reason for the unavoidable overlapping of art education and art therapy lies, as has already been suggested, in the intimate relationship of the arts to the needs of the developing personality. This natural connection explains why the use of art to help repair emotional damage and to compensate for failures of development often has much in common with its use in the education of less disturbed young people.

It appears that in early life an inner chaos of feelings and impulses is matched by a likewise overwhelming chaos of sensory impressions coming from without. Every child needs to be an artist insofar as he must find a means of conceiving of himself and of the world around him and of establishing a relation between the two. Susanne Langer concluded that the function of the arts is to give form to feeling.[5] It is only through the achievement of this form-giving process that the individual can understand and master his own feelings and that feelings can be shared among individuals.

Cultural history and the developmental history of each human being alike bear witness to a universal inclination toward the arts as a means of reconciling two conflicting demands: the need for emotional release and the need to discover order and impose organization. Art results from the dynamic interplay of forces too often kept in sterile, even dangerous, isolation from each other.

The artistic process calls on the widest range of human capacities. Like maturation in general, it demands the integration of many inescapably

4. Margaret Naumburg, "Spontaneous Art in Education and Psychotherapy," *Bulletin of Art Therapy*, Vol. 4, No. 2, 1965, pp. 51–69.
5. Susanne K. Langer, *Philosophy in a New Key*, Cambridge, Mass., Harvard University Press, 1942.

conflicting elements, among them impulse and control, aggression and love, feeling and thinking, fantasy and reality, the unconscious and the conscious. The goal of art education is to make available to the individual resources within himself and outside of himself, and the arts serve throughout life as a meeting ground for the inner and the outer worlds.

The function of the arts has been explained in terms of numerous theories, among them the Freudian, Jungian, and Gestalt psychologies. One writer may emphasize the organizing principle, another the liberation of feeling; both are essential to art and to optimum personality development. The common thread uniting these many views is recognition of the inherently integrative character of the arts, that is, their power to unite opposing forces within the personality and to help reconcile the needs of the individual with the demands of the outside world. Educators and therapists alike find here a key to understanding the value of art education in alleviating emotional disturbance.[6]

Stunted personalities may be characterized by excessively rigid controls, by chaotic inability to resist impulse, or by a frequent alternation between these two equally crippling states. True mastery of life's tasks depends on a disciplined freedom, whose model may be found in the artistic process.

Adaptation of Art Education

Art is natural to man, but its development beyond the most rudimentary beginnings is never automatic. The same principles which have guided progressive art educators since the early 1900s were later adapted to the special needs of the handicapped. Prominent among the basic tenets common to progressive art education and to what may be called, adopting Lowenfeld's terminology, an art education therapy are recognition that visual conception develops in an evolutionary manner and that each student's level of development should be respected; that motivation comes from within and should be encouraged, not imposed; that technique should be at the service of expression, not the other way round; and that the teacher's faith in the student does not militate against artistic quality but is an important factor in the development of artistic capacities.

The teacher of art to the emotionally disturbed, like all art teachers, needs to have had firsthand experience of the artistic process, for there is no other road to full understanding of the problems pupils face in their creative struggles. The teacher must also have expert knowledge of tools and materials; and he should be familiar with the developmental sequence in

6. Florence Cane, *The Artist in Each of Us*, New York, Pantheon, 1951; Kramer, *op. cit.*, 1958; Lowenfeld, *op. cit.*; Henry Schaefer-Simmern, *The Unfolding of Artistic Activity: Its Basis, Processes and Implications*, Berkeley, Calif., University of California Press, 1961; Elinor Ulman, "Art Therapy: Problems of Definition," *Bulletin of Art Therapy*, Vol. 1, No. 2, 1961, pp. 10–20.

visual conception that appears regularly in the visual arts and with the various methods art educators and therapists have evolved to stimulate the evocative use of art materials. Beyond this general equipment as an art educator, he may profit from whatever further knowledge of psychology, psychopathology, and psychotherapeutic principles he is able to acquire.

The function of the art educator dealing with a disturbed population varies according to the setting in which he works. In some situations the personal relationship between teacher and student, developed through the freedom of painting and the teacher's acceptance of its implied message, is one of the most important factors in the therapeutic effect. In psychiatric treatment centers the art teacher may supply information to the psychotherapists dealing with the children and may in turn receive guidance from them. Often, however, the art teacher must work in the special classes of regular schools where no psychological counsel is likely to be available to him.

If the teacher sees to it that the children's artwork is displayed, he enables art to fulfill its role as a form of communication by extending its influence into the whole community, including those who do not participate actively in the art program. When the children's artwork is also used directly in psychotherapy, however, conflict between its cultural and therapeutic usefulness may arise: when artwork is discussed analytically in the course of psychotherapy, the self-consciousness that results sometimes interferes with the artistic process.[7]

Useful Art Activities

In conducting art activities the teacher encourages the child to delve into his own experience and to order that experience according to his individual needs, wishes, and capabilities. In the child's work, as in any complete artistic production, content and form thus become inseparably intertwined. It follows that the kind of art suitable for an art education therapy should be as free from the self-expressive or abstract academicisms of today or tomorrow as from the imitative ones of yesterday.

Occasionally, art projects involving direct collaboration among members of a group may be useful. More often, however, art provides a refuge from the demands for group participation that permeate life in schools and institutions. Unlike activities which depend on immediate cooperation and sharing, art permits indirect movement into relationship with others by way of works so intimately representative of the artist that responses to a product are responses to its maker.

Genuine artistic work may be done, at however primitive a level, by persons suffering from severe intellectual, physical, or emotional handicaps.

---

7. Kramer, *op. cit.*, 1958; Leonard Bloom, "Aspects of the Use of Art in the Treatment of Maladjusted Children," *Mental Hygiene*, Vol. 41, No. 3, 1957, pp. 378–85.

Such limitations are not, therefore, a reason for short-circuiting the full artistic process. While the teacher may have to devise special methods to work within the limits of the child's capacities, he should never deliberately misuse art materials for the sake of easy success. The art educator opposes equally such old-fashioned home remedies as tracing or copying and modern commercial marvels like the numbered paint set. Successes that the child knows in his heart are phony undermine his belief in himself and foster his constraint and dependency. Pseudo-art may yield some immediate gratification but at a high price, for it tends to make the deeper satisfactions of independent work harder—even, at times, impossible—to attain. [8]

The distinction between fine art and applied art, however, is an artificial one. So long as the pupil continues to realize himself through the creation and development of form, applied art has a place in art education therapy. [9]

Crafts play a legitimate part in the education of the emotionally disturbed, but usually art and craft flourish best when they are kept separate, each being accorded its own dignity and special realm. The essential difference between art and craft is that, in the latter, form is imparted to matter not primarily for an expressive purpose but rather to produce, by following logical procedures, an object both beautiful and useful. In any particular activity, the elements of art and craft may be intermingled in varying proportions. [10]

No recommendation is being made here of such devices as prefabricated ceramic molds and kitcraft, whose use is often subsumed under the misleading rubric *arts and crafts*. In these activities, the element of choice so prominent in the arts is eliminated in favor of the assembly-line principle, and the loving workmanship common to both art and craft is bypassed. As with pseudo-art, justification is claimed for these procedures on the ground that a finished product is bound to result; unfortunately, it tends to be a product that is often useless and is almost always ugly.

The systematic exposure of the emotionally disturbed to art of high quality in the interest of art education may have both positive and negative effects. As with all immature artists, if disturbed children are to be inspired in their work and stimulated to appreciate art by viewing adult works, the teacher's choice of examples is of crucial importance. Students whose stage of visual conceiving has not reached the level demonstrated in artworks by sophisticated adults are often confused and inhibited when such art is held up to them as a model. Art and applied art deriving from primitive cultures or

8. Cane, *op. cit.*; James W. Crawford, "Art for the Mentally Retarded: Directed or Creative?" *Bulletin of Art Therapy*, Vol. 2, No. 2, 1962, pp. 67–72; Lowenfeld, *op. cit.*

9. "Therapeutic Art Programs Around the World—IV: Art and Applied Art by Mentally Defective Children," *Bulletin of Art Therapy*, Vol. 7, No. 1, 1967, pp. 29–33; Schaefer-Simmern, *op. cit.*

10. Edith Kramer, "Art and Craft," *Bulletin of Art Therapy*, Vol. 5, No. 4, 1966, pp. 149–52.

produced by naïve adults—artists who are relatively untouched by the artistic mainstream of their culture and whose stage of visual conceiving is akin to the child's—may, however, evoke the child's spontaneous response and help him solve his own immediate artistic problems.[11]

As for the teaching of esthetic principles, it should be remembered that the rules grew out of the analysis of works of art; no work of art was ever achieved by learning the principles of design and then applying them. Profound esthetic understanding may well depend on prior experience of the artistic process. Therefore, the focusing of attention on esthetic principles is useful mainly in a later educational context.

The materials appropriate to art education therapy are the same as those used with less disturbed children at similar developmental levels. Drawing, painting, and clay modeling are the basic activities which must be provided for. Among disturbed children, choices to be expected at a younger age than the actual chronological age will more often be encountered. With these children, the use of finger paints, which unnecessarily stimulates regressive messing, is highly questionable.[12]

Modifications of Teaching Method

Emotionally disturbed children tend to oscillate between rigidity and abandon, a factor which makes the art teacher's task, never an easy one, all the more difficult. Somehow he must maintain simultaneously the freedom and the order equally necessary to art.

The art teacher learns to expect that rigidity will be expressed by stereotyped modes of artistic production stubbornly clung to. In his attempt to help the disturbed student express himself more fully in art, the teacher must proceed with special caution, for fragile defenses may be all that stand in the way of complete breakdown.

The teacher must, at the same time, be prepared for more than the average turmoil as he leads children whose controls are exceedingly weak into experiences which may be threatening at the moment although their ultimate rewards are great. While the extremes of aggressive action must often be curbed, the expression of raw aggression in painting or sculpture should sometimes be welcomed as a first step toward the integrative use of art materials.[13]

Retardation, whether it is due to mental deficiency, psychological blocking, or a mixture of the two, often requires the teacher to introduce

11. Kramer, *op. cit.*, 1958; Schaefer-Simmern, *op. cit.*
12. Lena L. Gitter, "Montessori and the Compulsive Cleanliness of Severely Retarded Children," *Bulletin of Art Therapy*, Vol. 4, No. 4, 1965, pp. 139–48.
13. Kramer, *op. cit.*, 1958.

materials and processes slowly and in a carefully organized sequence. Various kinds of physical handicaps, which usually include an emotional component, make their own special demands on the teacher's understanding and ingenuity.[14]

History

The notion that art education can have special value for the emotionally disturbed has developed largely since the early 1940s. It was an outgrowth of an interest in the art of children, primitive peoples, and naïve adults that began in the early years of the twentieth century. As the results of the industrial revolution became consolidated, handicrafts lost their reason for being, and with them died the folk arts. Creative teachers of art, dismayed by the dearth of the man-made beauty that had formerly been taken for granted, discovered in children's art a new source of freshness and vitality.

Two innovative teachers, Franz Cizek in Austria and Marion Richardson in England, initiated the development of methods designed to make available to children the full psychological benefits of art activity.[15] In the 1940s, Florence Cane and Henry Schaefer-Simmern demonstrated that such ways of teaching could be extended to art education for adults, and each of them evolved a particular method of art education therapy.[16]

In her early years as an educator, Margaret Naumburg was keenly aware of the educative power of the arts.[17] Having left the field of education for that of psychotherapy, she published in 1947 a collection of papers about her pioneering work in the diagnosis and treatment of disturbed children through art.[18] Verbal exchange and psychoanalytic interpretation were important even in these early studies, but the therapeutic value of sublimation through art was also recognized.

Lowenfeld, whose *Creative and Mental Growth* was long the bible of art educators in the United States, experimented for many years with making art useful to the physically, mentally, and emotionally handicapped. His thinking reached its full development only in the last edition of his textbook to be published in his lifetime. His expanded chapter "Therapeutic Aspects

14. Crawford, *op. cit.*; Lena L. Gitter, "Art in a Class for Mentally Retarded Children," *Bulletin of Art Therapy*, Vol. 3, No. 3, 1964, pp. 83–95; Lowenfeld, *op. cit.*; Schaefer-Simmern, *op. cit.*; Rawley Silver; "Art and the Deaf," *American Journal of Art Therapy*, Vol. 9, No. 2, 1970, pp. 63–77.

15. Franz Cizek, *Children's Coloured Paper Work*, New York, Stechert, 1927; Marion Richardson, *Art and the Child*, Peoria, Ill., Bennett, 1948.

16. Cane, *op. cit.*; Schaefer-Simmern, *op. cit.*

17. Margaret Naumburg, *The Child and the World: Dialogues in Modern Education*, New York, Harcourt, 1928.

18. Margaret Naumburg, *Studies of the "Free" Art Expression of Behavior Problem Children and Adolescents as a Means of Diagnosis and Therapy*, Nervous and Mental Disease Monograph 71, New York, Coolidge Foundation, 1947.

of Art Education" has, however, been excised from the editions of *Creative and Mental Growth* published since his death. This deletion may indicate a wish on the part of the art education establishment to separate itself from the use of art as therapy.

Edith Kramer's writing has been primarily about art and art therapy; she was also an art teacher before she became an art therapist. As both theoretician and practitioner, she has demonstrated the harmonious integration of insights derived from experiences as an artist working with children in educational as well as psychotherapeutic settings.

Looking ahead, it appears that art education therapy, thus far used mainly with younger people, may find a growing currency in work with adults. It has been predicted that what I termed "the therapeutically oriented art class" may become a part of the treatment offered adults in the growing numbers of community mental health centers.[19]

---

19. Elinor Ulman, "Therapy Is Not Enough: The Contribution of Art to General Hospital Psychiatry," *Bulletin of Art Therapy*, Vol. 6, No. 1, 1966, pp. 3–21.

Theory and Practice of Art Therapy with the Mentally Retarded

Laurie Wilson

Art therapy with the mentally retarded has received relatively little attention. This study will discuss some general principles and theoretical ideas arising from several years of work in a newly established art therapy program at Brooklyn Developmental Center, a state residential facility for mentally retarded and multiply handicapped children and adults.

Since therapeutic methods are frequently best understood in relation to the pathology of the population for which they are designed, some features of pathology associated with mental retardation will be outlined. I shall discuss problems of particular concern to the art therapist and suggest the conceptual framework and some practical methods for their resolution through the use of art therapy. An extended case study will be used both to demonstrate techniques and to formulate some hypotheses concerning the iconography of child art in general as revealed in the art of the mentally retarded.

The Psychological Effects of Retardation

In recent years increasing attention has been paid to the psychological development of the mentally retarded. This has brought about attempts to understand the deviant personality traits accompanying the more obvious physiological disabilities of mental retardation. Most widely acknowledged are intellectual impairment, which limits the capacity for abstraction and consequently interferes with language development, symbol formation, imaginary play, and problem solving; and the slow and uneven rate of development in the physical and emotional as well as the intellectual spheres.

The disturbing effect these disabilities may have upon the psychological development of the mentally retarded has been summed up by Webster as a developmental disturbance with impairment in the differentiation of ego functions. The slow and incomplete unfolding of the personality is associated with partial fixations, which result in an infantile or immature personality structure. This particular style of ego development is accompanied by special descriptive features: a nonpsychotic autism, repetitiousness, inflexibility, passivity and simplicity in emotional life.[1]

While each of these features will be familiar to the art therapist working with the mentally retarded, it should be clear that the severity of the symptoms is usually related to the degree of retardation. Thus some retarded people have a quite complex emotional life involving intimate and enduring relationships, and where retardation is mild they may also be capable of autonomous and flexible behavior.

Although a number of studies have shown that the retarded are more likely to suffer from emotional disturbances in general than are the nonretarded, in this paper the discussion will be limited to the symptoms cited above. A further paper should explore the complex issues of deviant ego development and its relationship to severe emotional disturbances and the ways in which both of these impinge on the art therapist working with the mentally retarded.

Special Art Therapy Goals and Methods

The intellecutal impairment central to the pathology of the mentally retarded frequently takes the form of deficient language development. Since the art therapist is particularly adept with nonverbal approaches, this deficit does not present a substantial obstacle to treatment. In fact, the anxiety and sense of failure which face the mentally retarded person whenever his intellectual deficits make him unequal to the tasks life presents him with may be lessened in the art room. Here he may be encouraged and helped to manipulate the art materials in whatever way he is able to. Even if at first a retardate can only make random marks on paper with a crayon or lightly tap and squeeze some clay or hesitantly smear finger paint, an art therapist can display his work in the art room and praise his accomplishment, recognizing the retarded person's need for encouragement. Indeed the art therapist working with the severely and moderately retarded soon discovers that there is little need for words and that most of the clients' activity consists of exploring and manipulating materials that often are not art materials in a strict sense—e.g., water and sand.

The immediate goal with retarded people is to expand their sensory, perceptual, and motor horizons through this manipulation of materials. It is hoped that this will lead to some appropriate independent use of art

1. Thomas G. Webster, "Unique Aspects of Emotional Development in Mentally Retarded Children," in Frank Menolascino, editor, *Psychiatric Approaches to Mental Retardation,* New York, Basic Books, 1970, p. 22. See also Nancy M. Robinson and Halbert B. Robinson, *The Mentally Retarded Child: A Psychological Approach,* New York, McGraw-Hill Book Co., 1976, p. 189.

materials proper which would suggest that some real advances had been made in the development of ego functions. The early and intermediate steps in this line of treatment require that the art therapist be more than usually active in helping the client learn how to use these materials. For instance, in introducing clay one might at first hold the severely retarded person's hand and tap, squeeze, and roll the clay with him until he is able to carry out these maneuvers on his own. The art therapist's awareness of the retarded person's slow rate of development leads him not only to accept the infantile artwork but also to tolerate the seeming lack of progress through the expected developmental phases from kinesthetic experiences to organized imagery.

As has long been recognized by art educators, most retarded individuals are indeed capable of making some progress in this sequence, but it may take a very long time and be imperceptible to all but the most observant.[2] The art therapist working with retarded people should therefore be well acquainted with the earliest developmental phases of child art and be prepared to offer from time to time, in the appropriate order, the most fundamental steps toward higher functioning. Thus, working beside a random scribbler on a separate paper, the art therapist should periodically draw circles and vertical and horizontal lines.

Sometimes more active measures must be taken. A random scribbler may appear to be ready to form circles but he may have some visual or perceptual impairment that makes his next developmental step difficult.[3] In such a case the art therapist may place the child's arm on his own and make circular movements. The next step would be to continue such movements but instead with the therapist's hand on top of the child's, gradually releasing any pressure until the child continues the movement unaided. This must be done without coercion and it may have to be repeated from time to time. The art therapist is rewarded by being able to participate in and observe the acquisition of skills and concepts that are achieved with such lightning speed in normal children that the adult rarely is aware of it or understands its full meaning.

The Problem of Perseveration

The retarded person's development is made even slower by his tendency to be repetitious and inflexible. Webster noted that retarded children tend to repeat the familiar and avoid the unfamiliar and connected this characteristic

---

2. See, for example, C. D. Gaitskell and M. Gaitskell, *Art Education for Slow Learners*, Peoria, Ill., Charles A. Bennett, 1953.

3. Discrimination is made between sensory acuity, e.g., vision, and perception; the latter is understood to involve an interpretive response. See, for example, D. P. Hallahan and W. M. Cruickshank, *Psycho-Educational Foundations of Learning Disabilities*, Englewood Cliffs, N.J., Prentice-Hall, 1973.

to the quest for pleasure and contentment. He also pointed out that the retarded person does not actively exclude the unfamiliar but he rather fails to be interested in it.[4]

Thus a mentally retarded person will frequently repeat a pattern of lines or shapes hundreds of times with no sign of boredom but rather evident pleasure or reduced tension with each repetition. Even the same color may be used again and again.

The early work of Elena provides a particularly striking example of endless, unvarying repetition. This severely retarded young woman began art therapy sessions at the age of twenty-two.[5] She had been living in institutions for eighteen years. Aside from an undetermined degree of visual impairment, there were no signs of abnormal physical development. While Elena had been classified as nonverbal, some limited vocabulary was apparent to therapists who saw her regularly.

When Elena began art therapy sessions three years ago she was apparently fixated to one image: a circle with a pattern of radial lines imposed upon it (Figure 1). She repeated this pattern steadily in her art work for one and a half years. At first she would cover sheet after sheet with numerous examples of it, almost always using red. While she willingly varied the medium, using crayon, paint, or chalk, she would rarely alter the image or the color.

Other less extreme, more typical examples of such repetitiousness in the art of mentally retarded individuals may be seen in Figures 2 and 3. In Figure 2 the circular form is repeated, at first filling the original outline and then overflowing the larger shape apparently meant to contain it. In Figure 3 a vertical linear pattern fills the entire page. In both instances the moderately retarded people who made these drawings showed evident signs of pleasure while they were working. Having observed such repetitious behavior many times in the mentally retarded, I would agree with Webster that it serves some pleasurable function.[6]

How are we to understand this way of performing in the art room?

The retarded child lives through a prolonged infancy and is apt to be isolated because of his sensory, perceptual, and intellectual defects. His emotional immaturity causes him to be more isolated still, and the state of isolation, in turn, inevitably diminishes his opportunities for normal object relations that would stimulate the development of sensory, perceptual, and cognitive capacities. This unfortunate situation frequently results in either

4. Webster, *op. cit.*
5. Three art therapists have worked with Elena over a three-year period. First, Katherine Paras and I were cotherapists in both group and individual sessions. Later Ms. Paras assumed primary responsibility. In the past year Anne Morris has been working as cotherapist with Ms. Paras.
6. Webster, *op. cit.*

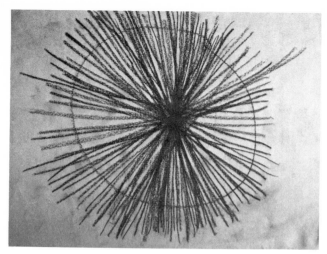

Figure 1

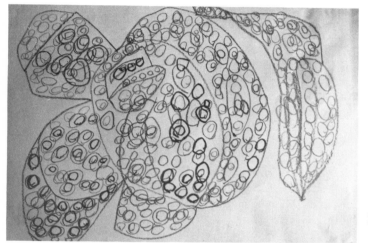

Figure 2

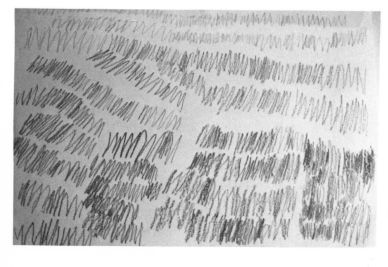

Figure 3

self-stimulating behavior, placidity, or both, and the end result is repetitiousness and inflexibility.

The retarded person's self-stimulating behavior is frequently autoerotic and takes such forms as rocking, massaging the face or other parts of the body, and manipulation of inanimate objects with the hand or mouth.[7] Rocking and facial massage are relatively acceptable public autoerotic behavior, while masturbation is not. Thus it may be that the repetitiousness seen in the art room and elsewhere has some of its roots in the early self-stimulating behavior of the retarded infant. In addition, retarded people urgently need a safe repertoire of satisfying behavior that is socially acceptable. If any piece of behavior serves both to relieve inner tensions and offer pleasure while not offending other people, its repetition will afford a safe haven.

In my opinion, repetitiousness or perseveration in the art of the mentally retarded is usually distinct from the stereotyped defensive art of higher-functioning people. The deficits in ego development common to the severely and moderately retarded frequently preclude the development of this type of defense. Sometimes, though, unwillingness to touch clay or finger paint may indeed be linked to the perhaps recently acquired or not fully stable accomplishments and controls of the anal phase.[8] It is thus a defense against the regressive pull of smearing and messing with art materials and is quite similar to the art-room behavior of some very young normal children.

However, I believe that early and prolonged deficits in the stimulus barrier of retarded children more often account for this repetitive behavior. It appears that these children frequently suffer from inadequate capacity for screening external stimuli. Either they are insufficiently protected from bombardment by sights, sounds, and other perceptual stimuli, or there is a pronounced blunting and blocking out of all or all but the most extreme sensations.

Children of the first type are highly distractible; they often enter the art room wide-eyed, tense, and fearful. Frequently they need physical comforting, a limited selection of art materials, and instruction in well-defined processes. It is often hard to predict whether materials conducive to regression, such as clay or finger paint, will comfort them and absorb their attention or overwhelm them. They are likely to want and need to use as many as three or four different materials in one art therapy session, and it is best to provide this variety until they discover those materials which are least threatening and most satisfying. The art therapist can then gradually persuade them to remain a bit longer with one material. Sometimes such a

7. *Cf.* Margaret Mahler, Fred Pine, and Anni Bergman, *The Psychological Birth of the Human Infant,* New York, Basic Books, 1975, p. 58.

8. *Cf.* Lena Gitter, "Montessori and the Compulsive Cleanliness of Severely Retarded Children," *Bulletin of Art Therapy,* Vol. 4., No. 4, 1965.

child may be satisfied with minor variations like change of paper or color rather than a change of medium.

Children who block out stimuli appear withdrawn, passive, or even autistic, and often fail to respond at first to regular art materials. They show features which characterize as well the normal autistic phase in which physiological rather than psychological processes dominate. They take action only in order to satisfy such inner needs as hunger or thirst. This emphasis on orality often results in overweight and sluggishness; such people often seem to maintain contact with the external world only through their mouths—by biting, swallowing, licking, and chewing.

Since their fixation seemed to be to such an early phase, we attempted to reach them through what is normally the infant's earliest pleasurable tactile experience outside of direct contact with the mother. We used play with warm soapy water. This was almost always successful and led through the progressive stages of sand play and sand-and-water play to play with tinted water to finger paint. As these children's initial resistance to external stimuli was relaxed through their experience of pleasurable sensations, we could gradually introduce them to more complex stimuli. Thus colored water was an intermediary stage between water play and finger paint. It is interesting that when such children are reached in this way the repetitious or perseverative behavior temporarily stops. One receives the clear impression that the entrance of the therapist via the newly perceived stimuli into this isolated and barren world stimulates growth. The retarded person may be persuaded to move by small steps to a more complex level of functioning.

The Developmental Significance of Configurations

It is evident that the stimulation of sensation and perception through the introduction of appropriate art materials and processes is one of the earliest goals of art therapy with the mentally retarded. The organization of these perceptions and the development of an increasingly flexible visual vocabulary are further goals. Because the visual vocabulary of the mentally retarded develops very slowly, we have an opportunity to examine the developmental process itself.

There is at present no general agreement as to the perceptual or psychological meaning of children's earliest habitual configurations. From her extensive study of child art, Kellogg claims to have found a regular sequence of configurations which leads from the early kinesthetic scribble to the human figure.[9] The crucial two steps before the figure she entitles mandala (Figure 4A) and sun (Figure 4B). She explains these as deriving from the earlier gestalts of circles and crosses and avoids any psychological interpretation, while also pointing out the absence of any statistical study

9. Rhoda Kellogg; *Analyzing Children's Art*, Palo Alto, Calif., National Press Books, 1970.

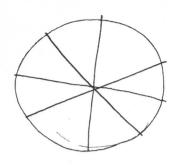

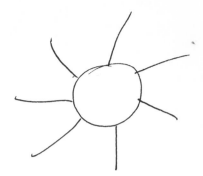

Figure 4 A   **Figure 4B**

confirming this sequential development. She places this sequence within the third and fourth years, which corroborates the findings of Gesell and others who place the child's ability to copy circles and crosses at thirty-six months.[10]

According to studies by Mahler and her collaborators, in normal development the infant begins to have a sense of himself as a separate being during the second half of the first year of life. This process is not usually completed until about the third year.[11] The sense of self and in particular the body image—that mental representation of one's own body as an object in space—is generally formed by this time. It seems to be constructed "from the visual perception and tactile exploration of the surface of one's body and sensations from the inner organs, skeleto-muscular system and the skin."[12] It is then to be expected that the mentally retarded person with his intellectual, sensory, and perceptual deficits and developmental lags will develop a distorted or deficient body image. In addition, he will probably achieve a body image more slowly than the normal child.

Since there have as yet been no studies linking the successive stages of ego development with the sequential development of child art, the inferences that will be made in this paper about such links should be understood at the outset to be general impressions. Furthermore, they are derived from observation of pathological rather than normal art production and behavior; however, just because the mentally retarded have a slow rate of development and disturbed ego functions, it may be possible to catch a glimpse of the underlying psychological meaning of some early schematic and pre-schematic art.

10. Arnold Gesell and C. S. Amatruda, *Developmental Diagnosis*, New York, Paul B. Hoeber, 1941; Joseph DiLeo, *Young Children and Their Drawings*, New York, Brunner/Mazel, 1970; Loretta Bender, *Child Psychiatric Techniques*, Springfield, Ill., Charles C Thomas, 1952, p. 50 ff.

11. Mahler *et al.*, *op. cit.*

12. Burness Moore and Bernard Fine, editors, *A Glossary of Psychoanalytic Terms and Concepts*, New York, American Psychoanalytic Association, 1968, p. 24.

An Illustrative Case

Striking evidence of a possible correlation between certain phases of ego development and the developmental sequence of child art imagery may be observed in a close examination of the art produced in therapy by Elena, the young woman briefly discussed earlier. It was pointed out that Elena had been fixated to a configuration (Figure 1) similar to Kellogg's mandala for a long time. In an effort to understand both the meaning of this image and Elena's behavior, the art therapy team studied the meagre information available about Elena's history.

Elena is classified as severely mentally retarded and profoundly socially retarded. Her Stanford-Binet scores yield a Mental Age of 3.6 and an I.Q. of 20. She is of average height, weight, and normal physical development except for poor vision. She was placed by her parents at Willowbrook, a large developmental center, at the age of four in 1956, at which point the clinical record states that she had an I.Q. of 15, suffered from hydrocephalus and epileptic seizures, and was hyperactive. The seizures have continued but the hydrocephalus was arrested. In 1970 she was again classified as profoundly mentally retarded, unable to care for herself or make herself understood, and in need of constant supervision. Elena remained at Willowbrook until 1973 when she was transferred to Brooklyn Developmental Center.

Institutional records indicate a prolonged fixation at the oral phase. She could not be weaned from the bottle until the age of five and shortly thereafter developed a habit of collecting and chewing or swallowing bits of string and buttons. By adolescence Elena still collected these objects but she no longer put them in her mouth. Upon arriving at Brooklyn Developmental Center she had abandoned this habit, developing instead a fixation upon a ball-like clump of metal jingle bells which she carried or wore around her neck on a chain. Elena herself wove the bells together with wire, increasing or decreasing the size of the cluster, and if they were taken from her or accidentally left behind she would cry inconsolably or angrily hit or overturn tables or chairs.

This fixation was already firmly established at the time of Elena's first art therapy session. She had, in addition, a repertoire of gestures which included rubbing her hands together, stroking her cheeks, mouth, and nose, or holding and rubbing her breasts. When she began to make these gestures her facial expression often signaled distress, which usually gave way to evident signs of pleasure or comfort. Elena appeared to be attempting to comfort herself with caresses that had in her past experience been given her by others.

Elena began art therapy as a member of a small group of residents who came to the art room once a week. She came willingly and seemed to enjoy using crayons, chalk, finger paint, and tempera paints. She energetically

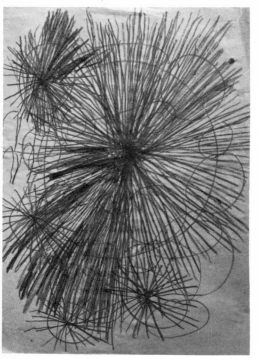

Figure 5

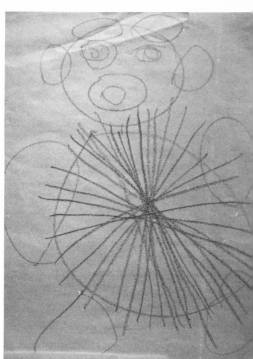

Figure 6

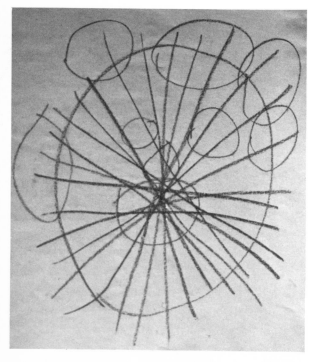

Figure 7

sought and responded to praise and verbal encouragement from the art therapists. (In the early phases of art therapy she was often dependent and clinging.) In addition, the few times she entered the art room without bells, she was despondent; but once persuaded to paint or draw, she calmed down and was able to concentrate.

As has been mentioned, her most persistent image was the radial configuration done in red (Figure 1). When an art therapist offered Elena a different color or shape such as a triangle, a zigzag line, or a letter, she was capable of repeating it but for many months she did not spontaneously initiate such variations. Typically she would oblige the art therapist with one example of the newly suggested idea and then revert for the remainder of the session to a succession of radial configurations which would ultimately obliterate the variant image (Figure 5).

After about six months, we felt that Elena was ready to extend her visual vocabulary. She had mastered some of the basic art-room procedures, such as washing her paint brush and taping her pictures to the wall. She was generally calmer than she had been at the start, and she was responsive to suggestions that she use a variety of media or make changes in her imagery.

It had become clear to us from observation of her behavior and knowledge of her history that Elena's clump of bells served as some kind of transitional object. We therefore concluded that Elena might be at the psychosexual stage preceding the moment in which an infant begins to perceive the mother as a separate person. Since the attainment of that step requires some sense of body image on the infant's part, we determined to work with Elena toward the development of her own body image.

We began by drawing in finger paint a simple face and simultaneously naming and pointing to each facial feature on the picture and on Elena. As before, when a new image was offered to her, Elena copied the face and then immediately superimposed a series of radial patterns upon it, thereby obliterating the new image. With the very attentive guidance just described, in the following two sessions Elena was able to draw a figure using her radial configurations as the component parts. At this point she began to alternate between two apparently interchangeable forms: the radial pattern and concentric circles. Elena continued to produce many examples of radial patterns between her attempts to depict body parts.

In a week following a session during which she would draw only the radial configuration, Elena corroborated the meaning we had hypothesized for that image. One of the art therapists drew a circle and two circular eyes and called it a face (see Figure 6). Elena was asked to draw the nose. Instead she drew a mouth and redrew the eyes. As the art therapist named them, Elena drew circular shapes representing the body, hair, ears, arms, legs, and neck. She then drew a radial configuration within the body, and when asked which body part it was, she held her breast. Next, when asked to draw a face, Elena began a radial pattern (Figure 7). The art therapist intervened and drew one eye within the configuration. Elena then completed the face, including eye, nose, mouth, hair, and ears. With similar guidance she proceeded to make more drawings of figures and faces.

Because of Elena's rapid progress toward acquisition of a body image, individual art therapy sessions were planned for her. We felt that she had shown more potential for growth than had been previously noted by the staff at the Developmental Center and that perhaps through art therapy she might be able to develop more advanced ego functioning and, therefore, more adaptive behavior.

For the next few weeks we proceeded as before, and Elena became increasingly able to identify and name the body parts as she alternately drew and touched them. She continued to use concentric circles as body parts but often added radial configurations to the drawings when left undirected. We noticed, however, that she was selective in her addition of the radial patterns and that they would usually appear in a few particular parts of the drawing. During her first individual session she provided us with another clue to her own iconography.

Following the suggestion of one of the art therapists to draw a "lady" she drew a number of circular shapes, again representing body parts and adding two radial forms below the "head" (Figure 8). She identified these by touching her chest. Immediately afterward she enthusiastically did a similar picture of herself (Figure 9) with a "head," "neck," "body," and "ears." To this picture she added a clump of circles at the figure's left which soon became radial configurations. She identified these as the bells which she held in her hand. There was indeed a visual similarity between the bells with their cut-out radial opening and her repeated graphic pattern. As we continued to help Elena distinguish among her own body parts through drawing and naming each one, the concentric circles replaced the radial pattern as her preferred configuration.

Elena continued at times to overload her drawing by repeating a particular shape. She might begin by making circles to suggest hair at the top of her head and would then keep on making circles all the way around the head. In the same way the shapes signifying arms and legs might come to encompass the whole body. Once this rhythmic repetition had begun, it threatened to engulf the entire page. She also reverted occasionally to the radial pattern. This usually occurred when she was in the art room as part of a group and was not receiving the considerable amount of praise, reassurance, and physical contact she sought. There appeared to be some correlation, as well, between the reappearance of the radial pattern and the use of regressive media such as finger paint.

On several occasions at the end of group sessions, Elena had tried to take pipe cleaners or wire with her as she left the art room. After she had drawn faces and figures for several months we decided to offer three-dimensional materials to Elena at her individual sessions. We felt that since her fixation

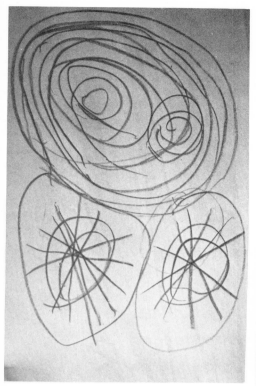
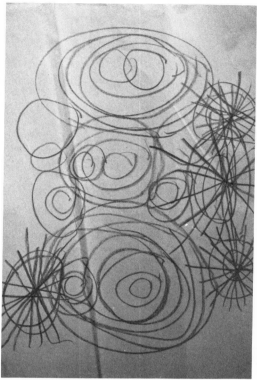

Figure 8　　　　　　　　**Figure 9**

was to a three-dimensional object constructed with wires, we might be able to reach her by offering similar materials and guiding her toward a more flexible use of them. She proved to have excellent fine-motor coordination and was evidently both comfortable and familiar with gluing and wiring. It was at this time that we discovered that Elena herself had wired together her clumps of bells.

Elena's first experience using these materials with us came at a time when she had recently been given a pocketbook in which she had placed her clump of bells. At the end of this session she again attempted to take some wire from the art room. When Elena returned to the art room on the same afternoon for a group session she did a finger painting of a clump of radial configurations. Then, for the first time, she left her bells behind her in the art room.

Since the development of body image has so much to do with the perception of the self in space, we decided to see whether Elena was ready to use her dexterity with three-dimensional materials to duplicate her achievements in the drawing of figures. For this purpose we chose clay. Two weeks after she had left her bells in the art room, an art therapist and Elena made a clay figure together, following the same procedure as had been used with drawing. She cooperated but was not enthusiastic. The clay body parts that she put on one side of the body to correspond with those placed by the art therapist on the other side were often smaller than those the art therapist had made. They were arranged similarly to the parts of the figures she had previously drawn.

The following week we returned to drawing the figure, again attempting to further Elena's ability to discriminate not only between parts of the body but also between herself and other people. These drawings were done on large paper taped to the wall. An art therapist began by drawing a "mommy." Elena added a mouth and two pairs of circles at the outside edges of the face and trunk. Her own drawing of a "mommy" (Figure 10), a word she clearly understood and could pronounce distinctly, included an excessive number of circles and the concentric circle configuration, but a head and trunk were clearly discernible. Following this the art therapist and Elena shared in making a drawing of a "girl" (Figure 11). Elena's contribution was the torso, which enclosed a number of circular shapes she called breasts, and a series of lines radiating outward from both sides of the body. This drawing was followed by a picture of a girl done entirely by Elena. The head and

Figure 10　　　　　　　　　　　**Figure 11**

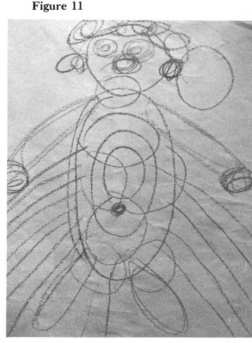

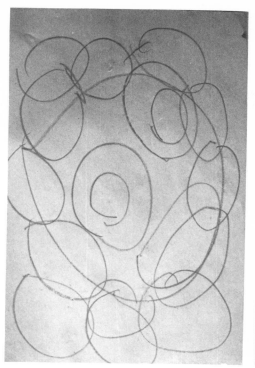

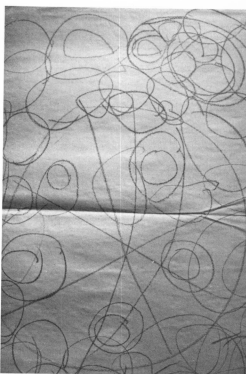

Figure 12   **Figure 13**

torso were more clearly depicted than before, and the overflow of circular shapes was restricted to an accumulation inside the torso and a border surrounding the figure. Remarkable was the total absence of radial patterns throughout this session—an unprecedented event.

At the start of the next week's session, Elena was offered clay. She experimented briefly with it, making spherical and cylindrical shapes which she built up as if they had been blocks and then squashed together. She then let us know she wanted to draw by drawing on the table with her finger. Given paper and crayon, she drew Figure 12, her first totally spontaneous depiction of a human being. She pointed in turn to her eyes, mouth, ears, hair, feet, and hands. The eyes and mouth were represented by the concentric circles within the larger circle: the hair surrounds that circle; and the feet and hands were placed below. Her pleasure with this achievement was obvious. Elena began her next drawing, Figure 13, by starting one of her radial configurations. One of the art therapists intervened and asked her what else she could do to make this picture mean something to herself. Elena placed concentric circles within each segment, and added a circumference of purple circles and a figure-like configuration at the upper right

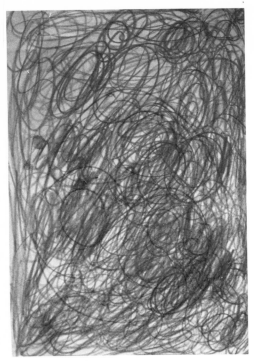

Figure 14

corner. As Elena began to work on her third picture, Figure 14, the art
therapist showed her (on a face the art therapist had drawn) how to make a
mass of color within the circular outline of an eye. Elena colored in the circle
representing the mouth and then, using red, orange, and purple crayons,
she covered the page with masses of color. This drawing was a source of
enormous satisfaction; when it was finished, Elena clapped her hands several
times and danced a few steps. Throughout the latter part of the session she
repeatedly said such things as "face" and "I did it." She clearly had
understood on some level that her accomplishment pointed the way toward
more flexible, coherent, and independent functioning.

In the group session on this same day the project offered was the making
of mobiles from a variety of materials that included wood, wire, pipe
cleaners, beads, and paper. Elena selected wire which she shaped into
circles, on which she strung a few beads. At her next individual session
Elena was given beads and wire thread because of the interest she had
shown in these materials. After some brief instruction and practice, she was
able to string beads of various size with great facility. She seemed to derive
tactile pleasure from this activity and had to be encouraged to look at what
she was doing rather than manipulate the materials only by touch. For the
next month Elena chose to work with beads at every individual session. She
was always offered a wide range of materials and sometimes chose to work, as

well, with clay or crayons. In the weekly group sessions she kept on making wire circles and stringing beads on them.

The next therapeutic intervention was the suggestion that she string the beads into a necklace for herself. She became very excited, as she showed by hugging both the therapist and herself. At the end of this session she purposely left her bells in the art room but showed some anxiety about them on her way to the classroom.

For the next three months Elena made necklaces and bracelets for herself at every individual session. At the same time she showed much less need to keep her clump of bells always with her. Although she brought them to the art room, she began to put them on the other side of the room rather than under her seat or in her lap. She frequently left them behind in the art room without a trace of anxiety. Her classroom teacher reported that more and more often she was not even bringing them to class from the residential unit. It appeared that she was in the process of very gradually giving up a conspicuous and unusual transitional object and replacing it with a more unobtrusive substitute. Several times, when she was visibly upset about her missing bells, she was calmed and reassured when the art therapist called her attention back to the bead necklaces and bracelets. It is interesting that there was also a correlation between Elena's occasional anxiety about the missing clump of bells and the reappearance of the radial pattern. Both usually occurred in group sessions when Elena did not have the full attention of an art therapist.

During this same three-month period Elena also demonstrated further progress in the graphic depiction of body image. She was strongly encouraged to draw at each individual session; and after she had made at least one bead necklace and bracelet for herself, she was willing to cooperate. Eventually, she would initiate the switch from beads to drawing. Her drawings at the beginning of this time were similar to those already illustrated: faces and figures made up of circles identified as body parts by Elena and finally overwhelmed by an overflowing excess of circles.

On one occasion Elena again made the connection between the overflow of circles and breasts. She began by drawing one of her usual pictures but identified the many circles as breasts and then, in response to a question from one of the art therapists, indicated that it was a picture of a woman she liked. Through a series of nonverbal clues, she identified the woman as a "mommy." The therapist spoke about people missing their "mommies" and Elena listened quietly. When the therapist suggested drawing a house in which a "mommy" would like to live, Elena excitedly began to draw a configuration of squares. When asked who else would live in the house, Elena said, "Me," and later as she continued to draw she said, "Baby." She was gently reminded that she was no longer a baby. She ended the session with a radial configuration enclosed in a square.

Following this session Elena's imagery became much richer and more flexible. She drew squares as well as circles, began to trace her hand and arm, spontaneously started to make triangles, and was much more independent in her efforts at drawing. She no longer had to begin every session with the bead jewelry but could shift freely between this activity and drawing.

During the next year Elena continued to take small steps forward, both in her artwork and her behavior. She learned in time to fill in life-size body tracings with a considerable number of details, including shoes, belly buttons, fingernails, and bracelets. The facial features and body parts became clearer and better differentiated as she learned to manipulate her expanded visual vocabulary. (See Figure 15.) She eventually began to include in her drawings new objects from her world, such as a baby doll which resided in the art room and a guitar she had been given. At first she traced these objects and then she drew them more spontaneously. The most significant behavioral changes were Elena's leaving the clump of bells in the residential wing whenever she came to the art room and, finally, her ability

Figure 15

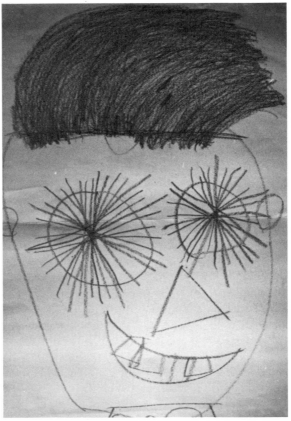

to make this trip without any assistance from staff. Her increased independence can clearly be seen in these two achievements.

Summary and Conclusions

Elena's course in art therapy epitomizes our more general findings. In two years of work with her we can see a gradual progression in both art expression and general behavior from an infantile dependency to greater maturity. When Elena began art therapy she was totally fixated upon both the clump of bells she carried and the radial configuration she drew. Her clinging and her need for constant reassurance and praise helped lead us to an understanding of the psychological meaning of her art. By partially satisfying some of her needs, both artistic and personal, and by leading her toward small but appropriate changes in these two areas, we gradually helped her to become more flexible and independent. Her graphic vocabulary expanded to include concentric circles, images of bodies, squares, and ultimately a relatively rich combination of circles, triangles, squares, and hybrid shapes which she used to depict full figures, clothing, and ornaments.

The changes in her behavior paralleled those in art. As she became less dependent on the art therapists, she displaced her fixation from the clump of bells to jewelry and a pocketbook. At the end of two years she had become able to travel unassisted to the art room.

Two points are significant. The only drawing in Elena's repertoire when she began art therapy sessions was an image in red resembling Kellogg's mandalas (Figure 1). This insistently repeated image was striking in that it was much more unvarying and at the same time more complex than the patterns habitually produced by other mentally retarded residents. Like the perseverative imagery of other retardates it did not have the quality of a defensive stereotyped image serving to ward off fear or anxiety,[13] but it seemed to be affording more than the pleasurable release of tension through repetition which we observed more generally. It seemed in fact to embody a particular meaning for Elena. We sought for clues in Elena's behavior both in the art room and elsewhere. One of the most conspicuous things about her was the clump of bells she wore around her neck. It gradually became evident that the bells served as a transitional object. This led to our conjecture that Elena's repeated image might signify a breast. Elena seemed to be arrested at the developmental stage between the second half of the first year and the third year, during which the infant begins to be a being distinct and separate from the mother but still needs a great deal of actual or

13. Edith Kramer, *Art as Therapy with Children*, New York, Schocken Books, 1971; Beverly Eftes Silverman, "Is It Possible to Differentiate Between Perseveration and Repetition Compulsion in Children's Drawings?" Unpublished master's thesis, Hahnemann Medical College, 1974.

symbolic contact with her. Elena's stroking of her own cheeks seemed to be an attempt to assimilate the mother's soothing gesture.

Transitional objects are usually soft, pliable, and warm to the touch like the mother's breast or warm neck, for which they substitute. In Elena's case, however, the similar *shape* of the bells, the repeated image, and a breast—round with a central focus—seems to serve as the link between substitute and remembered reality. Furthermore, Elena would frequently rub her cheeks or breasts while drawing this image or touching the bells. It is even more persuasive that Elena was able to give up both the bells and the radial pattern at almost the same time in the course of treatment.

All this leads us to the tantalizing notion that if the radial shape can stand for the breast at a moment when the artist is caught up with a transitional object similar in shape, there may in fact be a correlation between that particular shape as it generally appears in child art and the period in ego development when transitional phenomena occur. We know that the radial shape is usually drawn about two years after the phase where transitional objects are normally sought. One might expect then that the child's inner sense of a body image should become apparent in his art about two years after it has been achieved psychologically. According to psychological studies and studies of children's art, this is indeed the case. In the study cited above, Mahler and her collaborators observed that by the age of three children normally achieve an inner sense of a body image. Similarly a number of studies have indicated that most children can draw a human figure including head, trunk, and limbs by the age of five.[14]

Both of these achievements are products of slow maturational processes. Hard and fast conclusions about a causal relationship between the two await further research; however, we observed through this study of Elena's art therapy that progress in the graphic depiction of body image was accompanied by progress in ego development. The frequency of pathological or arrested ego development among the mentally retarded clearly supports a mode of treatment such as art therapy, which appears to foster ego development through the development of a mature body image.

14. DiLeo, *op. cit.*; Kellogg, *op. cit.*; Viktor Lowenfeld, *Creative and Mental Growth*, New York, Macmillan, 1957; Elizabeth M. Koppitz, *Psychological Evaluation of Children's Human Figure Drawings*, New York, Grune and Stratton, 1968.

Recovery, Repression, and Art

Stewart R. Smith, Lee B. Macht, and Carolyn C. Refsnes

The purpose of this paper is to study the relationship between a patient's recovery from psychiatric illness and his creativity. We will be interested both in the symbolism of the patient's artwork and its esthetic aspect as they are related to his psychological progress. In speaking of esthetic quality, we are concerned with the patient's command of composition and craft and his ability to imbue his images with feeling. We found it necessary to consider both symbolic content and formal qualities in attempting to understand changes in the productivity of a young man who was concerned lest he invest too deeply in art.

At the time when his disorganization assumed psychotic proportions, both the art therapist and the psychotherapist held the opinion that his artistic expression was of very fine quality. As his personality became more organized, his interest in the art sessions decreased, he spent less time over his drawings, and talked less with the art therapist about their meaning. When at his own wish he stopped attending art sessions altogether, he had produced forty-six drawings over a period of some two months.

The Patient's History

J. W. was a thirty-year-old Catholic Chinese man, never previously hospitalized, who, on admission to the Massachusetts Mental Health Center, said, "I need to see a doctor . . . there are voices . . . and there is the infrared." He was a slight, soft-spoken young man who appeared to be frightened and confused. He frequently interrupted his story to listen to voices which he recognized as hallucinatory. His illness was diagnosed as schizophrenic reaction, acute paranoid type.

J. W. had spent most of the first twenty-four years of his life on Formosa and had come alone to the United States, leaving behind his father, mother, and two older and two younger siblings. Six years later, he recalled his father, who was seventy-three at the time, as strict, scholarly, and demanding. His mother, ten years younger, was characterized as gentle, warm, and a devotee of poetry. She had suffered for years from a congestive heart condition.

In early childhood the patient was very close to his mother, but when he was five years old their relationship was seriously disturbed by her depression following the death of an older child. During the next eight years, the family's life was disrupted by the war, which drove them from the Chinese mainland to Formosa. The patient was sent to a Catholic grammar school away from home and here he converted to Catholicism.

Between the ages of thirteen and nineteen he attended a number of different high schools. In addition to some school art courses he had individual training in art. His leaning toward the arts was further evidenced at this time by his wanting to become a musician.

Later his ambition turned toward architecture, but because his father insisted on it, he attended military school after his high school studies were completed. He took a competitive examination for a government scholarship to study architecture, but did not win. After this he continued in military school and became involved in some gang vandalism. Father learned of this and lectured frequently to him about it. At approximately the same time, J. W. became engaged to a girl of whom father disapproved. He did not get married, ostensibly because he feared father would disown him and he felt that therefore he needed to be "practical" and get an education.

Six years before admission he came to a small Catholic college in this country on a scholarship granted by the church, still wanting to be an architect but lacking funds to study without outside support. He graduated at the end of five years. About a year earlier he had reacted with bitterness and depression to the news from Formosa that his former fiancée had married.

After graduation he studied electronics for a few months in order to learn a trade before returning home, but gave up for lack of funds. He then worked as a stock boy in several firms, and each time the same peculiar pattern was repeated. First, he claimed, he was accused of stealing; then he actually began to pilfer the stock, but returned the goods without being discovered. He left each of these jobs voluntarily. During this period he broke with the girl he had dated in his college days.

Next he worked as a short-order cook and began to feel that people were watching him, calling him stupid, and referring to him as "the Chinese queer." During the last three weeks before he entered the hospital he began to have episodes of hyperventilation and to hear voices outside his window, female and male voices speaking in English and in Chinese. It seemed to him that the people who lived next door could see him in the bathroom through the use of "infrared," and he believed that especially his hands and penis were thus illuminated. In addition, he was convinced that these people had used the infrared to burn his whole left side. When he called the police to ask for protection, he was taken to a general hospital and four days later was transferred to the Massachusetts Mental Health Center.

Course in Hospital

In the hospital, the patient was seen two or three times a week in individual psychotherapy by a male psychiatric resident, and twice weekly in individual art therapy and once weekly in classes by a female art therapist.

At first he was floridly psychotic and he quickly incorporated the hospital into his delusional system. He saw it as a prison, where the police were holding him for a nameless crime committed against his girlfriend. While he was still psychotic but somewhat improved he had the experience of feeling "newborn," as if he were "coming out of his shell."

Gradually he began to react to the world around him more realistically. As the doctor's relationship with the patient developed and the psychosis began to abate, therapy centered on reconstructing the events and feelings leading up to the psychosis. This work continued for approximately two months.

When he was no longer psychotic, retrospective exploration of the content of the psychosis ran into difficulty. Unconscious productions which had been plentiful were made unavailable by massive repression. As he reconstituted, repression took the place of denial, projection, and distortion.

The final phase of inpatient psychotherapy was ushered in by the patient's receiving a letter saying that father wished to have him return home and telling that mother's cardiac condition had become worse. The imminence of going home brought up questions of racial, national, and work identity. Reviewing his relationship with his parents, he looked especially at his struggle with father who wanted him to be practical and bring home a trade. Gradually, he also considered the dependency wishes and fears associated with his return to Formosa. In this context, he worked on his inner conflict over his artistic-creative side and his more practical side.

Therapy dealt little with fantasy; some clarification was achieved, but little insight of any depth. In time, J. W. arrived at a compromise, whereby he felt he could return home and not lose face with his father and could also satisfy some needs of his own. He planned to become a teacher in Formosa and to study further at the university—perhaps fine arts or architecture.

He was discharged three and one-half months after admission but continued individual psychotherapy for some time as an outpatient until he left for Formosa. Art therapy had been terminated on the patient's initiative one month before discharge.

Art Therapy

During his first week in the hospital, the patient, who was in an acute state of psychotic disorganization, voluntarily entered the art class held on the ward. Art work turned out to be the one constructive activity to which he was able to apply himself during these early days; it seemed to provide relief from the turmoil of his fragmented thinking and hallucinations. At first he worked on still lifes and the city views that could be seen from the hospital window. His work showed talent and sensitivity but he denied that he had any previous training. It was not until later that he admitted his earlier experience with art and mentioned his mother's esthetic interest.

Because of his sustained interest in drawing, the individual art therapy sessions were begun within two weeks of his admission. From then on the art therapist and the psychotherapist met weekly to share material and confer about treatment plans. On occasion the psychotherapist would initiate discussion with the patient about a picture produced in art therapy. J. W. knew that the two therapists communicated with each other.

The approach used in art therapy was based on the dynamic methods developed by Margaret Naumburg in her work with schizophrenics.[1] In the first individual session the patient was encouraged to draw whatever he wanted, to talk freely and fully about each picture, and further to say whatever occurred to him whether it seemed relevant to the picture or not. He was next introduced to the technique of scribbling and developing a picture from imagery projected into the scribble.

This helped circumvent his constriction, his conventional artistic standards, and his perfectionistic notions about technique. In spite of his initial timidity, this projective procedure allowed him almost immediately to find his own symbolic images and to channel his unconscious feelings directly into his artwork. This started a spontaneous flow of pictures, produced with or without the scribble, in individual art therapy sessions, the art class, and at other times.

In the second session the patient brought in a series of seven drawings which were his first pictorial formulation of his conflicts. We will begin here with three of these pictures, all of which were titled by the authors on the basis of the patient's comments. What he said about the first, *The Bridge* (Figure 1), is mainly descriptive; he pointed out the river flowing into the distance and the bridge connecting two hills, and said that it is stormy, dark, and ominous on one side, clear and light on the other.

The picture appears to express his healthy wish to make some connection between the opposing forces of his inner conflict. Some weeks later he recalled photographing his fiancée in Formosa on such a bridge, thus linking the picture with one of his recent losses.

In the second picture, *The Earthquake* (Figure 2), the ominous elements have prevailed. Jagged cliffs are broken up as if by an earthquake. The trees are dead and broken. All that he said about it was that it is somehow about death and that he is at peace when he can sit alone and contemplate nature.

We took the symbolism of this picture as a revelation of his anger projected into a fantasy of world destruction, and as an indication that his

1. Margaret Naumburg, *Schizophrenic Art: Its Meaning in Psychotherapy*, New York, Grune and Stratton, 1950.

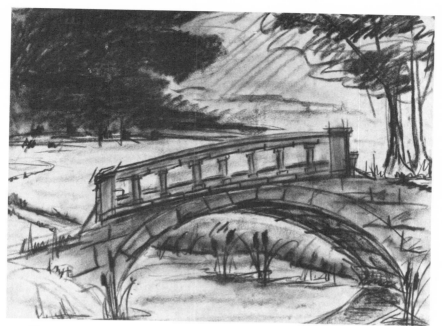

Figure 1

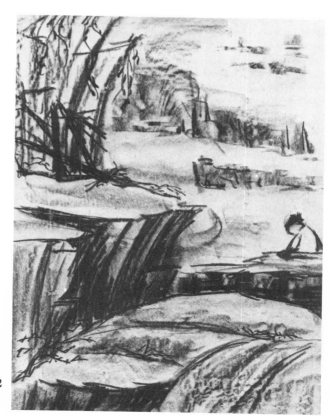

Figure 2

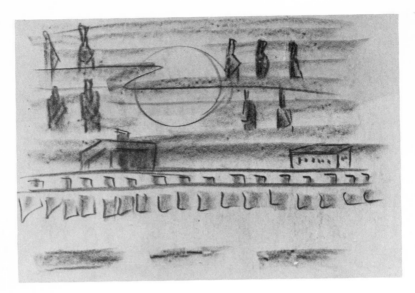

Figure 3

needed defenses had broken down. He appears to use the little figure, reminiscent of the contemplative scholar often seen in traditional Chinese landscape paintings, to convey his withdrawal and his helplessness. It seems that his effort to bridge the conflicting forces has failed; the breakdown is cataclysmic.

The series culminated in the picture of the *Hallucinated People in the Sky* (Figure 3). He said that while he was drawing it he heard voices telling him to jump off the building, and he was so disturbed by them that he had to stop drawing. The anger projected outward in the preceding picture is here turned against himself.

Figure 4

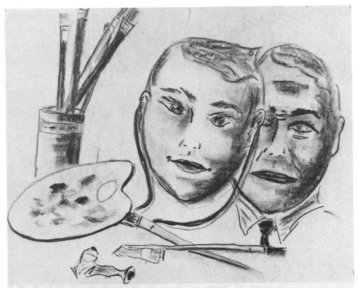

The male and female voices of his hallucination are indicated by figures of both sexes in the picture. The five figures on the right reminded us of his being one of five surviving children in the family. Pursuing the familial theme we noted that the two pairs of figures on the left might well stand for parents. If so, perhaps the repetition of them indicated his wish to replace the actual parents, whose conflicting demands he perceived as destructive to himself, with a more benign counterpart.

The themes of bridging (by means of arches), and death or destruction (frequently implied by crossing out all or part of a picture) occur again and again. Bridging and direct expressions about death each appear ten times, and canceling-out eleven times in the whole series of forty-six pictures. Bridging appears to symbolize the patient's healthy wish to resolve the pervasive conflict; death and canceling-out represent, of course, the negative aspects of his illness.

In talking about *The Mask and His Inner Self* (Figure 4), a self-portrait made five weeks after admission, the patient brought up explicitly the problem of his identity. He said, "People have an inner and an outer self. The outer is a mask, young and smiling. It looks all right. Painting is part of the mask. This is my inner self—I wanted to make it more ugly but I couldn't. I am not sure who I am."

In the two images his characteristics, actual and imagined, desired and undesired, are mixed and confused. The inner face, to which he gives Caucasian features, is the masculine one; he associated Americans with masculine and practical attributes. The expression of this face and its darkness suggest his inner tension and anxiety. To the mask he gives his own Oriental eyes and serene expression, but the features are pretty and feminine. The instruments of painting are linked with the mask, and painting was indeed associated in his life with feminine influence. We surmised as much from this picture and only later learned about his mother's encouragement of her son's artistic interests and his father's opposition to them. Possibly the crossed brushes in the picture indicate the canceling-out of his creative inclination, which yet seemed strong enough to have stood in the way of his working out the "practical" career demanded by his father.

It was at this time that we learned about his frustrated wish to become an architect; his dearest dream was to be a designer of churches. *The Church* (Figure 5) was painted on the same day as the preceding picture. Coming in the midst of his psychotic disorganization, its skill and sensitivity were amazing. Indeed, it was the high point of his artistic production while he was with us. We take this performance, so integrated in the face of acute illness, as suggesting that architecture presents the perfect symbol for the resolution of J. W.'s conflicts. It is the one profession which combines the artistic and the practical; achievement in it could therefore satisfy both the masculine and feminine components of his striving, at the same time enabling him to live as a responsible adult.

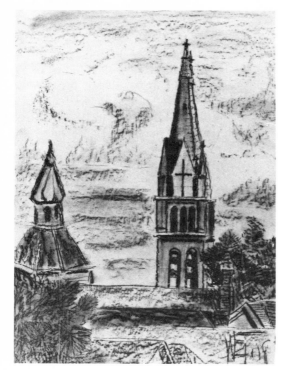

Figure 5

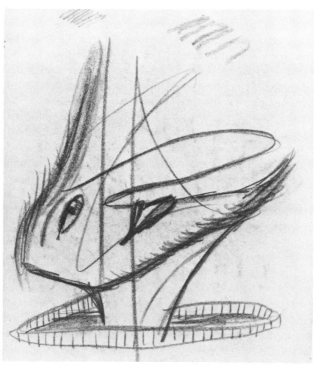

Figure 6

Figure 6, *The Nosy Beatnik,* was drawn two days later; it demonstrates the power of the scribble to elicit feelings that are beyond words. J. W. reacted to it at first with a mixture of harsh self-criticism and embarrassed amusement. He called the quality of the drawing childlike and bad, and said he felt as if his brain had dried up. The art therapist asked in vain who the image represented or what the patient's thoughts about his picture were, but in answer to her last question, "What does the fellow in the picture feel?" J. W. laughed and then spoke at length. He admired this person, who reminded him of a bearded homosexual patient on the ward. Of the pictured character, he said, "He enjoys life. He has a life of his own, like a beatnik. He has no thought for material things." He himself, he declared, would like to be like that. Actually, he was just the opposite.

The picture tells us about primitive fantasies which the patient, even assuming that he was aware of them, could not begin to share with the art therapist except through the picture. The ambiguous visual image permits the emergence of material whose verbal expression is forbidden. Indeed, feelings that are beyond words may at times be expressed in the "universal language" of visual art. In working with J. W., whose English was limited and who came from a culture which discourages directness, painting played a crucial part. Without it the linguistic and cultural gap between him and his therapists might have been impossible to bridge.

The erotic implications of the *Beatnik* were obvious to the art therapist although the patient did not verbalize them. The exaggerated nose is undeniably phallic and the smiling, open mouth readily suggests a vagina. The flat skull leaves little room for a brain, the organ of control, and it contributes a savage quality further enhanced by the bristling hair and beard. It all engenders the self-engrossed, lusty enthusiasm the beatnik exudes. We may think of this fellow as a personification of the pleasure principle.

J. W., however, told us indirectly that he could not accept the erotic side of himself. He pointed out the two lines cutting through the nose and face, saying he had put them there because he wanted to cancel out the image. He did not seem to notice that what he designated as the beatnik's turtleneck sweater might also suggest a platter; this could turn the image into a possible reference to the beheaded John the Baptist. Martyrdom might then be a symbol of punishment for forbidden wishes. We note further that only in such an outlandish image was J. W. able to express his erotic feelings. None of his pictures suggest adult heterosexual strivings.

It was not only his sexuality that the patient had difficulty accepting but also his aggressive and angry feelings. He was, however, able to make pictures of violent gestures, such as *The Smashing Fist* (Figure 7). Through such pictures the psychotherapist learned more about his patient than he was able to gain from direct experiences with him. He also understood his firsthand observations better in the light of the art therapy material.

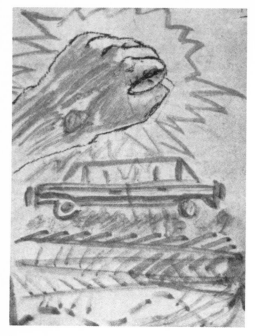

Figure 7

Although he could surmise that J. W. was angry, anger was never directly expressed in the psychotherapy.

But even in the face of his own imagery J. W. would deny the obvious. "It has no meaning," he said of the *Fist*. "I just wanted to draw a hand, just for the anatomy." He could only talk about the canceling-out elements, the crisscross lines and the car with the indistinguishable front and back, all of which, according to him, represented his confusion.

The confusion itself was probably a means to guard against the hostile urge expressed by the fist. In a later review of the picture, J. W. admitted that sometimes he felt angry, but he said that he controlled such feelings by putting them out of his mind. At this time he identified the automobile as a police car, and it therefore reminded him of his father's castigations at the time when he was in military school and his involvement in episodes of minor vandalism had resulted in trouble with the police. Thus we see that he was using denial to mask his intense anger and deep rebellion against his father. Buried anger also helped to account for his excessive politeness and reserve.

The turning point in his illness came a week later. J. W. said he was all right; he no longer heard voices or felt that people were talking about him. *The Upraised Hands and the Priest* (Figure 8) expressed symbolically what was happening within him. He told us, "The hands reaching up have to do with people's desires. The body is buried alive. The hands reach up in desperation. Young people do not know how to control their desires. Older people, like the priest, know how to control; they deny their desires and restrain them." J. W. was turning to repression as a defense. He had buried himself and his desires, all but the tortured hands.

The art therapist found many implications in the picture which the patient did not confirm in words and which she did not mention to him. We see that he had buried his erotic and aggressive impulses in submission to the controlling, punitive, and exemplary father. At the same time, what is intended as the priest's folded arms and praying hands gives the impression of breasts and, together with the long skirt, suggests the nurturing mother. The hands then may be raised in a gesture of supplication and dependence. We recall too his early notion that "infrared" made his hands and penis glow in the dark. This picture, consisting of hands and phallic-shaped figure, may echo that delusion but it has become less bizarre in the course of its transformation into an artistic symbol. The cut-off arms may reflect his castration fantasies and fears. We may also see the stark, black figure as a specter of death, to which the battered hands are raised in a gesture of surrender. Death is thus accepted as the ultimate punishment for hostile and destructive urges.

This picture also summarizes the basic conflicts which interfere with his settling on a career. The artist's hands are his tools. He uses them not only to

Figure 8

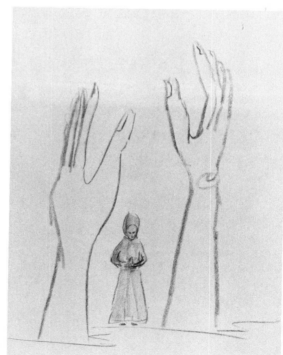

achieve the more ordinary human goals and gratifications, but as the instruments with which he creates. They can also be used to destroy, and this is the point of impasse for the patient. His conflicts force him to renounce his natural inclinations at all levels, from basic biological needs to the complex choice of a career. Father thwarts his artistic bent and at the same time drives him toward mother, whose femininity is associated with the world of the arts.

As his hallucinations subsided the patient tended to suppress more and more of his feelings. He complained of being bored. He had no ideas for pictures and at his request the art therapy sessions were reduced to one a week. Ten days before the last session, he did the picture shown in Figure 9, which we called simply *A Man*. He saw it as suggesting a detective with an upturned trenchcoat collar, and it also reminded him of Yul Brynner in *The King and I*, that is, of an American in the role of an Oriental. He pointed to the rectangular grid, saying, "If you think on a square, the mind will become square." His words have the ring of the sayings the Taoists repeat in their meditations. The play on words seemed like an attempt to think of himself as a "square" instead of a "queer."

The eye had been an important feature in his paranoid fantasies, which included the notion that people could see into his thoughts through his eyes. He said he was no longer concerned with this fear, and the picture gives us an idea of how he was coping with it. The art therapist observed that the grid

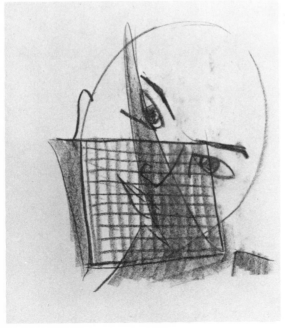

Figure 9

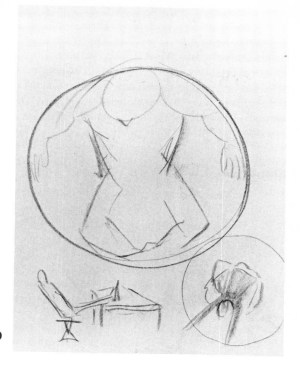

Figure 10

in front of his face screens the *Man* from the scrutiny of others and the collar also is extended so that it almost covers his mouth and one eye. The phallic or knifelike shape of the collar at the same time suggests sexuality and aggression. The square with its crisscross lines has, then, a second function: it partly hides this dangerous symbol and thus represents an attempt to cancel it out. As his own verbal formulation implied, if he himself focused on the square, he would be protected from knowing his own thoughts. He was now suppressing his feelings, hiding them from himself behind the abstract grid.

This is one of the last pictures that shows the tolerance for ambiguity often noted as characteristic of artists. We see here a subtle fusion of opposites, hiding and exposing, creating and destroying, masculine and feminine, all contained in a self-portrait at the same time sexually aggressive and egg-shaped!

As the patient continued to improve, he gave less and less attention to his artwork. He was impatient to leave the hospital, and his concerns centered on immediate and long-range plans for what he would do outside.

The Glass Ball (Figure 10) is one of the pictures from the last art therapy session. In connection with it, J. W. said that he felt frustrated, "like rolling around in a glass ball and can't get out." He was annoyed with his psychotherapist who, he felt, was sitting doing nothing, like the man in the picture reclining in the swivel chair with his feet propped on the desk. The circular theme is repeated at the lower right, where a man is bursting through a paper disk. We recall the fantasy of rebirth which was likened to a chick breaking out of its shell. Rebirth is both wished and feared; the end of his psychotic episode means that he must again face the world outside the hospital. From our vantage point, we see that he had not been reborn as a new and different person, but had rather reverted to his premorbid personality.

Summary and Discussion

This young man had been faced with tremendous changes in his lifetime. The flight of the whole family from the Chinese mainland to Formosa was followed by his lone emigration to the United States. His American studies were intended to prepare him for a career that would be to his father's liking.

His illness came at a time when his return to Formosa was imminent and he had to face up to the conflict with father about his career. At the same time the experience of losing his former fiancée was repeated in the loss of the young woman to whom he had more recently been attached. It appeared that he reacted to these stresses by provoking accusations that he had stolen and then by actually stealing.

At the time he was most ill he was preoccupied with homosexuality, castration, and death. As he began to emerge from his psychotic episode, he began to talk about and make pictures concerned with rebirth. The conflict between creating and destroying was represented pictorially by bridging and crossing out. His conflict about identity was most clearly shown when he represented himself as having two faces. The narcissistic element in his retreat from reality was evidenced in pictures showing his preoccupation with the parts of his own body, notably the phallus, eyes, mouth, and hands. The hands were also used to express either anger or supplication.

His ambivalence about sexual identity and career identity have to do with his relationship to his parents. The feminine side of himself was associated with his mother's interest in art and was seen as subverting the father's wish that the patient prepare himself for a more practical career.

When J. W. could once more begin to observe himself, he began to perceive his ability for artistic expression as potentially dangerous, for through it he risked self-exposure. In the earlier symbolism of his psychosis, exposure had been linked with "infrared," and in contemporary political terms the color red implies subversion. It appears that "infrared" thus connoted both self-exposure and Oedipal rebellion; the latter also came into the open at the height of his psychosis.

His ability to repress his rebellion against the father coincided with his gradual withdrawal from art therapy and with a distinct lessening of the artistic quality of his drawings. By reestablishing his repression he was able to bypass the conflict with his father to the extent that he could return to Formosa like an obedient and loyal son. This compromise, possible only on the basis of repression, exacted a sacrifice of his creative capacity. The relief from acute conflict may not last, but at least it gives him a respite.

As therapists we must acknowledge that repression plays a part in the healing process. Those of us who view repression mainly as a defensive limitation of awareness and who consider whether we should work to liberate the psychic energies by which repression is maintained know that these energies will not automatically be turned toward constructive goals. There are others who liken the mechanism of repression to an observing ego or superego; in the light of this second concept the therapist's task is to help direct repressive forces so that they will be used to achieve a desirable balance between inhibition and expression.[2]

The art therapist recognized that as J. W.'s condition improved he was becoming less expressive. She could not help being dismayed by the diminishing quality of his art, but she realized that with this particular young man creative freedom was tied up with rebellion that might have fatal consequences. The psychotherapist shared her feelings of disappointment, for his high hopes for far-reaching results from insight therapy were dashed by the reestablishment of repression, with its more prosaic reparative effects.

2. Murray Sherman, "Freud, Reik, and the Problem of Technique in Psychoanalysis," *Psychoanalytic Review*, Vol. 52, No. 3, 1965.

Discussion of "Recovery, Repression, and Art"

Margaret Naumburg

This is an interesting paper on the treatment of a difficult case. Its emphasis on "the relationship between a patient's recovery from psychiatric illness and his creativity," and on the vital importance of the meaning to the patient of his own symbolic images recapitulates the keynote of this entire symposium—a symposium which presages the growing application of art therapy in psychiatric treatment throughout the United States in the coming years.

Another important point made in this case report is that the therapist needs to understand the unconscious symbolism conveyed by patients in their projected images. J. W.'s pictorial symbols were not interpreted to him by any of the therapists, but were employed as a means of insight into his problems. One may wonder whether, without the aid of the spontaneous pictures, much could have been accomplished in the treatment of such a resistive and inarticulate schizophrenic patient. This case, I feel, is a dramatic exposition of how pictures can truly be symbolic speech which helps in the unraveling of unconscious conflicts. The authors have given due weight to the contribution of the pictures which lies in their expressing through symbolic imagery what the patient did not dare to tell in words.

Nothing is more frustrating to the psychotherapist than a patient who is so withdrawn that he will not or cannot speak. In treating J. W., not only the art therapist but the psychotherapist made ingenious use of the pictures to reconstruct the patient's early life, so as to understand his conflicts with the demanding, authoritarian father, as well as his dependence on the artistic and creative mother. The pictures thus helped greatly in his treatment by both art therapist and physician.

The case is thus of particular interest because of the close and perceptive collaboration between Dr. Smith, Dr. Macht, and Miss Refsnes. Only through such close teamwork could the most be made of the rich source of nonverbal communication contained in the patient's symbolic imagery. I hope that this fine example will stimulate many other psychotherapists in hospital settings to develop similar joint therapeutic procedures.

The authors' method of tracing how this Chinese patient gradually revealed, through his spontaneous images, the nature of his deep unconscious conflicts is impressive.

Let me review some of the pictures in order to emphasize their outstanding features. The drawings and paintings of this patient manifest great delicacy. In particular, the first picture, *The Bridge,* has an Oriental quality. It is stormy on one side, clear and light on the other; in this first symbolic statement J. W. thus expressed the intensity of his internal conflict. In this design, as in many others, he uses a form of symbolic speech to communicate with the art therapist. The second picture, *The Earthquake,* was a vivid symbolic expression of his explosive state. In picture 3, *Hallucinated People in the Sky,* he is telling the therapist that he, too, hallucinates.

Picture 5, *The Church,* presents a condensation of many of the patient's problems that were gradually worked through in psychotherapy. It not only symbolizes his unsatisfied longing to become an architect, but also shows how he has begun to fantasy himself particularly as a builder of churches. His wish to become an architect was, originally, related to using his creative ability in a way that was forbidden to him by his authoritarian father, but was encouraged by the sympathy and understanding of his creative mother. The authors find that this is his most unified drawing. Perhaps this is in part because, in this picture whose subject matter is ecclesiastical architecture, he shows that he has transferred his warm and dependent feelings toward his mother to the Catholic mother church.

In following the case of this young man, who was both Chinese and Catholic, I suddenly realized that the two Chinese whom I had known personally in recent years were also both Catholic. The original Oriental quality of these two young people had been appreciably dimmed by their Western education. Like J. W. they had received training in the United States through the financial aid of the Catholic church.

It appears that we are rarely able to know the pure strain of the Chinese culture in the students who come to our shores. J. W. had, it seems, been detached in several ways from his original life on the Chinese mainland, first by the removal of his family from China to Formosa in his boyhood, and then by an allegiance divided between his adopted Catholicism and his native religious background.

The Mask and His Inner Self (picture 4) is an interesting symbolization of this young man's conflict. By making the outer mask like his actual face, and giving the face representing his inner self a decidedly American appearance, he hints at his feeling that if he really belonged here as an American his problems would be solved. Such double images delineating a problem of identity by portraying two aspects of the self occur often in the treatment of patients by means of art therapy.

Picture 8, *The Upraised Hands and the Priest,* was very significant, and the patient was here able to say quite clearly what it meant to him. In this drawing he symbolizes his struggle against the older generation, particularly the father who stood in the way of his deep longing for creative expression.

Picture 6, *The Nosy Beatnik,* was crucial in the understanding of the patient and is an excellent example of how the "scribble" technique released unconscious conflicts that J. W. could not have verbalized.

I do, however, question some of the interpretations suggested for certain parts of this drawing, for which the patient had offered no associations of his own. I cite as an example the idea that the form below the Beatnik's neck might represent a platter and the head might therefore stand for John the Baptist. It is evident without imposing any such interpretations that this drawing, as well as the following one of the *Fist,* served to release the patient's long-repressed aggression which he had never before dared to express in either word or picture.

Despite the scarcity of information about the patient's early years, these therapists found in the pictures and his limited comments about them significant clues not only about his current problems but about his past life and its conflicts. I feel that the treatment of this young man became possible through a skillfully coordinated therapeutic program which in turn depended on recognition of the particular importance of the symbolic images. Insights gained from full use of the pictures by the therapists enabled them to help the patient adjust to returning to Formosa and his family.

In conclusion, I would like to raise one question about this interesting case. Why did the authors end their report with the statement, "As therapists we must acknowledge that repression plays a part in the healing process"? Do these therapists really believe this? Does not healing usually occur by the release of conflicts and, thereby, the gaining of insight?

In my opinion, the patient's acceptance of the plan to return to his family in Formosa should simply be regarded as an adjustment to a painful reality, an adjustment which may or may not work out successfully. It did not look to me like the healing of his fundamental conflicts.

Freud on the Nature of Art

Brian Halsey

Nowhere in his many books and essays does Sigmund Freud attempt to present a systematic or thorough account of his views on art. However, he seemed to be fully aware that his ideas—on such topics as the psychic needs out of which art arises, the psychic materials art uses, and the psychic purposes art may serve for both the artist and his audience—might contribute to a greater understanding of art.[1]

Freud was also aware of the implications of art for his own theories. When faced with the initial rejection of some of his ideas, he seized the opportunity to corroborate his findings by reference to similar ideas expressed in the works of such eminent literary artists as Sophocles, Shakespeare, and Goethe. It is rather surprising, then, to realize that some critics have insisted that Freud spoke of art with "contempt."[2] This assessment of Freud's views on art is even more astonishing when one considers that he regarded the psychological acuity of certain artists with the greatest respect. He wrote that ". . . works of art exercise a powerful effect on me, especially those of literature and sculpture, less often of painting."[3] He further spoke of being both "overawed" and "overwhelmed" by art.[4]

Freud praised artists for their insights into human nature and on occasion went so far as to give them credit for seeing psychological factors before they had become evident to himself or other scientists. Speaking to this very point, Freud wrote in his *Delusions and Dreams in Jensen's "Gradiva"*:

> . . . creative writers are valuable allies and their evidence is to be prized highly, for they are apt to know a whole host of things between heaven and earth of which our philosophy has not yet let us dream. In their knowledge of the mind they are far in advance of us everyday

---

1. See Louis Fraiberg, "Freud's Writings on Art," *International Journal of Psycho-Analysis*, Vol. 37, 1956, p. 82; and C. Crockett, "Psychoanalysis in Art Criticism," *Journal of Aesthetics and Art Criticism*, Vol. 17, 1958, pp. 34 ff.
2. See, for example, Lionel Trilling, "Freud and Art," *Kenyon Review*, 1940, pp. 152–73.
3. Sigmund Freud, *Standard Edition of the Complete Psychological Works of Sigmund Freud: The Moses of Michelangelo* (Vol. 13, 1955), translated and edited by James Strachey, London, Hogarth Press, p. 211. (All further references to and quotations from Freud's writings in this paper are derived from this edition.)
4. *Ibid.*

people, for they draw upon sources which we have not yet opened up for science.[5]

An obvious example of such insight into the psychological aspects of human experience in a literary work is the presentation by Sophocles of the Oedipus conflict. And there are other examples. Freud remarked that previous to himself E. T. A. Hoffmann had noted the source of his imaginative figures as being in some way derived from his childhood. An even more remarkable example is afforded by Wilhelm Jensen's *Gradiva: A Pompeiian Fancy*, which paralleled Freud's own theories as presented in *The Interpretation of Dreams*. Since Jensen's study was written independent of any knowledge of Freud's work, the latter found its close correspondence to his own theories so remarkable that he published a psychoanalytic study of its characters.

There is of course some truth to the observation that Freud was not greatly interested in the formal aspect of art. He himself wrote:

I have often observed that the subject matter of works of art has a stronger attraction for me than their formal and technical qualities, though to the artist their value lies first and foremost in these latter.[6]

And, at least initially, Freud freely admitted that he had approached the psychological insights of artists with the primary intention of confirming the findings he had made in examining unpoetic, neurotic human beings. In fact, he often used such material—gleaned from his study of artists and works of art—in much the same way as he used clinical records.[7] However, at the time of the writing of his "Postscript to the Second Edition (1912)" of *Delusions and Dreams in Jensen's* "Gradiva," Freud insisted that psychoanalysis had expanded its interest in art to the point of desiring to investigate ". . . the material of impressions and memories from which the author has built the work, and the methods and processes by which he has converted this material into a work of art.[8]

Somewhat surprisingly, Freud's important biographical studies of artists (Shakespeare, Goethe, da Vinci, and Dostoevsky) do not focus for the most part upon the major problems of art. The goal of these studies[9] (in addition to

5. *Delusions and Dreams in Jensen's* "Gradiva" (Vol. 9, 1959), p. 8.
6. *The Moses of Michelangelo*, p. 211.
7. See Fraiberg, *op. cit.*, p. 83; and Ludwig Marcuse, "Freud's Aesthetic," *Journal of Aesthetics and Art Criticism*, Vol. 17, September 1958, p. 14.
8. Freud, "Postscript to the Second Edition (1912)" [of *Delusions and Dreams in Jensen's* "Gradiva"] (Vol. 9, 1959), p. 94.

9. See *Leonardo da Vinci and a Memory of His Childhood* (Vol. 11, 1957), *Dostoevsky and Parricide* (Vol. 21, 1961), *A Childhood Recollection from "Dichtung and Wahrheit"* [Goethe] (Vol. 17, 1955). Freud treats the Oedipus theme in Sophocles and Shakespeare in several places but especially in *Extracts from the Fliess Papers* (Vol. 1, 1966), pp. 265–66, and *The Interpretation of Dreams* (Vols. 4 and 5, 1953).

that already mentioned) seemed to be, rather, to show that the implications of psychoanalysis extend far beyond the areas of its original concerns: the study of dreams and neuroses. Further, he seems to be engaged in an attempt to demonstrate that our most significant cultural achievements are rooted firmly in the unconscious.[10]

Generally speaking, the studies by Freud which treat artists or artworks directly emphasize the inner motivation and behavior of the creative man; they confirm his sensitive nature and the fact that he is, on the whole, governed by the forces which dominate all men: "The motive forces of artists are the same conflicts which drive other people into neurosis and have encouraged society to construct its institutions."[11] Of course these studies do underline significant differences between the creative artist and the majority of mankind, which differences will be discussed in a moment.

General Views on Art

If one is to understand Freud's more general views on art, he must patiently search out numerous insightful remarks that are sprinkled throughout his many books and essays—works which are, for the most part, dedicated to the treatment of other subjects.[12] It is in these isolated passages that Freud's theory of art can most clearly be comprehended.

His first significant definition of the nature of the artist is contained in his *Introductory Lectures on Psycho-Analysis* (1916–17). It is quoted here in its entirety because of its paramount importance in any attempt to understand Freud's concept of the creative artist. He has been discussing the general symptoms of neuroses and the type of fantasy life the neurotic must live to give vent to his repressed instincts:

> . . . I should like to direct your attention to a side of the life of fantasy which deserves the most general interest. For there is a path that leads back from fantasy to reality—the path, that is, of art. An artist is once more in rudiments an introvert, not far removed from neurosis. He is oppressed by excessively powerful instinctual needs. He desires to win honour, power, wealth, fame and the love of women; but he lacks the means for achieving these satisfactions. Consequently, like any other

10. See Richard Sterba, "The Problem of Art in Freud's Writing, *Psychoanalytic Quarterly*, Vol. 9, 1940, p. 257.

11. Freud, *The Claims of Psycho-Analysis to Scientific Interest* (Vol. 13), p. 187.

12. See Freud, *Jokes and Their Relation to the Unconscious* (Vol. 8, 1960), *Delusions and Dreams in Jensen's "Gradiva," The Occurrence in Dreams of Material from Fairy Tales* (Vol. 12, 1958), *The 'Uncanny'* (Vol. 17), *Humour* (Vol. 21), *The Geothe-Prize* (Vol. 21), *To Romain Rolland* (Vol. 20, 1959), *Thomas Mann on His Sixtieth Birthday* (Vol. 22, 1964), *Preface to Marie Bonaparte's* "The Life and Works of Edgar Allan Poe: A Psycho-Analytic Interpretation" (Vol. 22), *The Interpretation of Dreams, Introductory Lectures on Psycho-Analysis* (Vols. 15 and 16, 1963), *The Future of an Illusion* (Vol. 21), *Civilization and Its Discontents* (Vol. 21), *The Claims of Psycho-Analysis to Scientific Interest,* and *An Autobiographical Study* (Vol. 20).

unsatisfied man, he turns away from reality and transfers all his interest, and his libido too, to the wishful constructions of his life of fantasy, whence the path might lead to neurosis. There must be, no doubt, a convergence of all kinds of things if this is not to be the complete outcome of his development; it is well known, indeed, how often artists in particular suffer from a partial inhibition of their efficiency owing to neurosis. Their constitution probably includes a strong capacity for sublimation and a certain degree of laxity in the repressions which are decisive for a conflict. An artist, however, finds a path back to reality in the following manner. To be sure, he is not the only one who leads a life of fantasy. Access to the halfway region of fantasy is permitted by the universal assent of mankind, and everyone suffering from privation expects to derive alleviation and consolation from it. But for those who are not artists the yield of pleasure to be derived from the sources of fantasy is very limited. The ruthlessness of their repressions forces them to be content with such meagre day-dreams as are allowed to become conscious. A man who is a true artist has more at his disposal. In the first place, he understands how to work over his day-dreams in such a way as to make them lose what is too personal about them and repels strangers, and to make it possible for others to share in the enjoyment of them. He understands, too, how to tone them down so that they do not easily betray their origin from proscribed sources. Furthermore, he possesses the mysterious power of shaping some particular material until it has become a faithful image of his fantasy; and he knows, moreover, how to link so large a yield of pleasure to this representation of his unconscious fantasy that, for the time being at least, repressions are outweighed and lifted by it. If he is able to accomplish all this, he makes it possible for other people once more to derive consolation and alleviation from their own sources of pleasure in their unconscious which have become inaccessible to them; he earns their gratitude and admiration and he has thus achieved *through* his phantasy what originally he had achieved only *in* his fantasy—honour, power and the love of women.[13]

Like all men, then, the artist needs honor, fame, riches, and so forth, but unlike normal men and like the neurotic the artist is unable to attain these goals to any satisfactory extent. What do the neurotic and the artist have in common? They both turn to lives of fantasy. It is at this point, however, that Freud pinpoints the difference between the artist and the average neurotic:

The artist, like the neurotic, [has] withdrawn from an unsatisfying reality into this world of imagination; but, unlike the neurotic, he

---

13. *Introductory Lectures on Psycho-Analysis* (Vol. 16), pp. 375–77.

[knows] how to find a way back from it and once more to get a firm foothold in reality.[14]

The neurotic's fantasy life is and remains individual, and his repression eventually explodes in madness. The artist—who might otherwise become neurotic—is capable through sublimation of avoiding the harsh consequences of a life of fantasy. That is, he is able to turn his fantasies toward some social use by creating art. In the process the artist is able to objectify and universalize his mental life.

Although Freud never says, as some have assumed, that the artist *is* neurotic, he does say that the artist may become so if he is unable to release and transform pressing instinctual impulses through artistic activity. It would seem, then, that the artist's life could tend to be rather unstable, revolving around alternating periods of mounting tension and the relief gained through the creative act.[15]

Artistic Transformation of Fantasy

According to Freud, then, what separates the creative artist from the average individual is his ability to objectify and universalize his fantasies in his artworks. By doing so, he enables others to participate in his fantasy life. But just how is the artist able to do this? Freud suggests at least three aspects of the process of transformation.

First, the artist makes the fantasy into a work of art, in part, at least, by stripping the original fantasy or daydream of all that is personal and egocentric. At the same time he conceals the more offensive aspects of the original instinctual stimulus. This is accomplished by distorting the wish-fantasy so that what is offensive slips by the censorship of the artist's superego and the "superego" of society in a disguised and inoffensive manner. As Freud puts it, the artist,

> . . . represents his most personal wishful phantasies as fulfilled; but they only become a work of art when they have undergone a transformation which softens what is offensive in them, conceals their personal origin and, by obeying the laws of beauty, bribes other people with a bonus of pleasure.[16]

Thus the work of art, like the dream, can be seen in terms of two types of content: manifest content and latent content. The manifest content is merely a mask which conceals the real meaning and source of power of works of

14. *An Autobiographical Study*, p. 64.
15. Fraiberg, *op. cit.*, p. 94.
16. Freud, *The Claims of Psycho-Analysis to Scientific Interest*, p. 187.

art—in other words, the latent content. The latent content relates to those instinctual needs and drives which all men generally feel to some extent but which each usually represses, only to see them fulfilled in some substitute manner more acceptable to his own superego and that of society. The work of art can then be seen as a compromise between the unconscious desires and demands of the artist, as dictated by the pleasure principle, and the conscience or superego of the artist, which tries to keep these tendencies in check and to redirect them toward more socially acceptable goals. The ego, which works under the direction of the reality principle, must balance these two opposing tendencies.

This brings us to the second means by which the artist is able to transform his fantasies, i.e., through elaboration, so that the original fantasy appears as a new kind of reality. The original fantasy is formed according to the pleasure principle. However, if the fantasy is to provide the basis for a work of art, it must be molded into an image of reality, and this takes place in conformity with the reality principle. The creation of a work of art, then, involves the mental process of reconciling the pleasure principle and the reality principle.[17] In a way, the artist is much like a child at play who creates a fantasy world in the image of reality and then treats it with all seriousness. Members of a work's audience permit themselves an extensive identification with it because their belief in its reality corresponds to their own needs, on the one hand, and their consciousness that the work is only play, on the other.[18]

Freud's analysis of art and the process of artistic invention discussed thus far has a rather obvious relationship to his ideas concerning the nature of dreams. Like dreams the art work is an attempt to fulfill a wish, and like the dream art exhibits both a manifest and a latent content.[19] Just as "a dream is a (disguised) fulfillment of a (suppressed or repressed) wish"[20] so is the work of art. For both the artist and the dreamer, the Oedipus complex is an important element in the repressed material.[21] Freud not only saw the Oedipus complex as constituting the nucleus of all neurosis but he also stated that ". . . the beginnings of religion, morals, society and art converge in the Oedipus complex."[22]

Again like the dream, the art work involves the distortion of these instinctual fantasies in such a way that the conscious mind will not censor them when they are expressed. In short, it would seem that the artist is a public dreamer who successfully disguises and universalizes his fantasies through the mechanisms of artistic transformation. In so doing he disguises

---

17. See Sterba, *op. cit.*, p. 266.
18. See Freud, *Creative Writers and Day-Dreaming* (Vol. 9), pp. 141–53.
19. *The Interpretation of Dreams* (Vol. 4), pp. 122 ff. and 135 ff.
20. *Ibid.*, p. 160.
21. *Ibid.*, p. 261.
22. *Totem and Taboo* (Vol. 13), pp. 156–57.

their socially unacceptable source, but still manages to strike common chords with other men because his imaginary reality conforms to and expresses needs and instinctual wishes common to all.

Freud observed that the source of enjoyment in a work of art comes when the artist ". . . softens the character of his egotistic day-dream by altering and disguising it," and then ". . . bribes us by the purely formal—that is, aesthetic—yield of pleasure which he offers us in the presentation of his phantasies."[23] This "bribery" constitutes the third and final way the work of art breaks down the barrier between the artist's ego and those of others. Freud referred ". . . to a yield of pleasure such as this, which is offered to us so as to make possible the release of still greater pleasure arising from deeper psychical sources," as an "incentive bonus" or, more technically, "fore-pleasure."[24] Of course, the fundamental pleasure involved in the enjoyment of works of art relates to wish-fulfillment. The artist puts each member of his audience in a position to enjoy his own daydreams without reproach or a feeling of shame. In other words, the esthetic side to a work of art seduces us into enjoying the gratification of a forbidden instinctual wish and the resulting release of tension without our becoming conscious of the original source of the pleasure.

As one might expect, Freud's brief discussion of beauty parallels his ideas on esthetics at this point. He never underestimated the importance of beauty to human consciousness, but he did see its source primarily in mankind's sexual needs:

> Psycho-analysis, unfortunately, has scarcely anything to say about beauty either. All that seems certain is its derivation from the field of sexual feeling. The love of beauty seems a perfect example of an impulse inhibited in its aim.[25]

Freud saw no obvious use or cultural necessity for beauty, but insisted that civilization could not do without it. Although the appreciation of beauty could not shield one from the vicissitudes of life, the happiness it brought could compensate for a great deal of suffering.[26]

Freud admitted to frustration in his attempt to understand just what kind of peculiar sensibility enabled the artist to transform his fantasies into material form. This aspect of artistic invention was the artist's "innermost secret."[27] Freud eventually came to feel more optimistic about the possibility that the mystery of artistic creation might be defined "meta-psychologically"; in fact one partial solution to the problem lies in something Freud himself said.

23. *Creative Writers and Day-Dreaming*, p. 153.
24. *Ibid.*
25. *Civilization and Its Discontents*, p. 83.
26. *Ibid.*, p. 82.
27. *Creative Writers and Day-Dreaming*, p. 153.

Toward the end of one of his lectures on the anatomy of mental personality, Freud was careful to point out that the three spheres into which he had divided human personality—id, ego, and superego—did not have distinct, hard and fast boundaries and that their function might even vary from person to person. He then observed:

> It is easy to imagine, too, that certain mystical practices may succeed in upsetting regions of the mind, so that, for instance, perceptions may be able to grasp happenings in the depths of the ego and in the id which were otherwise inaccessible to it.[28]

Herbert Read, the well-known English art historian and critic, applied this seemingly casual suggestion of Freud's to the phenomenon of artistic genius and used it as a hypothesis to explain the lyrical intuition or inspiration of the artist. In this process, Read proposed that,

> . . . the sensational awareness of the ego is brought into direct contact with the id, and from that "seething cauldron" snatches some archetypal form, some instinctive association of words, images or sounds, which constitute the basis of the work of art.[29]

Perhaps the traditionally close relationship between art and religion (at least until modern times) is no mere coincidence since both the genius of the artist and that of the mystic might very well be related to the same psychic phenomenon.

From what has already been said about the nature of artistic creation, it is clear that one source for the latent content of works of art is that which is spontaneously created in a manner Freud related closely to daydreaming. Since he felt this phenomenon was a continuation of and substitution for the play of childhood, he also insisted that the memories of childhood weighed heavily in spontaneous artistic creation:

> The deepest and eternal nature of man, upon whose evocation in his hearers the poet is accustomed to rely, lies in those impulses of the mind which have their roots in a childhood that has since become prehistoric.[30]

The work of art would come about, Freud hypothesized, when some actual experience made a strong impression on the artist by stirring up earlier experiences generally related to his childhood, and they, in turn, would arouse a wish that would find its fulfillment in the work in question.[31]

28. *New Introductory Lectures on Psycho-Analysis* (Vol. 22), pp. 79–80.
29. Herbert Read, *Art and Society*, New York, Macmillan Co., 1937, pp. 202–203.
30. Freud, *The Interpretation of Dreams* (Vol. 4), p. 247. See also *The Claims of Psycho-Analysis to Scientific Interest*, p. 187.
31. *Creative Writers and Day-Dreaming*, p. 155.

A second source for the content of works of art is that which Freud designated as "ready-made" material—myths, legends, and fairy tales.[32] In this instance the artist simply refashions the existing material. Of course, he may assert a degree of independence in that he selects only the material he wishes to use and, as well, may introduce numerous changes to suit his own purposes. In reality these two sources of artistic content—myths and the like, and childhood experiences—are very similar because the fantasies of the race correspond directly to the fantasies of the individual.

Inasmuch as the objectification of personal and racial fantasies is so often highly valued by those who enjoy art, it is evident, Freud felt, that art performs an important social function. He wrote in *The Future of an Illusion:*

> . . . art offers substitutive satisfactions for the oldest and still most deeply felt cultural renunciations, and for that reason it serves as nothing else does to reconcile a man to the sacrifices he has made on behalf of civilization. On the other hand, the creations of art heighten his feelings of identification, of which every cultural unit stands in so much need, by providing an occasion for sharing highly valued emotional experiences. And when those creations picture the achievements of his particular culture and bring to his mind its ideals in an impressive manner, they also minister to his narcissistic satisfaction.[33]

Freud's Views on the Value of Art

On the whole, as we have seen, Freud had a very positive attitude toward art. He was strongly attracted to works of literature and art; he even wrote of being "overawed" by them. He appreciated as no one before him the psychologically positive effects that art affords both the artist (who thereby finds his way back to reality) and the member of the artist's audience (who gains pleasure from art through the vicarious fulfillment of instinctual wishes). Further, he generally considered the methods the artist uses as being a "higher" and "finer" means of confronting reality.[34] He also pointed to the important cultural role art has played. But in the final analysis his attitude about art is ambiguous. Why? Because whatever might be the positive aspects of using art to confront human experience, there were also serious limitations.

First, works of art as a rule are inaccessible to the masses who lack either the requisite education to fully appreciate the arts or are too bogged down with the preoccupations of daily life to pay them any notice.[35]

Second, the making of works of art as a means of personally confronting

---

32. *Ibid.*
33. *The Future of an Illusion,* p. 14.
34. *Civilization and Its Discontents,* p. 79.
35. *The Future of an Illusion,* p. 13.

reality is available only to that handful who have the necessary special gifts and dispositions—characteristics which are all too uncommonly found among us. And even for the artist art has its limitations; it can never provide complete protection from suffering and misfortune.[36]

Third, as a more general means of confronting reality, artistic experience involves a compromise. It occupies a middle ground ". . . between a reality which frustrates wishes and the wish-fulfilling world of the imagination. . . ."[37] This is both desirable and undesirable in Freud's view. On the one hand, it allows the artist or his audience to find momentary happiness, to escape from life's grim realities, and to find a means to temporarily relieve instinctual pressures. On the other hand, the effects are always transitory, reality has not been faced directly (something Freud would have preferred), and the relief art gives to our crude primary impulses is very mild compared to the relief derived from satisfying these drives in a more direct fashion.[38]

Finally, Freud wrote of one other limitation to artistic experience: in the last analysis art is "illusion."[39] As such, art might induce a "mild narcosis" and provide temporary relief from life when it proves too hard for us; still its effect is not strong enough to make us oblivious to real misery. Freud saw art as a "substitutive satisfaction," an illusion in contrast to reality; but, nonetheless, psychically effective in diminishing our sensitivity to the harsh realities of life. Freud's attitude at this point is again ambiguous. On the one hand, we need the "illusions" or "substitutive satisfactions" that art provides because we must have occasional vacations from the misery of reality, as well as some acceptable outlet for repressed instinctual energies. On the other hand, he felt that art, religion, and philosophy were not valid sources of knowledge about reality, because what they offered was only illusion—the fulfillment of wishful impulses. For Freud the only true source of knowledge about reality was scientific research, and science provided for him the only proper comprehensive hypothesis upon which to build a valid world view (*Weltanschauung*). Speaking to this very point in his *New Introductory Lectures on Psycho-Analysis,* Freud insisted that no matter how important to human life might be the products of art or systems of religion and philosophy or how satisfactorily they might meet mankind's emotional demands upon a *Weltanschauung,*

> . . . we cannot nevertheless overlook the fact that it would be illegitimate and highly inexpedient to allow these demands to be transferred to the sphere of knowledge. For this would lay open the paths which lead to psychosis, whether to individual or group psychosis,

36. *Civilization and Its Discontents,* pp. 79–80.
37. *The Claims of Psycho-Analysis to Scientific Interest,* p. 188.
38. *Civilization and Its Discontents,* pp. 79–80.
39. See *ibid.,* pp. 75, 80–81; and *New Introductory Lectures on Psycho-Analysis,* p. 160.

and would withdraw valuable amounts of energy from endeavors which are directed towards reality in order, so far as possible, to find satisfaction in it for wishes and needs.[40]

In essence Freud saw art as illusion and as denying reality. He would have preferred, no doubt, that man face reality directly, rationally, and stoically as he himself tried to do. However, since he knew man's limitations, he realized the necessity for escape. Since art was ". . . almost always harmless and beneficent . . .,"[41] it provided one of the most acceptable means for man to deal with human suffering and misfortune. Freud certainly preferred art to religion as a means of escape, even though both were ultimately illusions in his view. Why? Because art makes no attempt to present itself as reality; and perhaps because, as Ludwig Marcuse has suggested, Freud felt art could avoid certain of the bad consequences of religion; that is, man might kill in the name of Christ or Mohammed but not in the name of Picasso.[42]

Summary

This discussion of Freud's views on art has the aim of helping to clarify his general attitudes toward artistic experience. In particular I have attempted to show how his psychoanalytic theories have contributed toward a fuller understanding of art—the psychic needs from which it arises, the materials which it uses, and the purposes of artistic expression for both the artist and his audience. Then, too, some wider cultural implications of Freud's thinking on art have been suggested. Although Freud never treated these matters exhaustively or systematically, I believe his thought has numerous obvious implications for the creative arts. In any case, I think it has been shown that Freud's greatest service to the understanding of art is his convincing reminder to us that works of art cannot be fully comprehended without an awareness of the dynamic role psychological factors play in both their creation and their assimilation.

---

40. *New Introductory Lectures on Psycho-Analysis*, p. 160.
41. *Ibid.*
42. Marcuse, *op. cit.*, p. 4.

Postscript to Halsey's "Freud on the Nature of Art"

Edith Kramer and Elinor Ulman

Brian Halsey has done readers a great service with his scholarly article about Freud's writings on art. Most obviously he spares us the monumental task of gathering together from widely scattered sources both casual references and more considered discussions. He has provided an unbiased representation of Freud's published thoughts about artists and the arts. Through these selections and his discussion of them, Halsey successfully counters the view that Freud held art and artists in contempt. But in fairly giving us the full range of attitudes that Freud expressed, Halsey acquaints us not only with Freud's remarks indicating a respect for art bordering on awe, but also with certain of Freud's remarks that most artists and lovers of art sense as disparaging and react to with irritation and resentment.

Halsey recognizes and seeks to explain some of the ambiguities in Freud's estimation of the psychological and social value of art, but he does not fully explore the inconsistencies of the material he has presented us with. Thus his unbiased selection of quotations and his stimulating discussion of them supply valuable spadework that prompts further search.

We start this postscript with an attempt to discover a pattern in Freud's contradictory statements about artists and what they achieve in their work. It is interesting that the key seems to lie in the very area where Freud's explicit formulations stop short—that is, the *quality* of the art to which his various remarks referred. As Halsey points out, Freud disavowed interest in the formal character of art, and certainly he made very little effort to account for it. Worse still, he rather casually dismissed the "formal" and the "aesthetic" as the artist's means of deceiving his audience and seducing it into fantasies of unbridled self-indulgence.[1] There is evidence nonetheless that Freud responded—perhaps more than he realized—to those very aspects of art that, in the eyes of artists and critics, determine its value. How else explain his sensitive appreciation of great works in literature and even, occasionally, the visual arts?

1. Sigmund Freud, *Standard Edition of the Complete Psychological Works of Sigmund Freud: Creative Writers and Day-Dreaming* [written in 1907–08] (Vol. 9, 1959), edited by James Strachey, London, Hogarth Press, p. 153. (Further references to and quotations from Freud's writing in this paper are derived from this edition.)

Halsey presents as Freud's "first significant definition of the artist" a long passage (dated 1916–17) about the artist as public daydreamer whose work not only allows him to escape neurosis but also to earn worldly rewards from a public whose conscience he has lulled momentarily by means of a sort of secret bribery. It seems fair, however, to tie this passage together with a somewhat more diffuse statement on the same subject that appeared about nine years earlier. In *Creative Writers and Day-Dreaming* (1907–08) Freud asks,

> May we really attempt to compare the imaginative writer with the "dreamer in broad daylight" and his creations with day-dreams? . . . for the purposes of our comparison, we will choose not the writers most highly esteemed by critics, but the less pretentious authors of novels, romances and short stories, who nevertheless have the widest and most eager circle of readers of both sexes.

Having pointed out the obvious kinship with the daydream of stories in which an invincible, invulnerable, and sexually irresistible hero and his helpers, all characterized as "good," are pitted against enemies just as unqualifiedly "bad," Freud goes on to explain indirectly his choice of trash in preference to great art for the purposes of his discussion. "We are perfectly aware," he writes,

> that many imaginative writings are far removed from the model of the naive day-dream; and yet I cannot suppress the suspicion that even the most extreme deviations from that model could be linked with it through an uninterrupted series of transitional cases.[2]

Thus Freud early expressed his awareness that the better the quality of the art the more completely have its infantile origins been transformed and obscured. He did not, however, address himself directly to this question. Sixty years later, when many of Freud's earth-shaking discoveries have become commonplace and Freudian thinking itself has continued to develop in the hands of younger theorists, it is easy for us as art therapists to make a further step. Bad art *always* invites speculation about its author and good art never does. We have all known patients who move from raw, easy-to-decipher presentation of symptoms in their pictures and sculptures to works that tell no more about them than that at a given moment they were able to function fully in artistic terms. In the larger world of art too, daydream art, self-serving autobiographical apologias, and unintended revelations of pathology inevitably stimulate speculation about their authors' personal problems and motivations. Great art, on the other hand, invites us to think not about its author and his experiences but about our own experiences and

2. *Ibid.*, pp. 149–50.

ourselves. The great artist's life story and its relation to his art may be of interest for other reasons, but they are irrelevant to the appreciation of his works. Every great work of art has a life of its own quite separate from the biography of its maker.

In the literature of escape and wish-fulfillment, all kinds of misfortunes are used merely as titillating delays that add to the pleasure of eventual gratification. Gratification, however, remains shallow, and this is borne out by the endless need for repetition. Trashy novels are quickly consumed and the wish for new versions of the same theme is insatiable. This insatiable demand indeed provides the producers of such literature with (as Freud says and Halsey duly notes) "wealth, fame and the love of women"—again, wish-fulfillment of a shallow kind. Such art further resembles daydreams in that it falsifies man's experience, particularly by hiding or denying the inner conflict of forces which prevents wish-fulfillment. It disregards, as well, those aspects of outer reality which impede direct gratification of forbidden wishes.

Great art, on the other hand, encompasses a broader and a deeper truth. It does indeed permit artist and audience vicariously to experience the forbidden and repressed—but in its totality: the wish, the conflict, the consequences.

Freud did not address himself to these general distinctions inhering in art at its various levels of quality, but his appreciation of such differences is clearly implied in his discussion of numerous individual works of art. To cite only two out of many examples, in his article on "The Theme of the Three Caskets"[3] and in "Dostoevsky and Parricide"[4] Freud recognizes that art serves psychological needs far more complex than those that stimulate daydreams and their artistic equivalents. In his treatment of numerous works (including not only the great classics but also the art of good but minor writers) Freud points out in each instance that the work presents not only the fulfillment of forbidden wishes but also the psychic processes whereby the wish arises, the inner pressures which lead to transgression, and finally the tragic consequences of the transgression. We may add that all these aspects of experience are conveyed with equal intensity and clarity. As Freud points out in his analysis of *The Brothers Karamazov*, Dostoevsky indeed describes the fulfillment of a common—if usually unconscious—wish: the wish for a father's death. But he deals, as well, with communal guilt: ". . . all of the brothers . . . are equally guilty—the impulsive sensualist, the sceptical cynic and the epileptic criminal."[5] The great artist has paid the emotional price and is able to induce the audience to pay the emotional price for

3. Sigmund Freud, *The Theme of the Three Caskets* [written in 1913] (Vol. 12, 1958), pp. 291–301.
4. Sigmund Freud, *Dostoevsky and Parricide* [written in 1927–28] (Vol. 21, 1961), pp. 177–94.
5. *Ibid.*, p. 189.

uninhibited gratification. Readers are profoundly moved and deeply satisfied. They crave no further variations on the theme.

In spite of all we have noted about Freud's own implicit recognition of qualitative differences among works of art, he certainly directed his overt attention more to subject matter than to form, and during Freud's lifetime the contribution of psychoanalytic writing to the understanding of art remained limited. Publishing (in 1941) only two years after Freud's death, Susanne Langer justly appraised the situation. The analysis of secret sources of energy tapped by the artist in his work has, she said,

> . . . much to recommend it. . . . It does justice to the emotional interest, the seriousness with which we receive artistic experience. . . . it brings this baffling department of human activity into the compass of a general psychological system . . . based on the recognition of certain fundamental human needs, of the conflicts resulting from their mutual interference, and of the mechanism whereby they assert, disguise, and finally realize themselves.

Nevertheless, Langer concluded that

> . . . this theory (though probably valid) [does not throw] any real light on those issues which confront artists and critics. . . . For the Freudian interpretation . . . never offers even the rudest criterion of *artistic* excellence. It may explain why a poem was written, why it is popular, what . . . it hides . . . what secret ideas a picture combines, and why Leonardo's women smile mysteriously. . . . But it *makes no distinction between good and bad art.* . . . An analysis to which the artistic merit of a work is irrelevant . . . can look only to a hidden *content* of the work, and not to what every artist knows as the real problem—the perfection of *form.* . . .[6]

A more explicit psychoanalytic investigation of the determinants of quality in art had to await the development of psychoanalytic ego psychology.[7] In particular the concept of sublimation grew richer and more complex in later years. Freud himself made no clear distinction between simple displacement and sublimation, and he only hinted at the likelihood that sublimation might be an important element in art.

We will here outline very briefly some of the writings based on Freudian principles that have appeared since Freud's death in 1939. In the intervening years, psychoanalytic theorists have turned increasingly toward consid-

6. Susanne K. Langer, *Philosophy in a New Key* (Third Edition), Cambridge, Mass., Harvard University Press, 1957, pp. 207–208.

7. The seminal publication in this area is "Comments on the Formation of Psychic Structure," by Heinz Hartmann, Ernst Kris, and Rudolph Loewenstein, *Psychoanalytic Study of the Child*, Vol. 2, New York, International Universities Press, 1946.

eration of questions related to the formal aspects of art and, ultimately, to standards of artistic value.

One of the earliest attempts to bring the theory of the two sources of psychic energy—libido and aggression—to bear upon the problem of artistic form was made by Hans Sachs in his essay (published in 1942) on "Beauty, Life, and Death."[8]

While Sachs did much to develop a theory of art based on Freudian principles, he was hampered by the relatively primitive state of ego psychology at the time he was formulating his ideas. Ten years later Ernst Kris was on a firmer theoretical footing when he made his substantial contribution by introducing the concept of "regression in the service of the ego."[9] In 1961 Kurt Eissler further defined the psychological value of art:

> One of the objective functions of all great artistic achievements, particularly in the visual arts, is not only to give pleasure . . . but to stimulate new ego differentiations in the personality of the beholder.[10]

Finally, one of the authors of this postscript, Edith Kramer, has sought to apply psychoanalytic understanding to the very questions Langer is concerned with. She agrees with Langer that the basic task of the arts is "to give inward experiences form and thus to make them conceivable."[11] She also shares Langer's conviction that both the excellence of a work of art and its meaning are inextricably bound up with its formal character.

Kramer uses the insights of Freudian ego psychology to elucidate the problem of quality in art. In her work as artist and art therapist she has observed that *the unity of form and content*, which is the hallmark of art, is attained when the psychic apparatus functions in an integrated fashion under the supremacy of the ego. Formal quality is intimately linked to the particular kind of sublimation that is an essential element of the artistic process.[12]

Halsey mentions at the start Freud's conviction that psychoanalytic insights might one day help us understand art through investigations that

8. Hans Sachs, *The Creative Unconscious*, Cambridge, Mass., Science-Art, 1942.

9. Ernst Kris, *Psychoanalytic Explorations in Art*, New York, International Universities Press, 1952.

10. Kurt Eissler, *Leonardo da Vinci: Psychoanalytic Notes on the Enigma*, New York, International Universities Press, 1961.

11. Susanne K. Langer, *Problems of Art*, New York, Charles Scribner's Sons, 1957.

12. Edith Kramer, *Art Therapy in a Children's Community*, New York, Schocken Books, 1977 (first published in 1958); and *idem, Art as Therapy with Children*, New York, Schocken Books, 1971.

Freud himself never systematically attempted. Art therapists may be in a particularly good position to help Freud's prediction come true. Again and again the study of malfunction has led to greater understanding of physiological as well as psychological processes in general. In art therapy, where we witness not only many artistic miscarriages and abortions but also are occasionally present at the birth of art in the face of formidable obstacles, we have an unusual chance to look into the genesis of that unity of form and content which lies at the heart of art's mysterious power.

An Art Therapist Looks at Her Professional History

Margaret Howard

[*Editors' Note: The first three paragraphs below are, we are happy to say, dated: training for art therapy has improved and general recognition of the existence of art therapy has increased since the mid–1960s when this history was written. We wish the kind of "flexibility" demanded of the author more than fifteen years ago were also a thing of the past, but unfortunately an art therapist is still sometimes made to feel "like an interior decorator."*]

Anybody with a paint brush and a patient is likely to be called an art therapist. Often it is not the artist utilizing art in some form at a hospital or treatment center who has laid claim to the title. A reporter in a hurry for a good feature story lights upon such an artist, emotes on the "miracle" of paint and canvas bringing out the "integrated" personality, labels the worker in charge of the miracle "art therapist," and the name sticks.

Not only the general public but professional members of hospital staffs bracket as art therapy the use of art activity for occupation, recreation, and rehabilitation. I do not deny that such programs are valuable and that those who conduct them should receive due recognition. But I have come to believe that an *art therapist* must understand the use of art as a diagnostic and therapeutic tool in psychiatry.

The way to such understanding is not easy. Colleges and universities are barely beginning to offer courses on the undergraduate and graduate levels. No standards have been established; art therapy as a profession is so new that the field is wide open. It is no wonder that manipulation of art materials as something to keep hands and (perhaps) minds busy is not clearly distinguished even from the psychoanalytically oriented methods developed by Margaret Naumburg.

I didn't know the difference myself until I had conducted a long series of art programs each of which I sincerely thought at the time was art therapy. First, as an artist-teacher, I volunteered some time in an orthopedic hospital for convalescent children.

I was assigned to the occupational therapy department, given an orientation course, and turned loose on the wards. I made the rounds of bed patients, helping them to use coloring books, numbered pictures, and stencils. It was frustrating, but I was assured that this was therapy and that I was releasing a busy nurse or aide for more important duties.

It was a small crumb of comfort, though. My "art therapy" consisted of pure busy-work. Today I would class this as giving patients some degree of "occupation," making incidental use of art materials.

Next I became a paid "recreational" or "diversional" therapist with art classes on a scheduled program. I inoculated my captive class with the old art-school method of still life, graphic arts, oils, and art appreciation. Many of the children had never seen great paintings or even been inside a gallery. Their idea of art was mainly Christmas trees, pumpkins, and hearts.

Flexibility was the thing. I was called on to paint murals, posters, and little cards, or help select pictures and colors for staff members' homes. I became adept at recognizing a certain gleam in the eye. I felt more like an interior decorator than an artist.

A New Insight

The first insight dawned on me when I discovered that children recovering slowly from rheumatoid arthritis, burns, polio, the quadriplegics and paraplegics often had varying emotional problems. I recall, for example, a seventeen-year-old girl with both arms paralyzed from polio. She wanted to paint a picture in oils. Although such patients often learn to use their toes to hold a paint brush and even to write and type, this method was totally unacceptable to this particular girl.

Another way had to be devised. Both arms were elevated in slings attached to her wheelchair. Then she was enabled to move a brush by means of a wax impression which she could hold in her mouth, and both useless hands were placed on the brush to steady it. After much practice, she was able to more or less control the area she wished to color.

She knew exactly what she wanted to paint. It was a still life of two Raggedy Ann dolls, one sitting and the other fallen over on its side. It didn't take an art therapist, which I certainly was not at the time, to realize this was the way she felt about her own limp, useless body.

A fifteen-year-old quadriplegic also knew precisely what he wanted to paint. Injured in a diving accident, he had recovered some movement in his right arm and thumb. After an aluminum ring was fitted to his thumb as a brush holder, he guided the brush but couldn't reach a palette. He would direct me to put the desired colors on the canvas and then laboriously scumble them in. What gradually appeared was a mountain lake with a large rock in the foreground. It was a picture of the exact place where his accident had occurred.

Although I had begun trying to meet individual needs, the main thing still seemed to be the achievement of an end result. I encouraged the patients to produce something acceptable not only to themselves but to the viewers, and felt called on to offer any means to attain such results, from copying and tracing to actually painting on the patient's canvas.

This should be called "rehabilitation art" because it accomplishes two things: it eases the long hours of pain and boredom, and results in a sense of accomplishment. Nearly all these patients preferred oils; perhaps they felt they were truly becoming artists. Occasionally a patient does find a hobby through rehabilitation art, or even discovers a genuine talent. Usually, however, the artist using art in rehabilitation is confronted with people whose anger is born of the frustration resulting from being cheated of their right to be active. Often they are demanding, or even downright rude.

I came to expect symbols of emotional disturbance to appear in the work of physically damaged patients. A paraplegic strewed a broken cigarette, a cross, a knife, a bloody eye, and a claw across his canvas. A child severely crippled with rheumatoid arthritis "ruined" a rather nice still life by painting in a wineglass with a broken stem. In retrospect it seems as if it was she who sent me off to become a real art therapist, never to return again to my old role. It was so obvious that this symbol meant something important to the patient herself that I longed to understand it better even though I had no idea as yet how valuable such emotional projections can become in the course of psychotherapy.

At about this time the hospital was transformed into a neuropsychiatric treatment center for emotionally disturbed children. The wheelchairs and braces gradually disappeared; a new kind of patient was seen on the wards, and not the type that the recreation artist or the rehabilitation artist could help.

My first introduction to a psychiatric patient was somewhat upsetting to my preconceptions. Having heard that we emit love waves which are received and, one hopes, returned by the patient, I was very anxious to start sending. My first patient was a screaming, kicking eight-year-old who had broken two windows and bitten an aide rather severely. Literally dragged to her first art session, she announced in colorful language her desire to exterminate all art therapists. I did not doubt for one moment that she meant me in particular.

After I had been kicked several times, I began to wonder what had happened to the love waves. Apparently they hadn't reached land yet. Common sense took over. I held this whirlwind of rage and warned her that one more kick and I would reciprocate with a few of my own. It worked.

We were both rather unstrung when she put her arms around me and started to cry. She was so frightened of her own actions that she was asking for someone to take control.

Psychiatric Art Therapy

Then, for me, began a long period of training and study based on the teachings of Margaret Naumburg, the pioneer of psychoanalytically oriented art therapy. I returned from Naumburg's course at New York University as an art therapist at last. I had been called one many times, but now I felt that it really meant something. My official title hadn't changed but my methods were radically different. I discarded my old teaching techniques and I learned to elicit rather than direct.

Each patient provides a unique experience. There was the child who had witnessed a suicide. Although she was unable to talk about it, she finally drew the whole scene in great detail, including the blood, the gun, and the position of the body.

A schizophrenic saw horrible monsters come out of people's mouths and would run screaming from the room. After many sessions, he was able to put his monsters on paper and paint them on the wall. He explained that it didn't look so bad when he drew it. Eventually his hallucinations ceased.

A gifted girl with an I.Q. of 160 painted many faces in clashing purple, green, blue, and orange. She explained to me that people "were ugly underneath" and that she could see them in their "true colors." Only when she found a friend on the ward was she able to paint a portrait from memory with natural skin tones.

Art therapy gradually emerged as a field whose horizons for me and the emotionally ill child are unlimited. There is the constant challenge to grasp messages that are sometimes camouflaged and sometimes deliberately misleading—but always pathetic because basically the patient who sends them yearns for them to be understood. As people become more aware of their problems, the spontaneous productions change. Then it is gratifying to realize that, as a member of the psychiatric team, the art therapist has played a small but vital part in the patient's recovery.

Even today, however, each art therapist must face the task of convincing other professional workers in psychiatry that art therapy can make a special contribution to diagnosis and treatment. We still await the time when complete art therapy training, both academic and clinical, will become available and gain widespread recognition. Meantime, some art therapists who do not have the chance to attend any of the few courses now designed specially for their needs return to school for extra training in psychology, and on their own maintain familiarity with a growing body of literature concerning the use of art in psychiatry. Beyond that they can only continue to learn from the spontaneous productions of the patients they see daily, and try to keep in close touch with each other, exchanging new ideas and techniques.

The Evolution of an Art Therapy Intern's View of the Therapeutic Process

Henriette de Knegt

As a prospective art therapist interning at a mental health facility I encountered the ways other people—the people who had come there because of what society considers problems in living—perceive, think, and feel. I was confronted, as well, with my reactions to these alternative approaches to experience, with the result that I began to question myself. I stood at the point where all my life—personal experiences and formal education—had led me. I began my practical training filled to capacity with good intentions and idealistic plans for those I was about to "help." (I might add I was also a little afraid of so much responsibility for another person.) Yes, I knew ·the definitions of schizophrenia, hebephrenic type, and manic-depression, circular type. Also, I knew the best way to mix paints, soften clay, and glue paper. I believed that somehow, with art as the medium, I, the helper, would cure the "sick" person. I found I wasn't wrong to believe in the benefits of a therapeutic relationship, but I was wrong about who is helped and to what degree.

I came·into the therapeutic relationship expecting to be the friend the residents never had and by sheer willpower to gain their trust. They would produce artwork, suddenly notice things about themselves that they'd been unaware of before, and tell me things that I would understand. I would help them find themselves and at the same time, share of myself, thus keeping the energy flowing in our sessions. As I write this I have been having sessions with Bob for five months, and I find much is happening to me as well as to him.

Bob came as a voluntary patient to the county hospital where we met. On admission he was characterized as depressed, destructive, and confused. His mother reported that Bob had thrown things and injured her in the past, and she feared that it might happen again. She and his father hoped that he would become stable enough to live in a boarding home.

The Relationship

In the beginning we make hesitant eye contact, then exchange monosyllabic pleasantries. I am confronted with a tall, gangly young man whose clothes are too big. He moves in an awkward yet seemingly purposeful manner with long strides. He is all arms and legs and moves rapidly, stopping momentarily, then moving again—always with a rigid body posture. He reaches for things with his whole body. There are periods when he is overcome by inertia; he sits with head down, immobile, hard to awaken. His fingers nervously twist and retwist a lock of long hair.

Sometimes he searches quickly through magazines, flipping pages too fast to read them, stopping only when something catches his eye. At other times he touches the different textures in his environment. Two fingers alight briefly on the wall, then the tablecloth, then a pocketbook. His hands, seldom at rest, express the direction of his energy. At times his fingers, bent and clawlike, strain with tension.

He often fixes his eyes on something I cannot see. At other times he focuses intently on an object that interests him. In general his eyes register anxiety, anger, and mistrust. They dart sideways to look at a person. But as time goes by, trust develops; Bob finally begins to maintain eye contact with me.

With his pale complexion he looks as if he rarely goes outdoors. His face can be blank or contorted as if in pain. Bob keeps to himself. He says he is "okay," while the other residents of the hospital are "retarded, stupid, sick," and unworthy of his attention. He is very much alone and continues to interest me.

We begin twice-weekly individual art therapy sessions, approximately forty-five minutes in length, and have, at this writing, had twenty-nine. Bob and I have our own sub-basement room with bare, irregularly plastered walls and high ceiling. He prefers to stay in it rather than go outside; it is familiar and safe.

Our room contains a sink and a broken washing machine in addition to a long table. Each of us usually takes the same seat at the table catercorner to the other. A pot of hot water and tea supplies are kept at the sink. Getting ourselves a cup of tea is a way for us either to interact or to avoid each other. Sometimes we make the tea together; sometimes Bob leaves the table to make his own tea, spending as much time by himself as he needs to.

When Bob feels nervous, he paces about the room. Sometimes he skips and emits a high-pitched hum that sounds like a suppressed scream. If the room becomes too confining of his expanding energy, he opens the door and goes out into the hallway. At times I have worried that he might leave altogether, but he has always come back into the room. I want him to have as much physical space as he needs; only once in five months have I become so anxious that I needed to assert my authority and ask him to stay in the room.

I can think of various reasons why Bob continues to move away yet stay close by: (1) he has his own self-imposed standards of how far it is all right to remove himself from where he is supposed to be; (2) having tested me and found that I make no effort to detain him, he has lost interest in leaving; (3) he assumes that I will not let him roam too far. Of course, leaving the room serves Bob as a way to release energy, act out frustration, and avoid a threatening situation. Rocking fulfills some of the same needs. Bob rocks tensely while both sitting and standing. As the tempo increases, his face contorts and his fingers and hands tighten up. Thus is his fury contained.

When Bob feels too much pressure from the outside, he angrily shouts questions and demands relative to his hospitalization: "I want to get out of here. Get me out of here. I want to see a doctor. Now!" "I don't want to forget." "I'm not sick." "I'm getting worse." When I respond with a comment designed to provoke self-exploration, Bob clams up. When the reply is interpretive or supportive of what he says, Bob seems satisfied and stops shouting.

Sports, the Beatles, questions about Chaplin and Picasso are subjects Bob feels it is safe to talk about. He speaks of these subjects in a quick, low voice, prefacing his remarks with "Did you know . . . ?" or "Do you think . . . ?" Thus he creates a conventional opportunity to show what he knows, finds a way to take the initiative in breaking the silence, and sometimes avoids subjects of conversation that might make him uncomfortable.

As months go by, Bob begins to acknowledge some relation to the human race. He steps out of his self-imposed isolation to ask where my parents have gone on vacation. (His parents have just returned from their vacation.) On days when his curiosity is stronger than his defensiveness, he inquires, "How old are you?" "When does your internship end?" "Did you go to school for art?" He has his own reasons for asking these questions and the answers are important. After getting an answer he lapses into silence again. I don't know whether he is incapable of reacting spontaneously and continuing the conversation or whether he simply doesn't care to.

Bob is sensitive to questions. Sometimes an innocent remark on my part is met with a quick glance and a "What do you mean?" He retreats then after lashing out with "I'm not sick. My father put me here because he hates me and wants me to die here." In the presence of another man, Bob is passive and hesitant. When something he says is contested, he defaults. He sets up a barrier between himself and other people by running about, reading in a corner, hunching over his art work, or closing his eyes.

Some of Bob's questions are unanswerable. "Why am I always the one that everyone hates?" Years of rejection and hurt feelings are too complicated to unravel. Out of touch again, he slips into his delusions and hallucinations. They are private and fleeting; the sound of his name will call him back to the outer world again.

In his art work, Bob has a few standard images from which, after five months, he has strayed little. His usual routine is to get his art supplies from a bag, make an outline on the paper, color it in, initial it, and possibly add a few finishing touches. If he has time, he'll study his work from various angles by changing the paper's position.

Bob's pace and his manner of working are determined by his mood. In a state of uncontrollable anger he refuses to draw; he walks around instead. When he's feeling bad but in control, he works fast and furiously. His whole body is intent on his drawing; he grimaces, clenches his teeth, and exerts heavy pressure. He uses his energy assertively, pushing hard as if against great resistance. Lines are straight and he controls their length; spaces are filled in with crisscross strokes, first one small area, then the next. When Bob feels more relaxed, he works more slowly, glancing up at me occasionally, dawdling, and taking tea breaks. When I attempt to introduce an activity other than drawing (such as clay work or photography), Bob nervously moves to the other end of the table, seating himself as far away as possible from the new threat. Thus we keep to drawing.

Bob demonstrates his need for control by always choosing the smallest paper available and working on it systematically. The subject, firmly placed, must be contained within the bounds of the paper.

Over a period of five months Bob's drawings seem to get somewhat closer to the source of his problems. His work of the past three months is less sophisticated than the work he did during the first two months. At first he showed horizon lines, attempted three-dimensionality, and dealt with a greater variety of subject matter, such as a sports stadium (Figure 1), and a

Figure 1

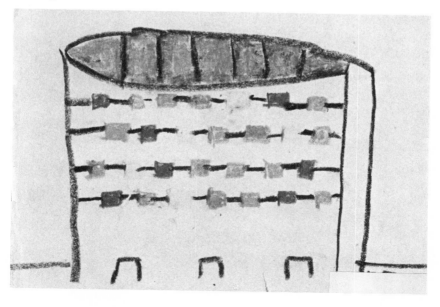

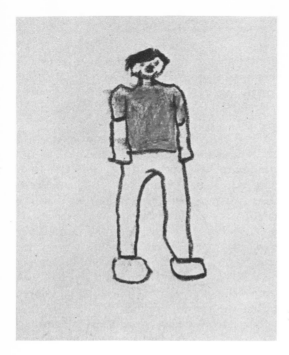

Figure 2

person (Figure 2). Other pictures showed a car, a tree, a house. Bob's more recent pictures are simpler; he uses the bottom edge of the paper as a baseline; subjects are two-dimensional; and an image of a house predominates (see Figure 3 for a representative work). One new subject has made its appearance; boat and fortress together (Figure 4). An innovation seen in this picture and some others is a small yellow sun added as a final touch. Always

Figure 3

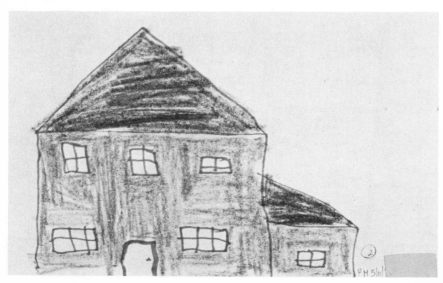

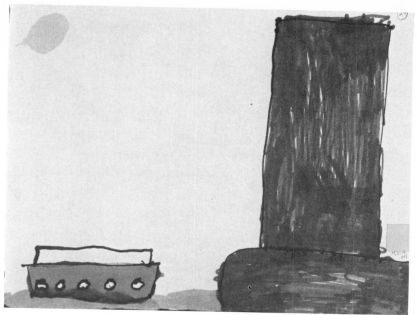

Figure 4

located in the corner, the sun does not seem to be a source of strength. Bob draws the boat-fortress motif once or twice a month and his behavior is relaxed while he does so. As it rests in the water, the boat, which Bob says carries only himself, seems to be heading for the impenetrable fortress. Although Bob used many colors in drawing boat, water, and fortress, the surrounding environment remains empty.

Repetition of the house theme shows the close ties Bob has to his home and parents. It is a place he hates and loves and wishes to return to. As we see in Figure 3 and Figure 5, Bob's close-up view of the house causes it to dominate one's vision both physically and mentally. Occasionally Bob attaches a small, one-windowed shed to the side of one of his simply rendered houses (Figure 3 is an example). The shed snuggles and leans close to the main house. Possibly it symbolizes Bob's dependence on his parents.

Doors to the outside world are closed, but they are large and have knobs. Bob gets upset if while he is coloring in the house he gets any color on the door. There are often three windows on the second floor and one on either side of the door. None of the windows gives any glimpse of life within the house, which always lacks a chimney, a symbol that might suggest warmth and life. Bob tends to place the house, which is symmetrical and balanced, to the left of center. He sometimes places a tree at one side of it (as in Figure 5) or two trees flanking it. The trees, despite their tall, thick trunks, have relatively sparse greenery. The crown is flattened, contained, kept small. It touches or goes off the top of the paper.

In all Bob's drawings, brown is the most used color. Since there is no

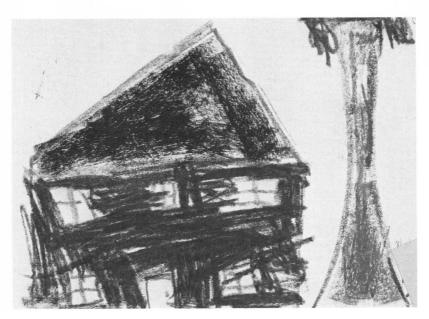

Figure 5

shading, the effect is one of flatness. Bob's drawings communicate his feelings of emptiness about his life. Imagery is isolated in great expanses of space; one senses that Bob feels vulnerable.

My knowledge of Bob thus far is based on his art work, his behavior, and the comments he makes while with me during sessions. I have learned how misleading each of these facets can be if taken separately and how revealing if taken together.

There are parallels between Bob's general behavior and his art work. He is compulsive and fastidious about how much physical space to take for pacing, rocking, and skipping. The same restraint and meticulousness are evident in his placement of images on paper. Depending on his anxiety level, the white borders in his pictures grow narrower (as tension increases) or wider (as tension decreases). (Compare Figure 3 and Figure 5.) During times of great stress Bob tends to exceed his self-imposed bounds; he may walk out of the room or color beyond an outline or off the paper. His movements are likely to be less controlled at such times; his rhythmic rocking may hesitate and he may draw a less neatly constructed house. Such behavior and such artwork both suggest fragmentation. Bob's characteristic rigidity in body posture can be related to his practice of outlining in his pictures. He defends fiercely against stimuli by blocking out impressions. He seems to say, "This is all I see, all I feel: there is nothing else."

Like his pictorial subject matter, Bob's conversational topics are limited and repetitive. Together with the endlessly repeated house drawings, his talk suggests that Bob is frozen in some moment of his past. He restricts his comments to statements about sports and his family, and he repeats such comments many times. I must introduce very subtly anything new, whether it is an art material or an idea. With time and patience Bob responds; my low-keyed, nonchalant comments and answers register with him, although he shows no immediate reaction. The idea is absorbed, germinates, and then, maybe three weeks later, Bob may respond to it. Very slowly he begins to come out from behind his wall. Although he retreats from time to time, a pattern has been established. Next time he ventures out a little further.

My Reaction

When I draw during our sessions, I use art to react emotionally to our relationship, to confront it intellectually, or simply to escape from it. Art is a way to make evident my current state of mind. My drawings proceed slowly in curves and masses, moving usually from the abstract into the realistic (Figure 6 is an example). This transition seems to parallel my movement away from private emotional concerns toward an attempt to communicate socially by means of recognizable imagery. I prefer to use a variety of media in order to blur outlines, disregard boundaries, let go of intellectual reasoning, and record my changes of mood. Instinct seems to guide my life; it sometimes leads me into a morass that I then feel the need to contain. I work right into each individual part of my drawing, then step back and organize the whole. It becomes more and more complex.

I find in my work a sense of withdrawal from a tense situation into a

Figure 6

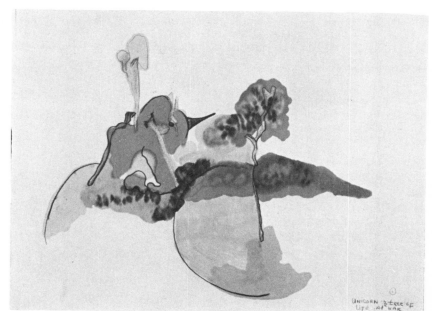

UNICORN & tree of
life at war

protected enclosure. My images are placed centrally on the paper. Mouths are closed and faces are pensive. Like Bob, I sometimes close myself off from what is happening. My predominant subject matter is countryside, mountains, and ocean. I satisfy my need for freedom and isolation by imagining myself there where life has a grand scale and idealism seems appropriate. When my immediate environment becomes too fragmented, nature restores a sense of peace and wholeness. For me my nature scenes, in vibrant color, are idyllic and magical. I try to keep in a corner of my mind a place for beauty, a place that is untouched by the sadness of Bob's plight. I hope to use this as a reservoir from which I can draw the strength to help him.

After each session, I review what has happened and roughly plan out a stimulus to art work or conversation by means of which Bob can release some energy and increase his self-awareness. In some of my drawings I consciously try to show him alternative ways of being. I vary my pencil strokes and use a wide range of color, willing him to change. As I learn to let him discover things for himself, my drawings become more spontaneous.

Some of my drawings record my doubts about being the therapist in this relationship. I feel that I am the one who carries the burden. I get so carried away that sometimes I shut Bob out (see Figure 7).

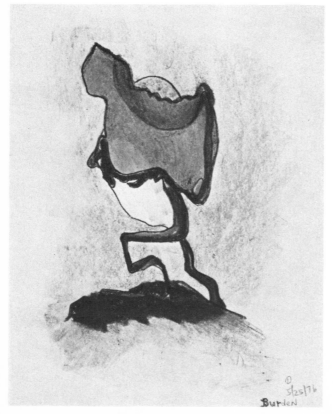

Figure 7

I have learned that there is more to my drawings than first meets the eye. Sometimes a picture looks calm on the surface, while beneath lie rage, agitation, and confusion. For both Bob and me our drawings are a reflection of our thoughts and moods—sometimes shifting—during a session. The present as it stands revealed in our pictures is a summation of the events that formed us through the years.

Theory Redefined by Practice

After five months' experience in a "therapeutic relationship" my understanding of this term has changed. The relationship can no longer be defined in terms of a person who helps and a person who is helped. Therapy is a joint venture into realization and change. Each partner in a relationship must develop a degree of trust in the other. Both must overcome fear of rejection and learn to take risks.

The therapist operates on the assumption that all human beings have a basic need to communicate and be understood. The therapist is in a position to gain an objective overview of the person who commits himself to her care. By observing the whole person—not just separate aspects that the client chooses to make known—the therapist becomes aware of what causes the client pain and what the stumbling blocks to his integration are. Since clients, like everyone else, are in continuing process, the possibility exists that the therapist can help them change.

Therapists deal with thoughts, feelings, and actions. Each of us is taught to see in specific ways. A client may not be ready to perceive the new; his needs may cause him to cling to old attitudes. What constitutes the client's reality at the moment is what the therapist must deal with; for her client's sake she must control her urge to force her view of reality on him. One cannot know all the reasons behind current problems so one must accept a person without reservation until he begins to reveal himself. A therapist must be careful to keep her facial expressions and comments nonjudgmental. Patience, stillness, and a nonexpectant attitude encourage therapeutic change.

A therapist must know her own weaknesses and be aware of how the biases of her background may affect her observations. Tolerance for the beliefs and lifestyles of others can help to overcome these biases. Since a client may profit from a range of healthy social interactions, possibly gaining thereby a broadened viewpoint and a new pattern of dealing with people, it is important that the therapist maintain a nonpossessive, nonauthoritarian attitude.

Honesty and a supportive attitude as a client struggles with his demons encourage a client's trust in his therapist. Being aware of the phenomenon of transference, the therapist realizes that sometimes a client's anger toward her is unwarranted and not to be taken at face value.

Mental illness is a refuge, an alternative way of dealing with life that our society cannot always understand. Each individual interacts differently with his environment. Art therapy can be the bridge between different perceptions of reality. The making of art satisfies a need to communicate and to impose order on chaos. The act has its wellsprings in the unconscious, and when successful, gives form to aspects of an individual's past, present, and future.

When a client keeps repeating a theme in his work, the theme relates to an area of unresolved conflict, yet even repetitious pictures can serve as a way to illustrate not easily expressed ambivalent feelings; making such images at least gives temporary relief from intense preoccupation with the conflict itself. And a picture can do more than merely reflect its maker's conflicts and ambivalences; it can also affect his attitude toward them and sometimes bring them close to resolution. The symbolic expression remains the same as long as the artist is satisfied with it. As he embellishes and makes changes in his work, his pictorial thinking is drawing upon the rich reservoir of the unconscious for answers. In learning to cope with pictorial problems, he may be slowly developing means to deal with life as well.

Instead of textbook theories, though, I work with a living, changing person. I realize that the way Bob behaves toward me is his characteristic manner of interacting with the world. I've stopped being so bewildered by his rejection of me. When he refuses help or sympathy, it is because he doesn't trust it, because he is unable to give and receive. He refuses to acknowledge openly that he might have a problem, that there may be some reason for his being in this hospital other than that his father hates him and wishes for his death.

Sometimes I am nervous about saying the wrong thing. But I try not to take the easy way out—which would be to help Bob avoid any confrontation with the unpleasant feelings that do arise. As times goes on and some good things have happened, I begin to gain confidence in myself, to feel more able to guide Bob over the rough spots. When he says "I am not sick," I gently remind him of his earlier, contradictory remark, "I am getting worse." I try to help him establish some continuity in his thought processes and to use deductive reasoning. I tell him that our perceptions of situations may not always be the same over time. Maybe he will one day come to understand the realities of other people.

Despite my need to structure situations and make sure of the results, I attempt to focus on and remain sensitive to what Bob is saying through his mood, posture, behavior, and art imagery. But even as I observe these aspects of Bob—and wish that I could concentrate exclusively on my observations—I try to be totally responsive to him in the current situation. Often Bob will block any effort to investigate the meaning of what he has expressed and I am left frustrated. I must store my observation with past ones, to be recalled when he is feeling less vulnerable. I accept the present resistance, try to empty myself of any expectation, and do not press for growth beyond his current abilities. I have to ask myself, "Does he want to be talked with? Am I intruding on his privacy? Am I even in touch with what he's trying to communicate? Am I regarding his needs or pushing my own hang-ups?" I wonder if something I do blocks his spontaneity. I try to keep far enough away from him to maintain my objectivity, yet close enough to be able to visualize what he sees.

I feel I am too removed at times. I become lost in my own thoughts, closing my eyes and ears to the monotony of the sessions. Sometimes days are quiet, and it may not be until Bob makes an unexpected move that I remember he is there.

To combat his feeling of being hated, I attempt to be consistently accepting in my attitude toward him. I do not reject him when he screams "You're stupid! I'm going to get out. Right now!" I continue to maintain an accepting attitude. Therapy no longer means to me only looking for a way to make someone not be schizophrenic. I talk a bit about myself, hoping he may recognize and share common ground. On two occasions other staff members join us. An art aide comes outside with us for an energetic game of Monkey-in-the-Middle. Bob maintains eye contact as the three of us discuss sports, travel, and Hitler. He is so interested in his surroundings that he almost stops rocking. Another time, a few staff members come to celebrate Bob's birthday. When Bob enters the room, we all yell "Surprise." He is taken aback and seems pleased: "Oh, this sure *is* a surprise." We sit around the table and for a few moments are a group of people without "roles" having fun and liking each other. But Bob isn't always willing to come into the present, to play any other role than that of second son in a family that he thinks hates him. Mostly it is all he can do to hold himself tautly together against the world.

If I ask Bob about the picture he is drawing, his replies are terse. He shows no insight or interest in exploration. If he withdraws into silence, we then work to handle his excess energy and his rigidity through physical movement. I matter-of-factly give him a piece of Plasticine and ask him to help me soften it. He rolls and pushes it and begins to slow down. As the material becomes easier to manipulate, I hand him more pieces to work on. This activity serves to keep Bob and me in contact; it helps Bob let off steam by expending energy; and, at the same time, it gets him used to handling Plasticine.

Bob escapes our shared reality by slipping into delusions, hallucinations, or autistic behavior. In his delusions, he is the "hated one" and the "one who is laughed at." This makes him angry. On a calmer day, apparently remembering, he asks, "Do you like me?" The opinion of another does matter; the delusion does not always keep him safe. Sometimes, starting to hallucinate, Bob says that he remembers something funny. He smiles, his eyes merrily fix on something I can't see; sometimes he responds to directives perceived by him alone with mechanical motions. I do not try to cut short his temporary escape because I no longer need his constant attention to feel that the session is succeeding. He soon returns to our reality voluntarily or upon hearing a word directed toward him. As I contemplate his easy mental escape from our room, I find myself jealous of whatever makes his face light up. He can smile and enjoy the invisible, while I remain tied to the reality around us—a reality that makes *him* grimace and glower.

At times objects in the room occupy him. I watch, fascinated, as he touches different things. He is like a child who sees something for the first time, yet does not take it in. When I ask him which "touch" he likes, he does not understand what I mean. He seems to touch for pure sensual pleasure and possibly to verify his own existence.

Bob needs the familiar. He finds security in sameness and repetition. I make no unexpected physical moves and I present him regularly with the same art materials.

Conclusion

My relationship with Bob is teaching me certain things that I hope will increase my ability as a therapist. Bob is compelling me to be less intense and to take the time to assimilate both spoken and unspoken messages. One of the most important things I am learning is the wisdom of letting a person set his own pace with no strings attached. My trust that he will one day leave the hospital seems to be rewarded twofold in Bob's more frequent moments of trust that enable him to let go of the past and his assumption of some responsibility for therapy. In our latest session Bob owns up to the pain he feels when he is rejected and he accepts my thanks for his voluntarily helping me to organize some art materials. He talks at length with me about travel and other topics. Because I let him be, he interacts with me on his own initiative—a far more effective strategy than futilely attempting to push him into responding. He is beginning to feel good enough to trust himself with another human being. For a moment, to him I am not one of his hated "schmucks" and to me he is not just someone who needs therapy. Instead, we are individuals daring to allow ourselves to be affected by each other.

PART TWO

PRACTICE OF ART THERAPY WITH ADULTS

A Student Group Art Therapy Experience*

Walter Carter, Drew Conger, Judith Finer, Suzanne Israel, Hanna Yaxa Kwiatkowska, Mildred Lachman-Chapin, Susan Castelluccio-Michal, Geraldine Nestingen, Linda St. Germain, Lauri Tanner, and Katherine Williams

[*Editor's Note:* The purpose of the group art experience reported below was to enable students in the Art Therapy Program at The George Washington University in Washington, D.C., to learn about group process and the use of art. The experience was in the context of a class, held in spring 1975. The course was designed in the belief that knowing firsthand the forces at work and what can happen in art therapy groups can be useful to students in their future work. Equally important was consideration and study of those experiences. A summary of what happened in each session and speculations on the significance of some of these events follows.]

First Session

The student members introduced themselves briefly. Hanna Kwiatkowska, one of the two leaders of the group, spoke of group rules: the group would meet in thirteen weekly two-hour sessions; each participant would be given the grade of A for the course and was encouraged to keep a journal.

During the first hour, various student members tried to gain a better understanding of what to expect since they had believed this to be a didactic class rather than an experiential "group grope." Many spoke of their anxiety over revealing themselves to the leaders who, after all, would be making judgments and giving other grades to the participants within the context of

*This report was adapted from a presentation made by students in The George Washington University Graduate Art Therapy Program at the Seventh Annual Conference of the American Art Therapy Association, held in Baltimore, Maryland, October 1976.

the Graduate Program. Lauri Tanner challenged the leaders to define their methods and goals. Mildred Lachman-Chapin, the other leader, responded along the lines of "wait and see." Some participants found her cryptic statements provocative and frustrating—especially in view of earlier interactions with Milly of a more open and supportive nature. The students wanted assurance that in view of their vulnerability, lack of group cohesion, and insecurity they could trust the authority figures.

At Katherine Williams's suggestion the group decided to do art work with no themes or definitions in mind. The pictures made had a searching, wandering quality characterized by many flowing, curved lines. Hanna singled out Lauri's picture, *Yearning*, for comment. She pointed out that Lauri had so positioned herself in the room as to suggest her isolation from the group. Her picture, Figure 1, reflects ambivalence over her desire for group closeness and involvement and her feeling of distrust.

Milly pointed out that Walter Carter had made a picture that differed in style from those of the rest of the group. His sketch had a rigid, straight-line quality, and Walter had difficulty confronting the picture. A discussion ensued over Walter's being the only man in the group as well as the only black person. A previously existing hostility between Walter and Lauri surfaced. Lauri did not feel comfortable talking about it, but Hanna encouraged work on this and other interpersonal matters.

Second Session

Many group members still felt like strangers to the others. The session began rather as a business meeting with discussion of scheduling and administrative decisions. Someone reflected on the group's willingness to

Figure 1

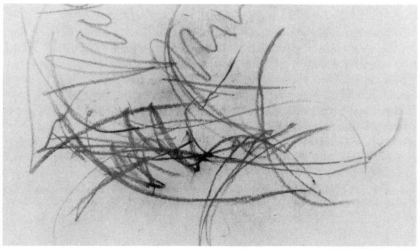

make decisions despite the absence of Judy Finer and Amy Gerson. [*Editor's Note: Amy Gerson was a fully participating member of the group, but she did not take part in the group's presentation at the American Art Therapy Association (AATA) Conference.*] This led to talk about ignoring minorities. That, in turn, led to the dissension between Walter and Lauri. Katherine joined the discussion, and the three of them talked at length of times when they had been angry at each other. Other group members became increasingly frustrated over merely looking on at the heated argument and made critical remarks among themselves. Hanna suggested doing some art, but this suggestion met with resistance. The group was working at cross-purposes because objectives were so vague.

It became evident that Walter, Lauri, and Katherine were arriving at a more harmonious feeling than existed among the other members of the group. Walter suggested that the three of them do a picture together, but Linda St. Germain and Suzie Israel objected strenuously. At this point the leaders talked about various ways to deal with anger, pointing out that most of the angry group members had chosen to remain passive rather than to interrupt the three members who occasioned their anger. Group frustration was a natural outcome.

Hanna again suggested that doing a picture might be helpful. Milly disagreed; she said that the group was focused on the current discussion and properly so. This glimpse of disagreement between the leaders, to whom group members were looking for guidance in solving the problem of animosity within the group, was disturbing to all concerned.

Third Session

Most members came to this session dreading more conflict, wanting to get it behind them and to arrive at a feeling of group solidarity. Milly raised the issue of the leaders' disagreement the week before. But instead of confronting this as a group concern, various members of the group addressed themselves to Hanna or Milly individually—sympathizing, criticizing, expressing disappointment. Suzie and Drew Conger left the group to do individual artwork. The other group members then rose simultaneously. Some chose to do individual work; but Susan Castelluccio-Michal, Gerry Nestingen, Linda, and Katherine worked on a mural (Figure 2)—perhaps as a way of symbolizing that the conflict had not affected their

Figure 2

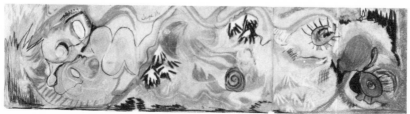

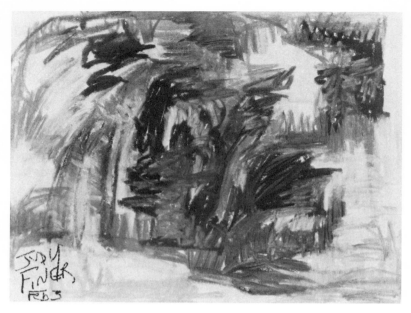

Figure 3

ability to function as a group. Whether initiated as a defense or not, the work on the mural took on a life of its own. There was much movement back and forth. Participants took pleasure in watching the mural grow almost effortlessly. Those working on the mural and those working individually did not constitute two opposing camps. All group members talked together easily while at work on their respective projects. After completing their individual works, Walter and Lauri joined in the mural-making. Afterward everyone commented on the strength, gaiety, and harmony of the mural— and especially on the separate forms blending together so well.

People suggested that Judy Finer's individual work, Figure 3, could fit in with the mural. Judy took exception to this idea; she saw her work as an individual statement. Figure 4, an individual work by Drew that she entitled *Framed*, symbolizes how Drew felt about being in a group that was supposed to be a class but was turning out to be far more emotionally demanding than any other class. Suzie, the first to get up to draw, called her picture *Cold Starry Night* (Figure 5). It is an icy statement of her feeling of aloneness and separateness from the group. After she completed this work she did not join in making the mural but instead made a red, tempestuous picture that suggested the passion and violence beneath the coldness.

Walter's individual picture (Figure 6; Plate III), is the one that attempted to deal with the issue of the leaders and their relationship to the group, the issue Milly raised at the beginning of the session. Walter's tree within enclosing lines suggests the leaders surrounded by the group.

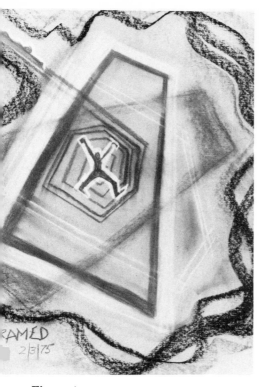

Figure 4

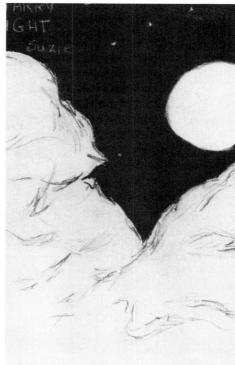

Figure 5

Figure 6

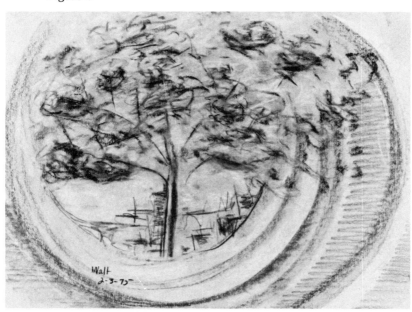

Fourth Session

Walter dominated the early part of the session. He placed his picture (Figure 6), begun in the last session and completed later at home, in the middle of the floor and spoke at some length about the role of the leaders and his desire for their protection. Many members resented Walter's domination of the session. Judy Finer suggested, as an indirect way of removing Walter from the spotlight, that the group turn to drawing. No one acted on her suggestion. Instead, various individuals expressed their resentment of Walter's behavior directly. This had the effect of enabling them to begin to talk about personal and deeply felt issues.

A school holiday scheduled for the next week meant that it would be two weeks before the group met again. Perhaps the awareness of the coming two-week break contributed a sense of urgency to many members' need to connect on deeper levels. By individuals' revealing themselves they might form bonds of sufficient strength to keep intact over the two-week break their still-emerging sense of being a part of a group.

The discussion centered around certain themes: personal loss, pain, illness, and death of loved people. Gerry talked about the recent death of her daughter; Drew, about her husband's death; and Susan, about the serious illness of a friend. Everyone was touched in some way by these expressions of genuine and profound emotion. Even those who remained silent identified with the others' grief out of their own experiences of sadness and loss.

This session marked the beginning of a sense of group identity—an identity that was more than the sum of all individual identities.

Fifth Session

Coming together after the two-week break, the group took up the question of scheduling a makeup session. The matter was complicated by the absence from this session of Gerry. Some members were concerned that something might have happened to her; others thought that perhaps she was anxious over having discussed her daughter's death and could not face the group. The group considered too its feelings about absenteeism and the frequent interruptions of the group process. Nothing was resolved, and after twenty minutes no date had been set for the makeup session.

The group turned to making pictures, most of which dealt with the themes that had emerged in the fourth session. Amy entitled her picture, Figure 7 (Plate IV), *Life's Juggler*. Amy could not talk about it, but it was apparent that she was representing a situation of some precariousness. The juggler is balanced on a thin, wavering horizontal line that does not look capable of supporting her weight. Of the juggler's ten balls, four are falling.

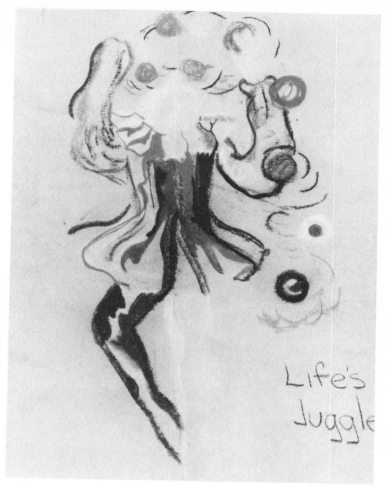

Life's
Juggle

Figure 7

Susan remained quiet throughout the session, but her picture, Figure 8, conveys through its somber and brooding quality her personal sense of foreboding over the fate of her very sick friend.

Sixth Session

Walter expressed his desire to discuss the picture he had started in the fifth session and completed later (Figure 9; Plate V). He related it to his childhood in the South—a childhood filled with fear, violence, and sorrow. He went on to talk about how he felt being a black man in a group whose other members were eleven white women. He said the group was tainted with racism and that Lauri in particular had a racist attitude. Lauri responded immediately. She spoke of her family's involvement in the Florida civil rights movement and of the discrimination she had been

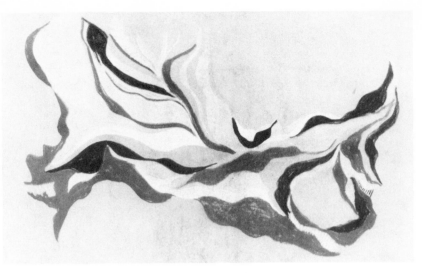

Figure 8

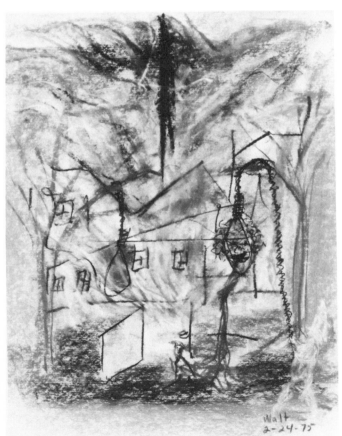

Figure 9

subjected to because of her position on this issue. Milly suggested that possibiy just because Lauri treated Walter the same way she treated anyone else she posed a particular threat to Walter. His early years had taught him to fear dealing with white women. When Lauri presented herself as someone he should deal with in an open, normal manner, Walter's early fears were reactivated. Walter acknowledged the likelihood of this, and Lauri responded by hugging him.

In speaking of his picture later during the AATA Conference presentation, Walter recalled—

. . . before creating this picture I was sweltering with anger. The fear of loss and the threat of death had become as real for me in this group as it had been during my childhood in a small southern town. The local Ku Klux Klan was a constant source of terror for all black people in the town. As an adolescent I lived with the constant fear that I would one day be hung from an oak tree and lynched if ever I was discovered looking at or talking with a white girl in a friendly manner. This group was both white and female. At the time this picture was made I did not feel that the group leaders would protect me from the hostile forces of this all-white group.

Of the picture directly, he said,

A dense black cross appears above a wood frame house engulfed with flames. The cross symbolizes childhood feelings that even God could not stop the Ku Klux Klan from burning our neighbor's house. Two oak trees with nooses stand to the left and right of the picture.

A beheaded figure hangs from the noose on the right. Notice that the noose to the left is permanently fixed to the branch. This anchored noose is symbolic of my constant fear of death.

Group acceptance and group support enabled me to open this issue and to deal with it. Had this group become rejecting, patronizing, or overly protective, I do not feel that I would have become trusting enough of them to work on such issues.

Amy then became the center of attention by instructing Walter to apply what he had learned in the group to his life. Soon several members accused Amy of being "teacherish," which, in turn, made Amy defensive. Amy was indeed a teacher, the only non-art therapist in the group. The conversation drifted to the picture Amy had made in the fifth session (Figure 7; Plate IV). At this time she revealed that she was in the midst of a painful divorce and that her picture reflected her feelings of loss and uncertainty. Of the six balls in the air, Amy said, "These are the new things in my life. The new is tenuous and uncertain, and I don't know if things will work out." The four falling balls are "old things" and consequently losses.

Shortly before the end of the session Suzie and Lauri together expressed their anger at the silent group members—Katherine, Linda, and Susan—charging them with withholding. The group's attention focused on Susan who said she did not feel that Lauri and Suzie were really concerned about her, that she was still attempting to sort out her feelings about the previous session and was not ready to talk. On the defensive because she felt Lauri and Suzie were attempting to dictate her responses, Susan went on to say that she was weary of Lauri's and Suzie's attempts to control the group. Hanna defended Susan's position several times, pointing out that Susan was stating her feelings as the group demanded.

At the end of the session everyone appeared to be confused and emotionally exhausted.

Seventh Session

Katherine opened the session by describing a dream or dreamlike incident in which she heard a woman screaming in the night. No dogs barked. Inquiring of her neighbors the next day she learned that no one else had heard the scream. This mixture of reality and fantasy seemed to set the theme of the session.

Gerry, speaking again of the death of her daughter, mentioned the comfort she found in her religion and expressed confidence that she would rejoin her daughter in heaven. Drew, speaking of her husband's death, said that religious beliefs she had once thought real had become fantasy to her now. She could not tell her son that his father was in heaven. Gerry and Drew shared the feeling of profound loss; Gerry tried to understand God, Drew to understand why medical science had proved inadequate.

Gerry spoke of her pain in trying to discuss her daughter's death with another daughter. Milly stepped outside her nondirective role at this point to advise Gerry to discuss the death with this girl. It seemed proper and natural for Milly to do so.

When everyone rose by common consent to draw, Hanna asked to join Drew in making a picture; Milly joined Gerry. Thus the two grieving participants were singled out by the leaders. Figure 10 is the joint picture made by Drew and Hanna. The flamelike shape on the left was drawn by Drew; Hanna added the (gray-and-black) wall on the right, which she described as a representation of the numbness of grief. Then the two attempted to unite the two very different sides of the picture with ribbons (of blue). They achieved some success. Speaking later at the conference presentation of this experience, Drew said that at the time she valued the companionship and consolation of working with Hanna, but that she never forgot Hanna was a teacher in her program as well as a leader of the group; Drew was afraid of losing control. While drawing, she expressed to Hanna some guilt about the group's concentration on topics of loss and grief. She

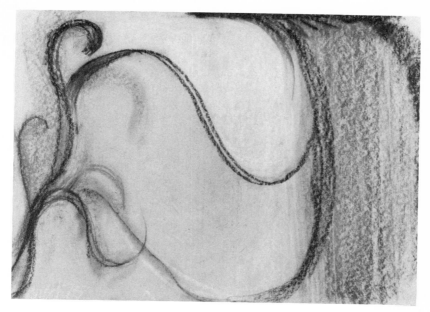

Figure 10

mentioned that the week before, Lauri had said she wanted to celebrate life, not death. Hanna suggested that Drew bring up her guilty feelings in the next session. The seventh session had proved very affecting; at its conclusion Drew, Gerry, and Katherine were in tears.

At the conference presentation, Drew spoke of what she had learned:

At that time I was art therapist with an adult group in which the subjects of separation, loss, and death often arose. Until my own experience with this group I had attempted to divert discussions from tragic stories. It was during this evening that I first felt real empathy in our group, that I realized how necessary it is for each person to tell his story in words as well as pictures. It was, so to speak, the difference between knowing the keyboard and understanding the music.

Eighth Session

Everyone had been through an emotional wringer, and it had drawn them together. Hanna was absent from this session, and Milly told the group that Hanna was ill and might have to miss a number of sessions. The group was very concerned, and a feeling of anxiety pervaded the rest of the session.

Drew and Gerry spoke of their misgivings about the group's reaction to being forced to concentrate on loss and grief. The general response was supportive. Almost everyone had suffered the loss of someone close and knew what it was to grieve. But all agreed to move on now to other concerns. Milly said that first she wanted to explain why the leaders had acted as they did in the last session—pairing off with two individuals rather than remaining available to the entire group. A number of members protested that compassion prevented them from feeling excluded by the leaders' behavior. Milly pointed out that the pictures made by the single individuals in the last session did, however, reflect feelings of isolation that the joint pictures did not. For example, Figure 11 by Linda showed a solitary camper sitting in front of a sheltering tent against a yawning, black background. Lauri and Judy said they objected to Milly's trying to use group dynamics to analyze an emotional situation, that Milly's assessment of the group's reaction was incorrect.

With this rejection of Milly's theory and with Hanna being absent, the group members began to vie among themselves to lead. Walter, Katherine, and Linda spoke excitedly about personal concerns. Susan expressed her objection to therapists who analyze pictures too deeply. Suzie said she wanted to discuss what it felt like to be discriminated against because she was a Jew. Everyone wanted to talk at once—not about sad concerns of the past, but about current personal frustrations. Lauri grew extremely agitated and then withdrew into silence for the rest of the session. Tension grew as Walter and Amy exchanged angry words. Katherine, too, spoke critically to Walter. (After some quiet reflection, she hugged him.)

Everything anybody said seemed to provoke a fight. Gerry surprised the group by making her first angry comment; it concerned the group's failure to support Suzie in her effort to talk about anti-Semitism.

Comments were made about Lauri's obvious withdrawal from the fray. Milly explained that there are many ways to handle rage, and this was probably Lauri's method.

Figure 11

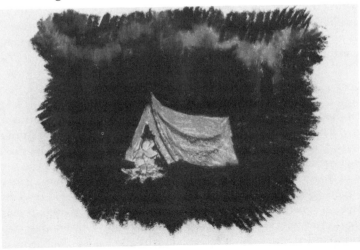

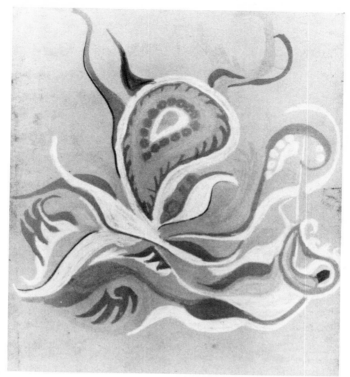

Figure 12

Perhaps the sudden effort on everyone's part to bring his or her concern to the center of the group's attention was triggered by Hanna's absence and by the approaching dissolution of the group when the course would be over at semester's end.

Ninth Session

Both leaders were present. An effort was made to acquaint Hanna with what had happened in the previous session, but it was not very successful. There was considerable difficulty in getting the session started. Judy, feeling frustrated and bored with what was going on, got up to draw. She drew with large body movements that she described as a body dance. Her picture seemed to reflect the group's dancing around sensitive issues. Now in the mood to draw, the other group members, with the exception of Amy, got up to make a mural, very likely as an attempt to deny underlying conflicts and to attain a superficial closeness. Amy, like Judy, chose to draw by herself. Her lovely, fluid picture, Figure 12, suggests emotional detachment from the rest of the group, a denial of the group.

After the group sat down once again, discussion of interracial relationships and religion ensued. Katherine talked of having had a black boyfriend when she was younger and of her parents' negative reaction. (It is interesting that the two women with whom Walter had the most difficulty—Lauri and Katherine—had earlier had close friendships with black people.)

This session seemed marred by troubling relationships between members outside the group. Although there was some talk about bringing to the group's attention things that happened between members outside, the discussion never quite came to grips with the underlying problems that were affecting what was going on in the group. In the same way, the art work produced in the session was primarily evasive.

Tenth Session

This session was recorded for Hanna, who was absent. Since this was the next-to-the-last session, one of the main topics discussed was terminating the existence of the group. Related to the theme of termination, Katherine brought up a personal dilemma: she needed to decide whether or not to terminate a pregnancy confirmed just that morning.

The group's reaction varied. Some wanted Katherine to have the baby. Others urged abortion. Still others remained silent. Everyone wanted desperately to help Katherine, to give something to her. The energy and depth of feeling the group exhibited in rallying to Katherine's side reflect the group's simultaneous, if unconscious, concern with the question of its own existence as well. In the midst of struggling with the problem of its termination, the group ironically was presented with the potential for new life. Katherine's pregnancy became the group's pregnancy. Even if the group's life must end, there was the hope that it might be perpetuated by an offspring. The prevailing mood became festive and hopeful. It was a welcome relief from earlier preoccupation with loss and separation.

Words seemed inadequate in this session, perhaps more so than in any of the group's experiences. It was only by making pictures that individuals faced their feelings about pregnancy and birth, thereby identifying with Katherine on a fundamental level.

Figure 13 is Katherine's picture. She described it at the conference presentation in these words:

> The two figures on the right are my daughters, whose school situation dictated a change. I knew I would have to finish my degree and get a job as soon as possible in order to finance private schooling. The black lines suggest other conflicts: my age (the feeling that this was my last chance to have a baby before 35, that magic age in birth defect statistics); the already frantic quality of my life with my husband (both of us working and in graduate school).
>
> Drawing the picture was a way of allowing myself an opportunity to express my longing for this baby. Without intending to make it so, the fetus I drew radiates a warmth and life that relegates the more rational considerations to the edges of the page. The next day these considerations again assumed great importance.

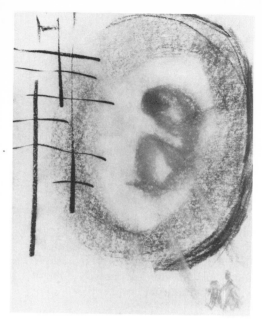

Figure 13

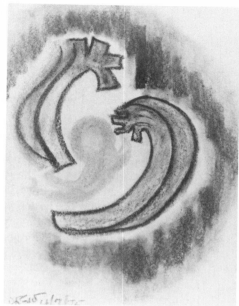

Figure 14

Both the potential for new life and the threat of termination figured in pictures made by other members of the group. In Figure 14, drawn by Drew, the fetuslike form is threatened by ominous forces that surround it. Walter's picture (Figure 15) is an expression of the mounting gaiety within the group. Members commented on its likeness to a congratulatory baby card. Walter described it as a bouquet of flowers he wanted to give to

Figure 15

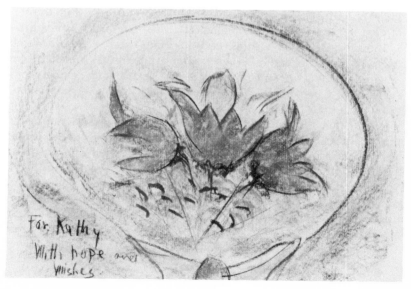

Katherine. He expressed his hope that Katherine would have the baby and joked about being called "Uncle Walter." He mentioned, too, his own desire to have a son.

The session ended with Katherine still undecided about what to do.

Eleventh and Twelfth Sessions

Both sessions were held in Hanna's absence on the same evening in a long, four-hour meeting. This was the group's final experiential meeting in which to share thoughts and feelings through talk and art. Another session for theoretical study and discussion would follow.

With the semester ending, many individuals were separating permanently from the people they had encountered in various clinical placements and, for the summer, from classmates and friends. For a while talk centered on these topics. Termination of clinical experiences was proving particularly difficult for both Susan and Suzie. The group was sympathetic and supportive of their feelings.

Lauri brought up her pain and bewilderment at separating from a man who had been a companion for many years. Amy recalled the shock and pain she had felt in separating from and divorcing her husband. At the same time she reminisced about the happiness she had known in the relationship.

Such discussion served to sidestep the dramatic question that had been the focus at the close of the last session: Ought Katherine to terminate her pregnancy? Almost everyone knew that Katherine had meantime ended the pregnancy, but no one wanted to introduce the subject in the group. Yet when the group did collectively acknowledge Katherine's abortion and what each individual had invested in the pregnancy, it was ready to confront the termination of the group as well. Discussion deepened and was enriched by the imagery in the drawings made in the session. The focus shifted from the act of creation expressed in its biological sense—pregnancy and birth—to exploration of the relationships between men and women. Members discovered similarities and differences among individuals, some anticipated and some surprising. Because he was a lone man among several women, Walter served as a catalyst to discoveries about women's competition for attention from men.

In a revelation that climaxed the session, Milly revealed that, as often happens in groups, the discussion that evening had reflected an event of central importance to *her* life: she had agreed that very afternoon not to prolong legal proceedings that stood in the way of her own divorce.

The group had arranged to hold this meeting at Gerry's home and to follow it with a meal for which everyone contributed a dish. The dinner together prolonged the experience of warmth and companionship the group had attained.

As a footnote to the group's involvement in Katherine's pregnancy, nine months after Katherine revealed her pregnancy the group met for a reunion and at that time gave birth to the idea of presenting a report on its experience at the AATA Conference.

Thirteenth Session

At this final (didactic) meeting, the group addressed itself to defining the issues that pervaded its earlier sessions and raising general questions about group process and art expression as suggested by the group's experience. The concerns identified can be summarized as follows:

1. Male/female relations, particularly as influenced by race.
2. Death, illness, and separation.
3. Creativity, especially in the biological sense of having a baby.
4. Group power. How much could group pressure influence individuals, affecting their decisions outside the group (as in the abortion question) or their role choice inside the group? Conversely, how much power could an individual retain despite group pressure? How much power was the group giving unnecessarily to its leaders?
5. Protection. Ought the leaders to protect individuals from group action, and to what extent? What ends are served by refusing to protect in training groups such as this? In patient groups?

In discussing broad questions about the art produced in the sessions, the group decided that for the most part the quality of the art was surprisingly good. This was especially the case with individual works; joint art works rarely achieved the integration and evocativeness of the work done alone. It was decided that at times making art represented a way for participants to avoid group and personal issues, and at other times making art served to intensify participants' explorations. Other questions were considered: How did the art of individual participants affect other participants? What use was made of joint art work? Who made the decisions to do art? When did making such a decision become an important group issue? Under what circumstances? With what motivation?

The group asked itself the questions that arise in all groups: To what extent were the themes the group came to concentrate on and the ensuing course of events determined by the makeup of the group, the group's being a class for credit, the personalities of the leaders, the relationship between them? Group members discussed how they felt toward each other now that the experience was over. Perhaps the group's wish to preserve this experience by presenting it at an AATA Conference, and now by publication, was a way of achieving the immortality that many groups yearn for.

Using Slides of Patients' Work in Art Therapy

Jane Teller

To demonstrate my way of using slides as a special device in art therapy, I shall concentrate on the course in treatment of a single patient, Alice. She is twenty-eight years old, the second of three daughters of a rural teacher. Married and a lawyer's secretary, she works hard—and without enthusiasm—in both roles, finding it hard to get along with either husband or boss. At the time she was referred to me, her moods were extreme and changed frequently, swinging from states of virtual immobility to the kind of explosive tantrums she had thrown as a child. She feared these violent outbursts and the physical harm she might inflict on others, and they left her depressed and confused.

Alice is a patient of E. S. Weber, a psychiatrist in Princeton, New Jersey. Dr. Weber refers to me patients who, he feels, can benefit from adjunctive treatment. We confer frequently, and he sometimes makes general suggestions about areas to be explored. Alice had mentioned to him an interest in art and she seemed anxious to try art therapy. When I wrote this report, I had been working with her once a week for about fourteen months spread over a two-year period.

My General Approach to Art Therapy

My work with Alice is typical of my method. To gain useful results, I believe the art work must be done as spontaneously as possible. I can usually guide a patient to unpremeditated, noncognitive work by a simple exercise that uses kinesthesis as a springboard for the expression of affect. This procedure helps those who are sure they "can't draw" get started and demonstrates to each individual that when he abandons deliberation he is better able to express both how *he* sees something and how *he* really feels about it.

"Try moving vigorously," I say. "As you do, look around the studio and single out one thing that somehow interests you. Tune your bodily movement to describe the stance and rhythm of the object you are looking at. Repeat and repeat this descriptive movement—dance it if you like—until you feel it all through you, toes to fingertips. Now, hold a short piece of charcoal, the extension of your hand. It is easy to continue that movement, letting the charcoal record it on a big piece of paper flat on the table or on the wall."

After a few tries this becomes as natural as breathing and as individual as a person's walk. His line describes the quality of what he sees, how he sees it, his current mood, and his unique movement pattern. It releases him from conventions of drawing and from preconceived notions about art, and it frees him for the expression of how he feels. As Alice put it, "I had to get over painting *good*, and pretty."

Discussing her experience with art therapy after a few weeks' work, she said further, "I felt happy after it. Now, at home and at work, I often use it as a release if I'm tense. It helps. So do the exercises.[1] I do them at home, too. They make me feel comfortable. Now I have an awareness of my body and I'm happy about having it with me. That makes me more socially at ease and free in a way.

"In art therapy I found out what my concerns are and it prepared me to face them. It's the so-there-it-is quality when they're all down on paper. I saw them, and they didn't bite me. There were things I didn't realize— things I couldn't talk about to Dr. Weber until I drew them and got used to them a little—like my whole confusion about sex."

In studying the work, I try to stay away from subjective interpretation, leaving that for the patient. At the same time I watch for certain *qualities* in the painting to see if comment and quality jibe. How a painting is organized describes, I believe, the actual state of mind of the patient at the time.

Size and placement of subject matter, for instance, appear to indicate the patient's attitude toward its importance. I have found too that vagueness or lack of focus shows lack of awareness, while closure and general increase of clarity indicate progress.

I look at quality of line for an indication of current mood and degree of affect. Are lines generally heavy and sagging, or strong and incisive, or light and aimless? How much pressure is exerted?

What medium has the patient chosen for what subject matter, and how has it been used? Charcoal and poster paint are soft and are usually selected for easy, free expression. Wax crayons, or other media offering resistance, require more pressure. Alice said she could feel the crayon grate against the paper. Drawings done in these resistant media are frequently the difficult ones; their subjects more often than not elicit anger.

And last, how are abstract and realistic forms used? It is helpful to recognize each patient's attitude toward these modes of expression, and even, on occasion, to suggest the use of one or the other as, for example, Dr. Weber did toward the end of Alice's therapy. In her case the abstract

1. In combination with drawing, I use a system of body movement evolved by Bess M. Mensendieck, M.D., who has written extensively on this subject.

paintings were kinesthetic records of her inner state. She called these "my signature paintings,' and in them she felt her greatest strength (see, for example, Figure 12). Her more realistic work pinpoints problems, describing them more clearly as she gained the courage "to go after them."

How Slides Are Used

Slides can be useful at various times in therapy, depending on the patient and his requirements. Confronting one's own work in such a magnified form is sometimes shocking, and the shock may be compounded by a sudden realization of what it is all about. An emotionally resilient patient may be ready for such a confrontation early, when seeing even one or two slides can serve to speed the course of treatment. During later phases, viewing slides of past work may help when treatment has reached an impasse. Toward the end of therapy, slides provide a survey that makes it possible to digest or consolidate a long period of work.

In my work with Alice, it happened that after eighteen months of therapy she wanted to be on her own for a while and then return to get a fresh look and to assess her past work. I suggested that looking at slides would be the best way to get a comprehensive view of her productions, and Alice was delighted with the idea. During her five-month absence I made 125 color slides of work selected from Alice's total production of about 175 pieces. Figures 1, 3, 5, 6, 10, 12, and 13 were black crayon drawings; the rest of the illustrations were crayon or watercolor paintings, often in strong color.

When Alice returned we rapidly ran twice through all 125 slides in chronological order. This fast look clearly revealed her extreme emotional lability. She noticed "all the ups and downs," and said they were something to be aware of and to try to temper in her daily life. She also noticed that her early work was faint as contrasted with the decisiveness and vitality of the last forty slides. In addition, she mentioned some special advantages of viewing her work on slides.

"There isn't the distraction of moving around. Sitting in one place in a dark room, I really got absorbed. I forgot myself—let myself be transported. I felt a detachment." She said she got a concentrated picture of the work because of a kind of layering of the images, yet each one stayed with her longer, as well. She felt the intrusion of the medium was removed: that is, dry or cracked paint and unsatisfactory drawing were absorbed into the general view of the slide as a whole.

A few days later I gave Alice control of the projector. As we viewed the slides again, both she and I were struck by the persistent repetition of paintings dealing with her greatest concerns. Alice lingered over these slides. We separated them from those that either had never been of great interest to her or had lost their former importance.

We then concentrated on the eighty-four pictures that currently held the most meaning for Alice, and I asked her to group together those dealing with similar concerns. These groups we came to refer to as her "themes." Of course there was some overlapping, but more often than not each slide very clearly belonged in one of the seven categories we called Mother (eight slides); Father (six); Sexual Confusion (twelve); Self-Images: Very Young (four), Woman (eight), Man-Hater (eight), Wife (eight); Organic [growth symbols] (thirteen); Containment (ten); and Escape (seven). Alice noticed that in the first twenty-five drawings all seven themes appeared, although some were vague, "like the ones about my father and my attitude toward men in general, which I guess I couldn't face at first." Six of the seven themes are illustrated; the "Escape" drawings were so faint as to be unsuitable for reproduction.

In some instances comments made both at the time of painting and when the slides were studied are given so that changes in her appraisals become apparent. Where titles are used, they are taken from Alice's remarks. A college graduate and highly articulate, Alice talked at each session about the work she had done that day. Immediately after she left I wrote on the back of each painting her comments about it. When we projected the slides, I made notes (with her permission) as she commented on them.

Major Themes

Mother

Figure 1, *Puppy and Turtle,* made in the sixteenth month of treatment, is the sixth picture assigned to the "Mother" theme. Vaguely at first but with increasing force and definition, mother was seen as a monster crushing her helpless offspring. Alice, however, viewed this configuration of turtle and puppy in a more ambiguous fashion. "The dog steps on the turtle's head. Mother and I are puppy and turtle, or turtle and puppy. The turtle has a hard shell and little legs. Me?"

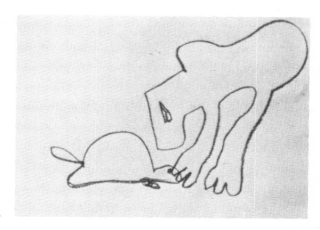

Figure 1

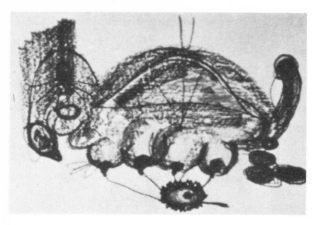

Figure 2

Figure 2 was made in the same session and was developed from a line drawing similar to Figure 1. "It looks like a turtle," Alice said. "That overpowering female again. Smothering. It is nursing that dried-up thing with the warm colors in the center and a dried-up shell, which is being victimized." She connected these last remarks with her feelings about sex.

Seven months later she commented on the slide: "I realize the animal is mother. It somehow reminds me of that gross female." (The last sentence refers to Figure 9.)

"When I was about thirteen," she then recalled, "Mother gave me a lecture about the 'priceless treasure of my virginity' and warned me that 'men might make me want to.' I was revolted and terrified by men from then on. At first [in therapy] I couldn't take the idea that there was anything wrong with my mother. Then I went through a period of anger and hostility toward her. Now it's O.K. I see her as a person and understand more about her attitudes—and that lecture."

Father

Figure 3, dating from the fourth month of treatment, is the earliest representation of Alice's father. "He's looking a little scared, teaching," she said at the time she drew it. "That's his little chair."

Viewing the slide nineteen months later, she remarked, "He looks like me."

Father was represented and spoken about with a kind of derisive bitterness. Guilt, evil, and impossible demands for goodness are the substance of the religiosity associated with him. In Figure 4, made in the seventeenth month of treatment and the last of this series, "a female is being squashed." She called the man "gleeful, silly."

Six months later, looking at the slide, Alice spoke more directly. "This is my father. Silly. Frilly. I think my attitude toward men stems from these Mother and Father drawings." She also noticed the reappearance of the

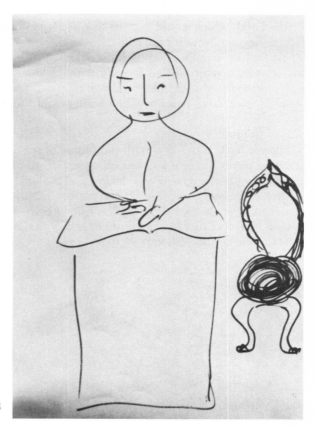

Figure 3

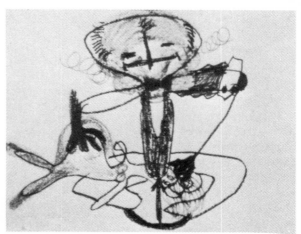

Figure 4

turtle shape, which would suggest that her wit is turned equally against her father, her mother, and herself.

"At first I was impressed by his sensitivity," Alice recalled, "but later, in the drawings, realized that I *really* thought him silly and weak. I also see how oppressive to me the religious references are. Now I see my real attitude toward my parents—their failures and the hostile feelings in me."

Sexual Confusion

Figures 5, 6, and 7 deal with the theme of sexual confusion. As with the previous series, there is growing clarity and focus in the course of treatment. The conflict between fear and desire, and the unclear choice of sexual role, at first expressed indirectly, come out toward the last in more open and powerful form. Notice the progress from Figure 5, a drawing done in the second month of therapy and more or less typical of Alice's early work. In it "a male-female fish" is angrily crossed out.

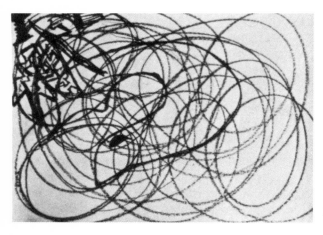

Figure 5

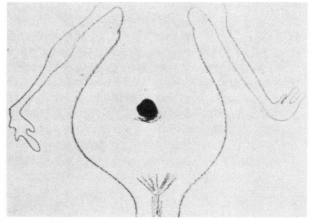

Figure 6

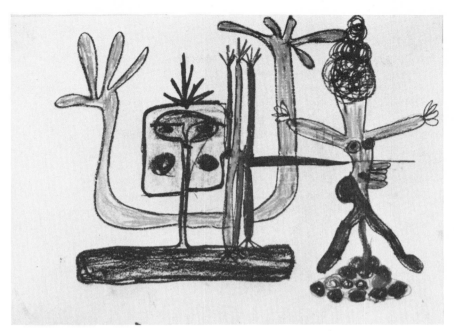

Figure 7

Alice said that Figure 6, drawn eleven months later, "started with a man and in drawing it, changed into a woman."

Figure 7, dating from the seventeenth month of treatment, was made in reaction to comments of some men in group therapy to the effect that Alice and her husband ought to separate. At that time she said of her painting, "I feel impaled, vulnerable, scared shitless and threatened by men. This is a woman being ridiculed and tortured. Dangled by her hair. Gory. The man is fiendish; he has breasts. The woman has penises on her stomach."

Commenting six months later on the slide, she said, "Here, at least, the figures are separate, not like in the first slide of this theme [Figure 5] both in one figure. The woman is having a miscarriage—that's a denial-of-motherhood business!"

Self-Images

The self-images, as mentioned earlier, fall into four categories: *Very Young, Woman, Man-Hater*, and *Wife*. Figure 8 (Plate VI), drawn in the eleventh month of therapy, is of the "very young" self. Of the puppy Alice said, "Pour things out. . . . That's how I felt when my husband went away [on a trip]." Viewing the slide a year later, she said, "It's functioning, peeing . . . it could be me."

Figure 9, drawn at the end of one year of treatment, is the last picture assigned to the series of the self as woman. Earlier attempts to draw the female figure were unconvincing or were crossed out. At the time the

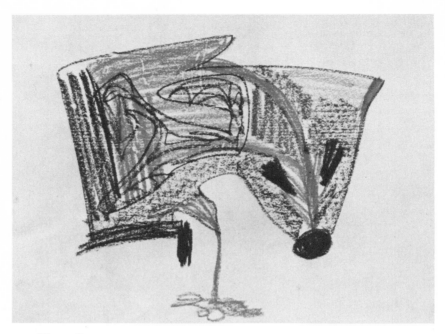

Figure 8

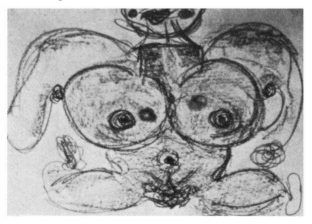

Figure 9

picture was made, Alice remarked that she had already ridiculed the male and now was treating the female in the same way. "I'm afraid of femaleness. But I can imagine the female body being presented in a beautiful way." Viewing the slide almost a year later, she was appalled at what she considered her "excessive" representation, and titled the picture *Whore*.

Figure 10, *Choked Collar*, was made in the thirteenth month of therapy and is the first picture of the self as "man-hater." In it she taunts the male.

This picture was important to Alice. She complained that she lacked wit and imagination, but here she saw that she really had these qualities after all.

In the self-images focusing on her role as wife, Alice gradually faced the realities of her marriage. In Figure 11, from the fourth month of treatment, she sees her husband as a guard, her marriage as a prison. Of Figure 12, a gesture painting made seven months later, she said, "We go in different directions," referring to herself and her husband.

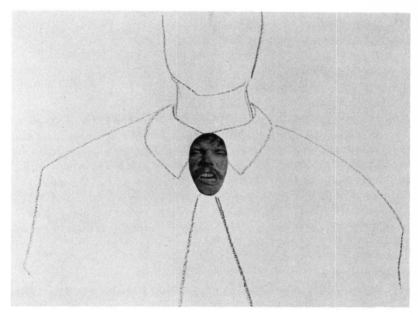

Figure 10

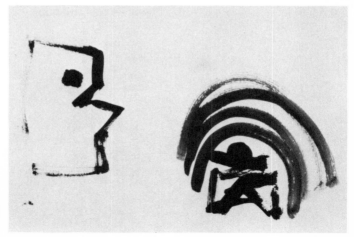

Figure 11

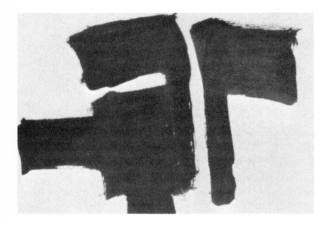

Figure 12

The last of the "wife" pictures, Figure 13, from the sixteenth month, made a deep impression on Alice. Its subject was "clinging vines," and Alice was distressed at the time to find that she had drawn them wilted. Although she was sad about the vines, she noted that they had been choking a little flower (lower left), and she saw herself in both the flower and the vines.

When she saw the slide seven months later, she remarked of the clinging vines that "Their day had come." Then she added, "I feel frightened but excited." She had begun to grapple with the problem of her dependence on her husband.

Organic

The pictures classified as "organic" consist of symbols, mainly abstract, of growth—earth, seeds, eggs. She liked Figure 14, from the fourth month of treatment, an abstraction of a seed, always for her a sign of integration. "It has a nice roundness," she said. Commenting on the slide more than a year and a half later, she remarked, "The male and the female combined, minus the hostility."

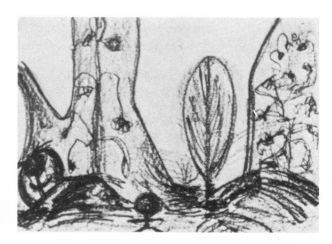

Figure 13

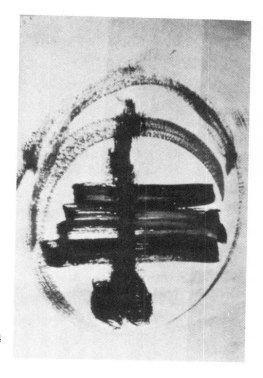

Figure 14

Containment

Assigned to this theme were ten crowded "claustrophobic" pictures obviously connoting emotional constriction. They often included an archway that symbolized a "goal." But what this series "contained" was a mystery to both Alice and me at that time. Figure 15, from the eleventh month of therapy, has the quality of a backdrop. One of the two doors in it was for her husband, the other for herself, indicating the separateness of their lives. Between these doors is the "center, where it might be glowing and good." A year later, she said of the slide, "Perhaps it leads in the direction of acceptance of the unknown. These 'containment' pictures seem to me like cities and have a dry, unpleasant look. Am I saying that I want to get away from the city and live in the country? Is this why there is so much organic symbolism in my work?"

Figure 16 (Plate VII), from the twelfth month of therapy, is prophetic. In it she developed the center section she had spoken of. "Here I stepped *through* a door," she said joyfully. "I pulled it shut behind me and am in a world of hills."

Six months after termination of therapy, Alice wrote me that she had left her husband and their city apartment and was living in Colorado. What her paintings foreshadowed had come true.

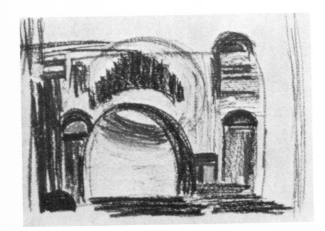

Figure 15

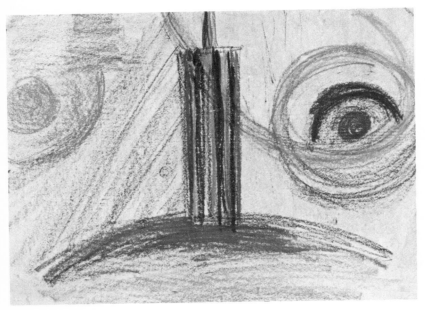

Figure 16

Alice's Assessment of Herself

Where did Alice stand at the end of her review of these pictures?

"A lot of things are clearer from the slides," she said. "I'm on the way toward untangling my sex attitudes and I'm somewhat braver in social situations. But I need very much to work further on both of them—and on my relationship with my husband."

Alice also saw that her confusion had been due to unrealistic appraisal of her parents. She recognized how her real feelings about them (which came out so clearly in her work), rather than the ones she thought she had, had set the pattern for her disdainful hatred and fear of men. She saw this attitude as connected with a lack of any sense-of-herself and thought these intertwined negatives explained her inadequacy in social relationships.

Knowing this much, she was aware that she needed to establish new attitudes. Therefore it was of utmost importance for Alice to recognize her growing strength. Now she could see it in her work, and she felt profoundly encouraged. This was a different kind of strength, not the strength of her violent outbursts or the violence she had equated with virility, but the strength of a developing self-confidence. I knew she could own her strength now and begin to use it to do the further work that, as she herself had said, still needed to be done.

Therapists' Assessment of Alice's Progress

Reviewing the work, Dr. Weber and I saw much fluctuation in thought and mood, evident in changes of both line quality and theme. Throughout there is much energy and conflict, showing inherent strength and a valiant, determined struggle for coherence. Thus, toward the end of therapy, Dr. Weber suggested to Alice that she make abstractions of some of the puppy drawings (or other subjects associated with weakness), since it was in the abstractions that she felt her greatest strength.

In the course of therapy Alice mentioned specific paintings to Dr. Weber. Since he had usually already seen them in the context of her other work, he was prepared to help her use them constructively.

On the whole he found that the usefulness of Alice's paintings did not stem from their revealing anything about her that was strikingly new to him; seeing slides of the paintings did, however, enrich and clarify what she had already told him. Further, her behavior showed that her own study of the slides powerfully reinforced insights gained in psychotherapy and helped her make the most of them.

Conclusion

Slides, we find, can be used as an effective therapeutic tool, not merely as a convenience in showing patients' work to an outside audience. The slow handling of many paintings has a way of isolating each piece of work—both for the patient and for others seeing it—rather than allowing significant patterns to become apparent; themes cannot manifest themselves so quickly and so clearly. Slides, on the other hand, serve to summarize the course of therapy, making it possible for the gestalt to emerge.

Work transposed into projected slides is one step away from the originals.

Because it is thus more distant, it demands objective appraisal; because it is greatly magnified, it demands attention.

Seeing and discussing slides at sensitively selected points in treatment can have great impact. The work of the patient's own hands, transmuted into such a different medium, most tellingly describes him to himself. Psychotherapy and art therapy have prepared him for this confrontation, which often appears to shorten the course of treatment. With the shock of self-recognition comes insight.

This process can help set the patient free to move. His new sense of himself is confirmed by his unequivocally presented visual work. The insights he has gained help him relate thematic constellations to problems that stand in the way of change and integration.

Art Therapy in the Psychotherapy of a Mother and Her Son

Mildred Lachman, Elizabeth Cohn Stuntz, and Norman Jones

A therapy system in which parent and child are treated separately is likely to generate certain problems. Child and parent often worry about the other's therapist. This may be due to fantasies constructed around pathological relationships in their past lives or it may stem from justified doubts about the therapist's competence or about his or her way of exercising power.

In the case we present here, the therapists treating parent and child were uncomfortable about the compartmentalized therapeutic relationships and together searched for a solution. Through a new way of looking at this therapeutic endeavor—as a system involving not only both patients but also both therapists—they were able to resolve some of their difficulty.

Ms. Stuntz, a psychiatric social worker doing therapy with a young child, and Mr. Jones, a psychologist working with the child's mother, called in an art therapist, Ms. Lachman, to conduct two art sessions during a seven-month treatment period. Our initial goals were to further our diagnostic understanding of the patients, to see how mother and child behaved toward each other, and to deal directly with some of the cross-therapeutic issues by actively involving the two therapists.

Background of the Case

Gregory, a seven-and-a-half-year-old boy, was referred to our child-focused outpatient clinic because, it was reported, he was behaving at a four- or five-year-old level, had learning difficulties, periodically withdrew into a trancelike state, and, until just before the evaluation, had been soiling his pants. Gregory's mother reported that he was made a ward of the court at age two, when she and her husband separated, and was placed in a foster home where he stayed until he was six years old. At the time of the referral he was living with his mother (who had not remarried) and a younger sister fathered by a man other than Gregory's father.

At the clinic, Gregory was found to be mentally retarded and quite depressed. He was very angry, suffered from unmet dependency needs, and did not know what to do with his own aggression. He also had poor powers of concentration and was hyperactive and restless.

In once-a-week individual therapy with Ms. Stuntz, Gregory immediately sought to define his boundaries, to determine whom he could rely on, to discover how much aggression he could safely show and what actions would make someone leave him. The permanence of object relationships seemed paramount to Gregory. He struggled to define the concept of father and to figure out what this concept had to do with the men his mother was seeing. There was very keen rivalry with his younger sister, and here again Gregory was uncertain how honestly he could show his feelings about her without negative consequences. Fear of fire, and the destruction of a house by fire or flood were other themes that Gregory brought up from time to time.

The mother's once-a-week therapy with Mr. Jones focused almost exclusively on Gregory's problems. She rarely discussed her relationships to any other people and, to our surprise, didn't ask what was happening in Gregory's therapy.

After two months both therapists began to wonder how this mother and her son actually got along with each other. Ms. Stuntz wanted to have a clear view of their relationship to further her understanding of Gregory. She also felt that the mother should be using her own counseling to make her child's therapy more effective. Mr. Jones felt that since the mother seemed so preoccupied with Gregory she must have many questions about what was happening between him and this other woman, Ms. Stuntz, who played with him and whom he obviously liked very much. Mr. Jones suggested a joint art therapy session where an art therapist who stood outside of the case would meet with all four members of this therapeutic group. Such a neutral person, he thought, could provide an appropriate structure and establish a non-threatening atmosphere for such a meeting.

Mr. Jones and Ms. Stuntz met very briefly with Ms. Lachman before the art session to give her a brief summary of the diagnostic information and a synopsis of the main features of the case that had emerged in the two months of therapy. They asked Ms. Lachman to focus on the relationship between mother and child as well as the patients' reactions to the two main therapists.

First Art Session

The session was scheduled to last one hour. The room had been prepared with two easels, white drawing paper eighteen inches by twenty-four inches, two boxes of assorted pastels, and two black felt-tipped pens. Gregory and his mother came in with the two therapists. Gregory clung to his mother in a jittery manner, while she was shy and inarticulate. Ms.

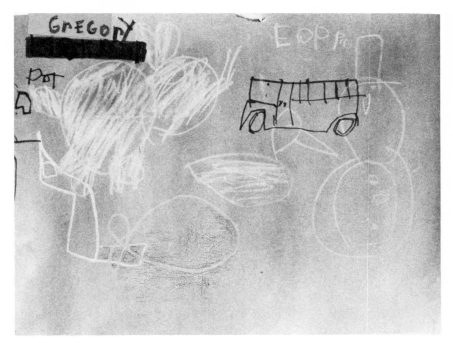

Figure 1

Lachman showed them what she had prepared for the session, explaining very briefly that she had been asked by Ms. Stuntz and Mr. Jones to help them. She said she was an art therapist and that she thought they might enjoy making some pictures and might also find it useful. She suggested that they each make a picture of whatever they liked.

While Gregory began right away using chalk to make animals and then switched to a felt-tipped pen to make a car, his mother found it difficult to get started. Gregory, observing this, went to her and began whispering suggestions. He suggested she make a snowman and then, when she had done so, returned to his own picture and made one himself. Gregory moved back and forth as he suggested ideas to his mother and then copied what she had drawn. The task seemed too unstructured for mother to feel comfortable with it, and she relied a great deal on Gregory's help and advice.

In Gregory's first picture (Figure 1) the car, the snowman, and a number of other images—a fish, some animals, a "shoe"—are loosely arranged in space. They are floating, not tied down by any indication of ground; some are drawn right over others; and they have no clear connection with each other.

While mother slowly proceeded to finish her first picture, *Snowman* (Figure 2), Gregory made three more pictures, each a comment on one of the elements in her picture. He did this silently, quickly, as if he had something important to say and wanted to say it.

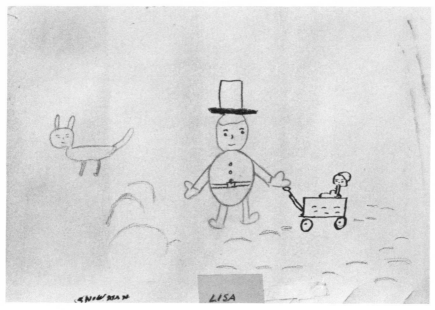

Figure 2

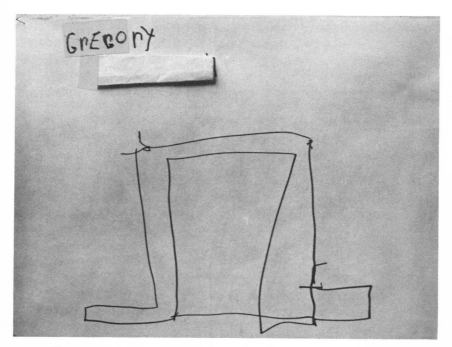

Figure 3

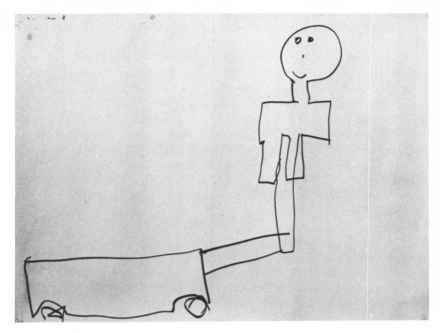

Figure 4

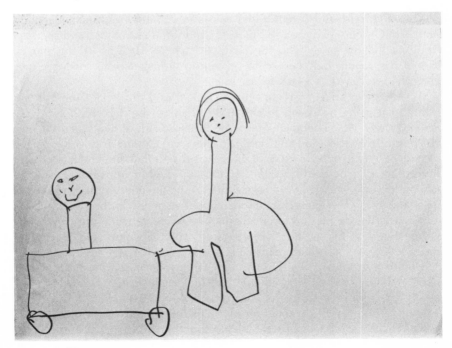

Figure 5

When mother finished her picture she sat down, and we all began to talk about the pictures. Gregory was agitated, alternately curling up on his mother's lap, whispering to her, and moving about the room restlessly, examining the toys on the shelves. When Ms. Lachman stopped him from playing with the toys, Gregory either hid behind one of the boards on the easels or again curled up beside his mother.

He identified the hat in his second picture (Figure 3) and then went on to explain that the boy in the next picture (Figure 4) was pulling the wagon. About Figure 5, he said the boy was inside the wagon. Ms. Lachman wondered whether the boy in Figure 5 was happy to be in the wagon and to have someone else pull him, like the boy in the mother's picture (Figure 2). Gregory said he wanted to pull the wagon himself, and this led to a discussion about being grown-up and doing things oneself and about deciding what one wants to do oneself.

Ms. Lachman then asked Gregory and his mother each to do a picture about "mothers and children." Mother titled her drawing, Figure 6, *Kids at Play*. Done in black ink, it shows a house, a mother, and several children playing. Gregory suggested that she sign this "Mom" rather than "Lisa," her first name, which she had used on her first picture.

Gregory drew his next picture, Figure 7, quickly and impulsively. He began to squeeze his legs together as if he needed to urinate, and kept this up until he began the next task.

When Figures 6 and 7 were under discussion, mother said she had made a picture of Gregory playing with his sister and some playmates, and she kept prodding him to guess who the characters were. He was jittery, moved around the room, and seemed to be more interested in his own picture, which he identified as a jack-in-the-box.

Ms. Lachman said to Gregory that it looked as if the jack-in-the-box was hiding, just as he had been hiding earlier behind the drawing boards. He listened shyly. Ms. Lachman wondered if he did things like that a lot, like whispering so we couldn't hear him, or maybe slipping inside the wagon instead of going outside to pull it. She sensed that he understood her implication that he could decide for himself whether he would "wear the hat" or "pull the wagon." As a logical next step, she offered him a chance to make a decision by suggesting that he choose someone in the room to work at the easel beside his and to make a picture while he made one. He began whispering with his mother, seemingly to ask permission. Finally mother said, "*You* say it," at which point he chose Mr. Jones. They each went to an easel, and Mr. Jones asked Gregory what he would like to make. Gregory said, "A house." They worked side by side, each on his own house, not talking to each other until after the pictures were finished.

Gregory said very little about his house picture, Figure 8. Note that again he had chosen an element from one of his mother's former pictures (Figure 6). Like her, he also added a smaller structure to the main house.

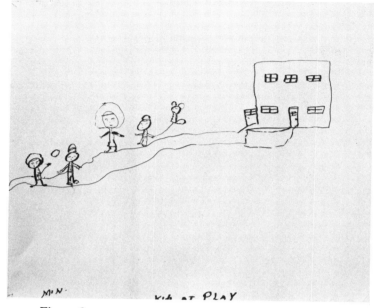

Figure 6

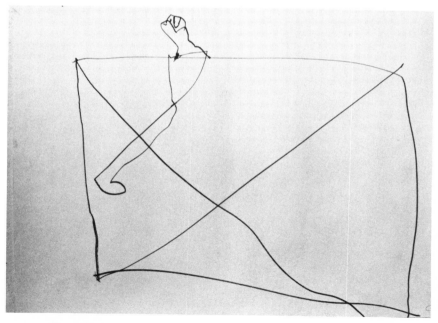

Figure 7

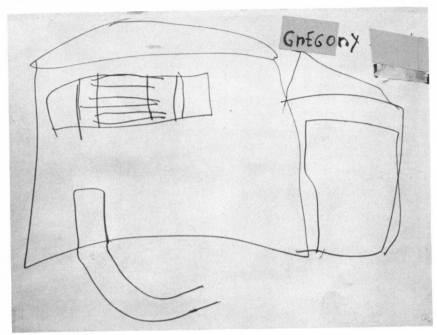

Figure 8

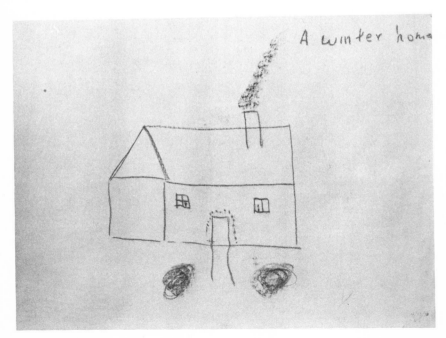

Figure 9

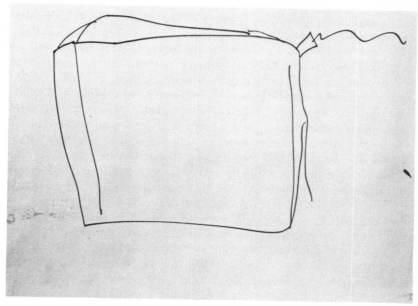

Figure 10

Mr. Jones titled his picture, Figure 9, *A Winter Home*. He explained to Gregory that it was winter in his picture, the candles were burning in the windows, the Christmas lights were decorating the door, and smoke was coming out of the chimney. He said also that the smoke meant there were people inside.

After Mr. Jones had talked about his own picture, Gregory got another piece of paper and, without saying a word, drew Figure 10, the bare outline of a house, to which he added a chimney and smoke; both had been missing from his last picture.

At this point, Gregory seemed much more relaxed and outgoing, apparently very eager to continue his conversation with Mr. Jones. Gregory spoke with normal loudness and did not pay a great deal of attention to his mother or act as if he had to urinate. Mr. Jones pointed out that Gregory had copied the chimney and smoke from his picture and said that he guessed Gregory thought it was a good idea to have it warm inside the house.

Discussion of First Art Session

Throughout most of the session, Gregory showed great dependency on his mother, wanting to hide behind her from encounters with others, whispering to her, squeezing in beside her on the chair, directing most of his remarks to her as if he needed her to do the talking for him. The mother, at the same time, seemed to need Gregory to suggest ideas for her pictures, asking for and taking his advice. Gregory picked up elements in his mother's pictures on which he commented pictorially. These had to do with authority (the hat) and who has it, and dependency (who pulls the wagon and who rides in it). There seemed to be a symbiotic relationship between the two, each dependent on the other. Gregory was asking himself, in effect, "Am I the father or can I be the little boy?" The mother, meanwhile, was shifting back and forth between treating him as adult and child. Gregory's hiding and the ambiguous nature of his jack-in-the-box also seemed to bear out his preoccupation with the uncertainties of authority and dependency. It was during the discussion of the wagon pictures that Gregory began to show concern with his genital area by squeezing his legs together as if he had to go to the bathroom. This would suggest that castration fears entered into his uncertainty about the question of male authority.

Following a discussion touching on these issues, Gregory showed a clear interest in developing a relationship with the man in the group, choosing him to work with, making his own decision about what to draw, and behaving in a much more independent way than he had with his mother. He chose to comment pictorially on the chimney and smoke, possibly symbolic of what was missing from his own life—phallic identification and warmth. After the session was over, Ms. Stuntz suggested that the houses he drew with Mr. Jones might also have been Gregory's way of symbolizing a new relationship. Earlier in therapy, she noted, he had used a house to mean a new mother. (Subsequently, when Gregory was transferred to a new therapist, he immediately established the new relationship by building a house.)

Ms. Stuntz and Mr. Jones were relatively passive during this session, entering into the discussion from time to time but leaving most of the initiatives and interpretations to Ms. Lachman. It was she who told Gregory what he was and was not permitted to do. This made for a situation in which the authority was clearly vested in one person, avoiding ambiguities and freeing the child to examine questions of authority more openly. Neither mother nor Ms. Stuntz had to exercise the usual maternal function of setting limits. Also, through a friendly exchange with Mr. Jones, Gregory could begin to consider the qualities and strengths of male authority and the meaning of his own maleness as well.

Between the Two Art Sessions

As a consequence of the joint art therapy session, Gregory learned that art was a way to get his concerns understood, and in the next four months he used pictures much more extensively. The themes of the art therapy session were picked up and worked through in his sessions alone with Ms. Stuntz—particularly the theme of his ambivalence concerning whether he wanted to be a big boy or a baby. He began to experiment, placing himself in both of these roles and trying to determine what he might lose or gain in each. He did, however, regress somewhat, needing much reassurance that neither mother nor sister would be allowed to invade the therapy room.

After a while, Gregory began to be much more openly concerned about men: how they acted, how he would act as a big boy, and how men affected him. For a time the man in whose office he and Ms. Stuntz met became an absent father and a representative of a man's unknown qualities. Not only was Gregory concerned with what this man was like—which things in the room belonged to him? what would he do if Gregory did so and so?—but he also developed a rich fantasy about Ms. Stuntz's relationship with this man. He apparently feared that the mysterious man might be able to disrupt the sessions in some way. Gregory seemed to be working out some of the problems which had been brought to the surface by Mr. Jones's presence in the joint session.

Ms. Stuntz began to work more directly with Gregory on the need to distinguish her from a mother. She also wanted to evaluate his progress in his relationship with his mother. In addition, she thought that some of his questions about maleness and his own maturity might be answered if he could deal further with his feelings about a man in his mother's life. Another contact with Mr. Jones might be helpful at this juncture.

The mother, meanwhile, was beginning to ask some direct questions about what was happening in Gregory's therapy. Therefore, Ms. Stuntz and Mr. Jones requested another joint art session, saying that they wanted to take part more actively this time.

Ms. Stuntz paved the way for the session during a home visit. In the home she could work with child and mother in a more natural setting, but it is likely that this visit brought out some of the mother's fears that Ms. Stuntz might be taking over her role as the foster mother had done. Gregory, too, may have had some negative feelings about the upcoming art session, but Ms. Stuntz had no chance to discuss his apprehensions with him.

Second Art Session

This session, like the first one, lasted an hour. Gregory was noticeably less jittery upon entering the art room the second time, looking Ms. Lachman in the eye and greeting her directly. Four easels were in readiness. After alluding briefly to the former session, Ms. Lachman said that Ms. Stuntz and Mr. Jones had asked her to see if they could all work together this time. She asked each to do a "together" picture. Gregory did two untitled pictures, Figures 11 and 12; mother's picture (also untitled) is shown in Figure 13; Mr. Jones named his picture, Figure 14, *The Egg Hunt*; and Ms. Stuntz labeled hers, Figure 15, *Gregory and Mom Out for a Walk*.

Gregory's first picture, of a truck towing a car (Figure 11), shows marked developmental progress compared to the pictures he had done four months

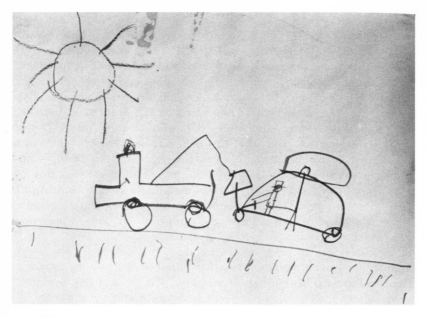

Figure 11

earlier. Here we see a baseline and a clear indication of the ground, providing a framework for spatial organization of the pictured world. The pictorial elements are clearly related to each other so that we can understand Gregory's intentions. The first picture he made in the earlier drawing session (Figure 1), with its floating, unrelated images, like his behavior at the time, resembled what is to be expected from a child of four or five, while Figure 11 is age-appropriate. It seems likely that this change reflects maturation due at least in part to his therapy. In addition, we see that a large sun is a very important feature of the picture. The sun is generally associated with father, and we surmise that Gregory is beginning to include father elements in his world, and that this supports him and helps him to organize his world.

Gregory's next picture, Figure 12, includes a house, two airplanes, a car, and two children. Again, the elements are organized in space, there is considerable detail, the house has a chimney and smoke, and the two children are playing together (jumping rope?). This may suggest that he has come to accept his sister in what is now a more complete, warmer home with elements of masculine power (car, airplanes) around it.

We talked about Gregory's pictures first, with Ms. Lachman bringing up the idea of being helped (in connection with his picture of the tow truck). She talked about asking people for help and how we all have to do that from time to time—like asking for the tow truck to help the car. Gregory suggested that fire engines put out fires. Ms. Lachman said that another kind

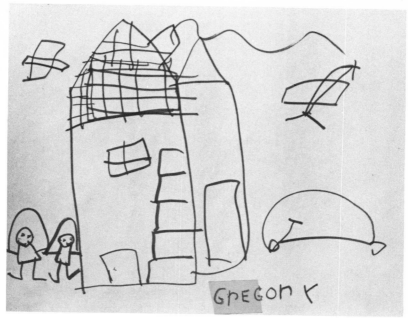

Figure 12

of helping was the way Ms. Stuntz helped him. About his second picture, Ms. Lachman merely remarked that smoke was coming out of the chimney this time.

Gregory talked rather easily about his two pictures. He spoke loudly and clearly and did not turn to his mother for help or approval. However, as his mother and then Mr. Jones began to talk about their pictures, he became restless and wanted to go back and draw some more. Ms. Lachman did not permit him to do this, and Gregory then sat quietly, paying attention to the discussion.

In discussing Figure 13, mother said simply that it had to do with herself, Gregory, and two kids from the neighborhood. She identified herself as the figure on the right. She tried to tease out of Gregory the names of the other two kids.

The figure on the extreme left is done with pink lines; the self-figure (on the right) and also the table are done with red lines. The two center figures are very lightly drawn in black, with faint pressure and feathery strokes. In studying this picture later, we felt that beyond her conscious intention it may well have portrayed the actual group of four working together. Through the choice of color and by means of varied line pressure, the mother seemed to be making a statement about the figures. We also noted the heavily scribbled-over table, with particular emphasis given to the section directly under the pink figure on the left. Thus, if our surmise is correct, she portrays herself as facing a person of another color—and indeed she is white and Mr.

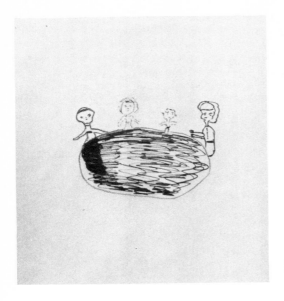

Figure 13

Jones is black. It seems that she makes herself and Mr. Jones the two most important people, drawing them with firm lines, while the two figures in between (Gregory and Ms. Stuntz) are faintly delineated, with the smallest figure (Gregory) placed next to herself. This picture may represent how she was viewing relations among the four principals at this joint session, the scribbling of the table expressing the tension she was feeling about this group's working together and her particularly strong concern about Mr. Jones.

Figure 14

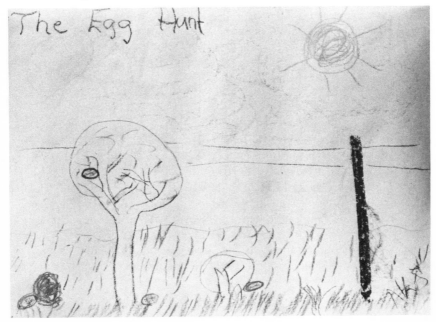

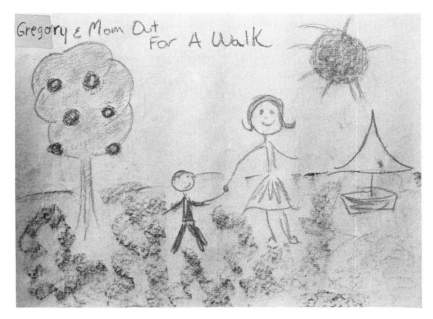

Gregory & Mom Out For A Walk

Figure 15

Mr. Jones said Figure 14 represented an egg hunt in which everybody's eggs are hidden in different places and have to be found. He said the egg in the tree represented Gregory, "the focus of us all." Mother thought that the egg in the tree was Mr. Jones, presumably the focus of *her* interest.

When it came time for discussion of Ms. Stuntz's picture (Figure 15), she asked Gregory to read the title. He read, "Gregory and Miss Stuntz Out for a Walk." Mother told him he had made a mistake and asked him to read it again. He repeated what he had said. Mother grew agitated and angrily insisted that he read it again. He grew restless and uncomfortable but finally read correctly, "Gregory and Mom Out for a Walk." Mother remarked later, "I didn't know that Gregory and Miss Stuntz went out for walks."

The atmosphere was very tense. At this point Mr. Jones suggested that all four do a joint picture and volunteered to leave the room to get a big piece of paper. Ms. Lachman suggested that Gregory go with him to the supply closet. She then spoke directly to the mother in the presence of Ms. Stuntz, saying that it must have felt unpleasant to have Gregory make the mistake about the title. She also suggested that it must feel funny that Gregory gets help from someone else who may seem like a mother to him at times. Mother agreed. This led to talk of how we all get help from others and sometimes we feel close to the people who help us, just as Gregory must sometimes feel that Ms. Stuntz seems close like a mother even though she does different things with him.

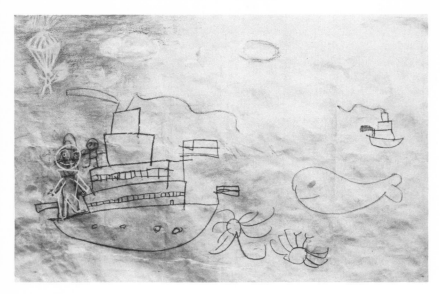

Figure 16

When Mr. Jones and Gregory returned, all four began working jointly on a large piece of paper (Figure 16). Everybody asked Gregory to make decisions and suggestions, and all the adults followed his directions, adding ideas of their own to develop his chosen themes. The mother always waited for Gregory's directions. He drew a boat; others added water, sky, fish, etc. Mr. Jones drew a parachuting man, asking Gregory whether or not the man was coming down to help. Gregory wasn't sure, but added fire around him.

Interest became focused on the boat, as Gregory made a man with black chalk and then tried to erase him (see Figure 17, the small figure to the right of the larger figure). He told Ms. Stuntz he found this man "scary," then added a larger man on the left (note the concentration on the phallic hat, which he redrew several times). He spoke to the other three (the art therapist was passive and quiet at this point) about this larger man who was also scary, and, finally, using blue chalk, he covered the figure over with still another man (see light lines superimposed over larger figure). When Ms. Stuntz asked him if the blue man was scary like the black man, Gregory said yes, he was.

When everyone sat down to discuss the group picture, Ms. Lachman spoke to Gregory about all the help he had gotten in making it. She asked who had helped him. He looked around but said nothing. Ms. Lachman said, "You got help from one white woman, one black man, and your mother." There was a long silence as all present seemed to be acknowledging identification of the scary "black" man of the picture with Mr. Jones. This was not spelled out further and the session ended shortly afterward.

Discussion of Second Art Session

The mother's unexpressed feelings of rivalry with the child's therapist were opened up unexpectedly through Gregory's misreading of a picture's title. The mother was directly confronted with his closeness to Ms. Stuntz. The art therapist here was able to verbalize the parent's feelings, which the child's therapist found herself unable to do. Ms. Stuntz was trying to assure the mother that she did not want to take over her role, but she was caught in feelings of guilt about her own countertransference. She was also inhibited because of her obligation to keep certain matters confidential. She hesitated to talk to the mother directly about her own relationship with the child, since in all therapeutic relationships there is a promise that the relationship will be a private one.

It was also possible, through the drama that took place around Ms. Stuntz's picture, for the child himself to become more openly aware that he was confusing Ms. Stuntz with mother and that his mother was jealous of Ms. Stuntz.

The understanding that therapy is essentially a helping relationship was clarified for both child and parent. Gregory's pictures concerned with help may have been a statement that he feels torn about becoming a big boy. It is something he yearns for, yet it is very threatening and, instead of mixed messages from mother, he needs some help in sorting out his feelings.

Figure 17

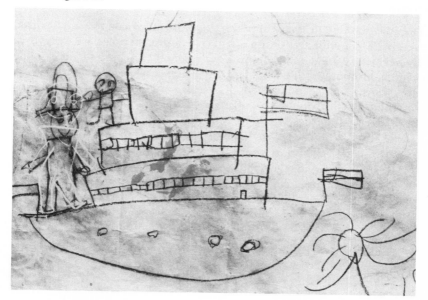

In the previous art session, Gregory had chosen Mr. Jones to work with and had clearly expressed his overriding concern about male authority and male identification. He had, at that time, experienced some of the positive aspects of a relationship with a man. In the second session, however, through his drawings he revealed his fears and focused on Mr. Jones as one of those mysterious men who had dealings with his mother—and his mother was indeed interested in Mr. Jones. In the joint picture, Gregory conveyed feelings about being afraid of men—in particular, of black men.

Mr. Jones found it difficult to deal with the child directly. He was not prepared for the intensity of Gregory's negative feelings toward him. Perhaps his uneasiness was compounded because Gregory's symbolic reference to him was so meagerly concealed and so specific with regard to race. It would have been difficult for Mr. Jones to make clarifying statements to the child at that moment since he was having a very strong reaction to Gregory's hitherto unrecognized hostility. The art therapist, as a detached participant, could make the racial interpretation in terms of the symbolism of the picture. That is, instead of saying "You must find Mr. Jones scary," she could say simply that the helping people in the group included a black man, making a connection which the child understood and could work through later with Ms. Stuntz. This session also alerted the mother to the necessity of dealing with her child's worries about the men she sees and how these men might be related to him—Are they his father? Are they like his father?

General Discussion

Let us now examine the ways in which this work enhanced the usual pattern of therapy. Most often transference and countertransference are worked out solely between patient and therapist. For example, Gregory's feelings about the men in his mother's life would usually be dealt with in sessions with Ms. Stuntz. The mother's feelings about Gregory's having a special relationship with another woman would be worked out with Mr. Jones. These concerns would come up after a time and be talked about or played out.

In this case, however, each therapist was able to help the other deal constructively with the transference. Instead of Gregory's working with Ms. Stuntz to face his feelings about the men in his mother's life, he worked directly with Mr. Jones, an actual man who was actually in his mother's life. The mother was also able to confront her jealousy of Ms. Stuntz directly during the art session instead of merely talking about it to her therapist. Thus, the anxious fantasies were changed into direct interaction, accelerating for both mother and child the process of coming to terms with their fears. As the "other" therapist became a real person, each patient's focus of anxiety changed somewhat, paving the way for further dissipation of unrealistic fears and recognition of real-life situations that sparked the fantasies.

Similarly, countertransference was dealt with differently here. Normally, it would be handled in supervision, where the therapist would work toward self-awareness. In the art therapy sessions, countertransference was confronted directly. Art allowed the therapists to take an active part in the session, so that they could address the problem of their countertransference then and there. Pictures by the two therapists which illuminated their countertransference will shortly be analyzed in detail.

Working on problems of transference and countertransference as publicly as this does hold risks. As we have seen, Gregory's fears were aroused, fears that his increasingly trusting relationship with his therapist might be invaded. Each case must be considered carefully so that such maneuvers are undertaken only when *both* patients are ready for them. In this instance we feel that the benefits derived from the two collaborative encounters justified the risks and outweighed the minor difficulties that were brought to the fore.

The usual pattern of therapy was further expanded by the introduction of a third therapist, previously not active in the case. Unlike the conventional behind-the-scenes supervisor or consultant,[1] the third therapist introduced a new medium, art, with which the key therapists and their patients worked together. This new person was included because of her expertise in a special modality. She was not seen as supervisory or judgmental; her authority derived from the modality itself. Since definition of roles and of boundaries of authority were very important in this case, the clarity of the art therapist's position was important. During the hour in art therapy, doubt about who had the power was eliminated for Gregory and his mother, thus freeing them to confront the authority problems they had with each other.

The use of art in joint diagnostic and therapeutic sessions has been developed by Kwiatkowska in her pioneering work with families.[2] She has demonstrated that art facilitates interaction and speeds the development of insight. It is often less threatening than the use of words. Furthermore, it provides parent and child with a more equal means of expression (the child is

1. See Paul L. Adams, "The Pediatric Consultation," in *Handbook of Psychiatric Consultation* (edited by J. Schwab), New York, Appleton-Century-Crofts, 1968, pp. 107–23; G. Caplan, *Concepts of Mental Health and Consultation*, Washington, D.C., U.S. Children's Bureau, 1959; Alberta B. Szalita, "Psychotherapy and Family Interviews," in *The World Biennial of Psychiatry and Psychotherapy*, Vol. 1 (edited by S. Arieti), New York, Basic Books, 1970, pp. 312–35; Jerome V. Treusch and Martin Grotjahn, "Psychiatric Family Consultations," *Annals of Internal Medicine*, Vol. 66, No. 2, 1967, pp. 295–300; Gertrude L. Wyatt, "Illustration of the Therapeutic Process," in *Language Learning and Communication Disorders in Children*, New York, Free Press, 1969, pp. 139–72.

2. Hanna Y. Kwiatkowska, "Family Art Therapy: Experiments with a New Technique," *Bulletin of Art Therapy*, Vol. 1, No. 3, 1962, pp. 3–15; *idem*, "The Use of Families' Art Productions for Psychiatric Evaluation," *Bulletin of Art Therapy*, Vol. 6, No. 2, 1967, pp. 52–69.

usually at a disadvantage with words), and it saves time since a great deal can be accomplished rather quickly (each of our two sessions lasted only an hour). Similar benefits have been reported by Rubin[3] and Landgarten[4] in their work with parents and children drawing and painting together, and by Wadeson[5] in her work with couples.

The special usefulness of art stems in part from the nature of visual symbols, which often have a richer cluster of meanings than do words; words tend to be more specific and therefore more limited. Moreover, by expressing emotional concepts in visual symbols, the patient can choose how much uncovering he is ready for. When Gregory drew the hat and the wagon (Figures 3, 4, and 5) and the art therapist, having been offered these symbolic messages, reflected back to him in words that part of their meaning which he might be ready to look at—i.e., worries about authority and dependency—Gregory chose to understand what "wearing the hat" and "pulling the wagon" really meant. He acted on this knowledge by deciding by himself to work with Mr. Jones. Had Gregory not been ready to face the issue of dependency versus self-assertion, he would have failed to see the symbolism of his hat and wagon and failed subsequently to make a decision by himself.

When emotional concepts are vaguely suggested in the assignment of an art task, the participants then express through visual symbols the interpretation they are most concerned with. As an example, let us look at one of the tasks of the second session. The art therapist asked the four participants to do a "together" picture. This ambiguous assignment was handled differently by each participant. Each focused on the aspect of the relationships among them that he or she was seeking to explore. Let us see how each one responded.

Gregory did a picture (Figure 11) about helping and being helped—tow truck and car. For him, help was the essential element of this "together" experience. The art therapist verbalized this for him.

It appeared to us that mother's picture (Figure 13) focused on her confrontation with the man of another color. This was not interpreted to her, but there was much evidence that her relationship with Mr. Jones was uppermost in her mind. She placed her faintly delineated child next to her, but her jealousy of his relationship with Ms. Stuntz did not come to the fore at this time.

Mr. Jones focused in Figure 14 on the mysterious, hidden, searching

3. Judith Rubin, "Mother–Child Art Sessions: I. Treatment in the Clinic" and "Mother–Child Art Sessions: II. Education in the Community," *American Journal of Art Therapy*, Vol. 13, 1974, pp. 165–81 and 219–27.
   4. Helen Landgarten, "Group Art Therapy for Mothers and Daughters," *American Journal of Art Therapy*, Vol. 13, 1975. pp. 31–35.
   5. Harriet Wadeson, "Art Techniques Used in Conjoint Marital Therapy," *American Journal of Art Therapy*, Vol. 12, 1973, pp. 147–64.

aspect of the therapeutic relationship, the group's concentration on Gregory, and the assertion of masculine presence and authority. Indeed, he was the one grown man in the room and it was Gregory's relationship with him that he wanted to explore. The countertransference revealed here centered around Gregory, but in retrospect Mr. Jones recognized that the prominent dark-brown telegraph pole may have reflected his wish to be viewed positively as a black masculine presence not only by Gregory but also by the group as a whole.

Ms. Stuntz's picture, Figure 15, seemed to focus on the relationship between the mother and her child, but it also had something to do with herself. She wanted to get across her recognition of the special relationship between Gregory and his mother, but an aspect of countertransference— Ms. Stuntz's competitive feelings toward mother—was also revealed. Ms. Stuntz came to recognize her own part in arousing the mother's fears that Ms. Stuntz was going to take over her role.

Each of the four participants extracted from the word *together* what he or she needed in order to make a picture that reflected his own most pressing concern.

The final way in which our joint sessions enhanced individual therapy was to provide material that could be explored and dealt with in subsequent individual sessions. Gregory, having begun, through drawing the hat and the wagon, to encounter his problem with authority and dependence, continued to work on it with Ms. Stuntz. These concerns became clearer to him after the initial symbolic opening up. He was also able to use art increasingly in his individual sessions.

The mother, somewhat uncomfortable at first about using art and unable to focus on her own productions and what they might mean, did see this as an opportunity to try to understand Gregory better. She paid careful attention to his behavior in the joint sessions and to the art therapist's interpretations of his drawings. The sessions, therefore, provided her with some clues to Gregory's major areas of concern which he had not talked about to her. In addition, the therapists' responses to Gregory provided a model she might find useful in her future dealings with him.

In conclusion, we feel that occasional joint art therapy sessions to supplement individual counseling can be an effective way to further the therapeutic progress of mother and child. Combining the skills of an art therapist with those of the therapists working with the two closely interlinked patients can help resolve transference and countertransference problems and can also accelerate the development of insight in subsequent individual sessions.

Rehabilitative Use of Art in a Community Mental Health Center

Saul Lishinsky

The John Thompson Center is the social rehabilitation unit of the Sound View Throggs Neck Community Mental Health Center, Bronx, New York. The art program I conduct there is based on my conviction that art is a wholesome, socially necessary form of work. I try to imbue the patient with respect for his effort, on whatever level he is able to perform and whether he thinks of it as play or as serious work. As in other forms of work and play, consistency, persistence, and purposeful striving must be nourished. The essential nature of art, however, gives genuine artistic work special pertinence to mental health.

All the arts characteristically employ metaphor, a mental construct made by transforming one image or idea into another. Unlike the representative symbol or the simile, metaphor does not constitute a static relationship but embodies a sense of movement or change. In painting, the sense of movement grows from the push and pull of shapes against one another. This becomes a language of gesture. It is developed as a sophisticated discipline in the highest order of art, but it may be intuitively grasped even in the most primitive attempts to draw and paint, for it is based on the universal experience of one's own bodily movement.

Through such tension of forms in space the visual arts transform representations by setting objects in motion, articulating the emotions with which things are charged. Thus a still life of apples by Cézanne may embody a sense of human drama comparable to that of Michelangelo's *Moses*. By means of a sense of movement and the language of gesture, art creates an amalgam of provocations from external life with projections from within ourselves. How art can thus reveal the very roots of consciousness, can develop and communicate a sense of identity, is a theme too large for the scope of the present article. But that is why I believe that the therapy offered by art work is often a first step toward helping the mental patient rediscover himself and begin to find or recover ways of using work to build self-esteem.

The Art Program

I work with patients whose psychopathology ranges from mild to severe. My approach to art therapy will be illustrated below by discussion of some paintings by selected patients.

I am qualified for this work by experience as a practicing artist and teacher of art. A professional artist, especially if he also has the teacher's feeling for the needs of his students, is aware of the particular problems of artistic expression. He will also convey to the student his own respect for and love of his working materials, and his awareness of the essentially social nature of art, although it may often appear to be a solitary activity. I have therefore insisted as much as possible on decent materials and respectful mounting and exhibition of selected work.

I try to induce people who are largely aimless and unproductive to engage in an activity that is purposeful, absorbing, and expressive of themselves, and I serve as a model and guide on the road to this goal. I do not try to elicit free association or interpretation of symbols, nor do I use art to stimulate talk. Conversation is primarily directed toward promoting the creation of art work.

The finest results of such work are pictures that reflect the full complexity of life with all its contradictions. A particular piece of subject matter (e.g., dark, jagged rocks or barren, broken trees) by itself might be a sign of illness, but if it is linked with contrasting elements in a picture its meaning is transformed, just as the components of any struggle are reshaped when a new equilibrium has been achieved. Thus a good painting creates a fundamental affirmation of human value even if it depicts desolate alienation; we look in the work not merely for evidence of symptoms but rather for the attempt to understand and resolve conflict.

The difference between art and the handicraft usually practiced in occupational therapy will be further clarified by examining the pictures to be discussed below. Look at the wide range of differences among them, reflecting the range of personalities. Works done according to a wholly preconceived procedure tend to be essentially alike, whoever the maker is or whatever his mood. And yet such stereotyped work serves a necessary human purpose: the sharing implied by imitation (being like everyone else or producing according to an approved or desired standard) is as indispensable as the distinction of individuality. The ultimate objective is to achieve the paradoxical union of these contradictory means.

I start by offering some rules and methods of craft, composition, and observation. I encourage their use for a result that is personally significant.

Most of our patients are inexperienced beginners. I often instruct them to start by doodling at random with the art materials at hand, in order to try out ways of creating various textures, shadings, and colors. At the same time this may help the student to discover a rudimentary sense of rhythm and balance. Next, the student is instructed to plan his picture: the relative sizes and positions of whatever is to be drawn. Following this, the particular shapes, shades, and colors are developed. The progression is from roughness and simplification to clarity and detail. The precise way to get a result is not shown; given only a general method, each individual must struggle with the problem, using his own senses and intelligence.

Difficulties often arise: the experimental approach of doodling may be threatening, and the patient may demand some rigid formula. Almost always beginners plunge directly at the exact shape, eschewing the abstraction involved in roughing out. The resulting frustrations due to disproportion and incoherence of form may somehow intuitively be compensated if the student keeps working.

The difficulties must never be taken at face value. I play it by ear and modify my tactics accordingly. With the right mixture of praise and critical comment or suggestion, each person's effort may be enlisted. The ultimate goal is sustained attention and work that will lead to the full development of his independent capabilities.

In the examples that follow, I shall try to explain briefly how these patients became productive and will refer to the affective content of their work mainly in general terms. More specific interpretations or stories will be recounted only where they were spontaneously offered by the painter. Conditions of class work militated against any effort to probe for such responses.

A Self-Disparaging Old Man

Frank L., a man in his seventies, came with only grade-school experience in drawing behind him. Only by giving him the closest attention and constant encouragement could I persuade him to try now. He kept repeating that he was "totally inept in all mechanical work."

His first attempt was extremely schematic: one look at snake plants growing in a box, and he produced in a few minutes a row of short, diamond-shaped spikes about the same height as the representation of the box (Figure 1, top). I asked him to take a second look, to note that the plant blades are much taller than the box, to observe their sinuous twists and changes of width, their varying tilt. I demonstrated by drawing one plant blade (upper left). Then I praised his next attempt (lower left) and he made some corrections as I repeated my earlier criticisms.

The next step was to note how the plant existed within surroundings, to fill the whole page, thus making a picture; in response he drew the boxed plant in the window (Figure 2). He gradually sustained his efforts for longer periods and set to work as soon as he came to class, needing less and less reassurance before beginning.

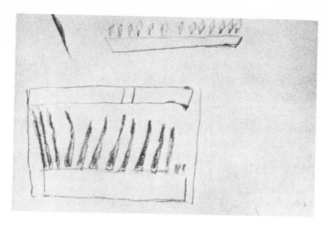

Figure 1

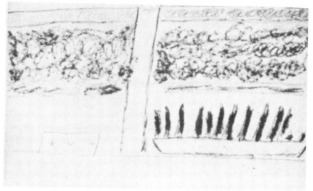

Figure 2

Figure 3

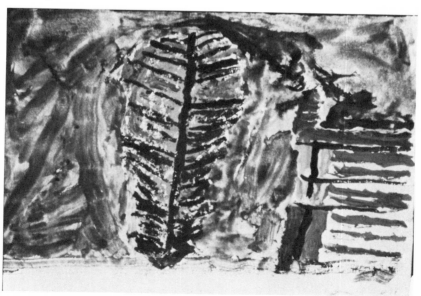

After about two months he had made remarkable progress, as shown in Figure 3 (Plate VIII), a watercolor. Often his pictures feature a single object, at first detached and floating but eventually contained and balanced by background; the effect is stark but this starkness is relieved by the use of color, shading, and subsidiary objects in which the main object is both echoed and opposed. Despite faltering execution, the form is clearly assertive. A primitive, symmetrical schema remains the basis of the way an object is rendered, like the tree in Figure 3 (Plate VIII); but the way the tree leans, its deviations from symmetry, give a sense of life.

I sometimes saw Frank L. take a very intent look at what he was trying to draw. He said to me more than once, "You got me doing things I never did before," and he told me that he was exhausted at the end of the class. I pointed out how worthwhile his efforts were, for although his pictures are primitive and fairly crude, they have vivid, lively qualities. Although he drew admiring comments from other students, he still maintained that he was "totally inept." His willingness to take instruction seemed to rest on a habit of obedience as well as his trust in my authority.

I used the same methods, with variations, in the examples that follow. The effort in each instance is to engage the patient in work, to teach him, and to reinforce his self-confidence and sense of power in accomplishment.

Initial Recalcitrance Gives Way

When I asked Harry D. if he had ever tried any art before, he answered, "Oh, sure," in a hostile, offensive manner. He then flippantly produced, as he had in past hospital experience, a rigid, constricted "free doodle" (Figure 4). I said that it was good for what it was, that the selection and distribution of colors were interesting, but pointed out how little care and thought he had put into it and suggested a more serious attempt. His answer was obscene.

In a later session, when his anger had simmered down, like Frank L. he produced a picture of the snake plants in front of the window (Figure 5). Note the persistence of certain elements that appear in the doodle: the extension of forms from one edge of the picture to the other, the crisscross opposition. The colors are not in absolute opposition, some being softly harmonious, but their arrangement gives the general impression of glaring brightness.

Perhaps without being aware of it, in this effort to describe the objective reality of a boxed plant in a room, he had made a lucid, eloquent statement about his inner life with which we may empathize. The weight of the room against the plant seems overwhelming, and yet the softer colors whisper of longed-for serenity. The schematic doodle, on the other hand, is merely something to hide behind.

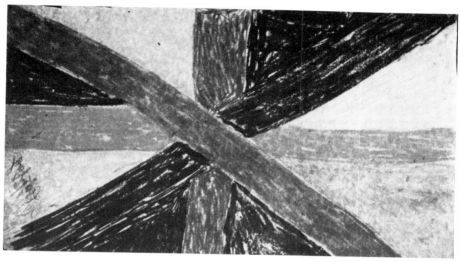

Figure 4

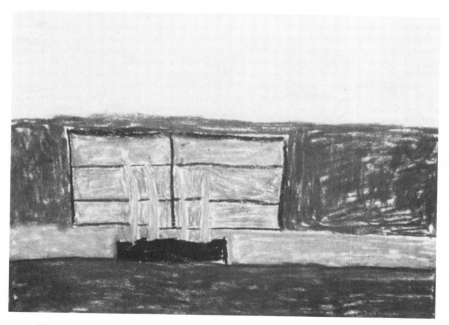

Figure 5

From Verbal Fencing to Art

Max S. had a tendency to fill the whole picture space with sweeping forms. The exuberance of his first try, shown in Figure 6, belies his avowed insecurity which I overcame only with much coaxing and reassurance. He said he knew nothing of art and hadn't drawn since grade school, but he did appreciate music. He focused on the fruit basket, and at the end of the class period, finding leftover space on one side, he added the framing border. He admitted that this first attempt didn't look bad.

While working on his next few pictures, he engaged me in constant argument. I kept trying to convince him that perfect photographic reproduction is not the absolute standard of art, that his own attempts were not beyond the pale, that it was all right to heighten the colors he saw since he disliked their drabness, that there was nothing wrong with his simplified versions of a complicated form he could not yet draw. Since he was dissatisfied with his serious efforts, I urged him to take a break and slop around childishly, just for fun. I told him that if he thought this was beneath him and felt he must strive for perfection, then he would have to cultivate patience and tolerance for step-by-step learning.

These violent arguments and his inner contradictions find expression in sharp contrasts of color and strongly opposed forms (see, for example, Figure

Figure 6

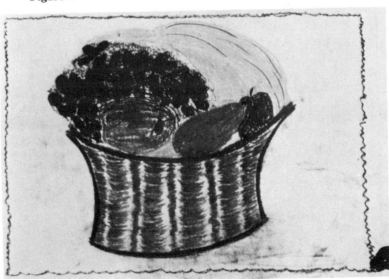

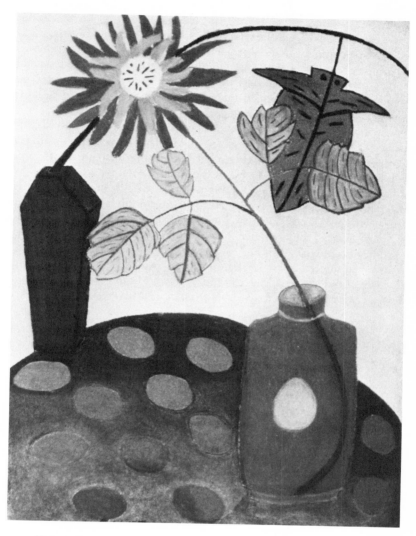

Figure 7

7, Plate IX). But the forms are also strongly tied together by color harmonies, curving arabesques, repeated motifs. These are often carried out with great subtlety.

As he worked slowly and painstakingly for many weekly sessions on this picture of a glass jar with large flowers, he began to talk of the symbolism that came to his mind: the red jar pregnant with a yellow egg-shape is woman; the blue table, earth. I didn't instigate this line of talk but encouraged it when it came up. I did instigate a search for balance in the picture, so he added the black jar at the far edge of the table, transforming the jar into a coffin. A branch projecting from this across the top has a dead leaf dangling from its end; this he modified slightly to suggest a hanged man. (The leaves outside our window had turned brown and fallen since he had begun his picture.) This hanged-man-dead-leaf doesn't look so dead; it seems to swing vigorously, like an animated sword of Damocles.

When somebody wanted to buy this particular pastel, Max told him that he had put so much of himself into the picture that he would not sell it "even for a hundred dollars"; he would give it for nothing, instead. I intervened at this point because I wanted to save the picture for this article.

I have only begun to suggest this picture's wealth of expression. In his subsequent work Max amply proved his considerable ability to learn and to grapple with problems, but always tortuously and using me as an argumentative prop. I don't believe that his habitual wrangling over a problem is wasted in his art work; it rather contributes to deepening his expression. But he never wanted to understand it that way, always bemoaning his difficulties. I did succeed in getting him to experiment with slopping paint a little, but otherwise he retained his pristine rigidity.

Figure 8

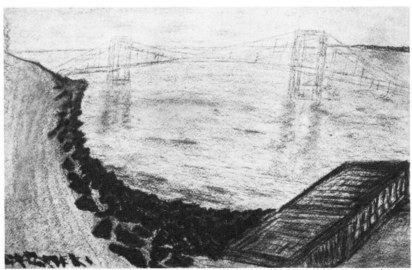

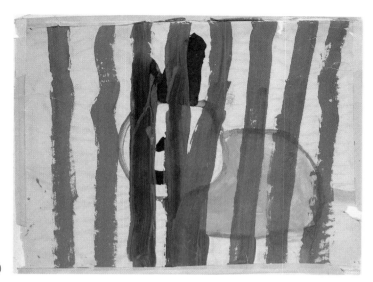

Plate I
(see p. 18)

"Margaret . . . painted strong red bars across the whole paper . . . because 'the lion is dangerous and might hurt people.'"

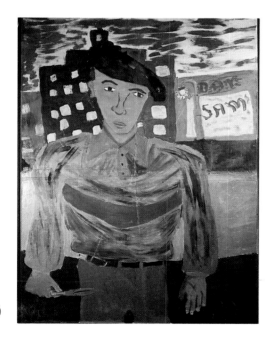

Plate II
(see p. 22)

". . . dominating the scene in narcissistic pride, yet shut in by the city, weak . . . but dangerous to himself and others."

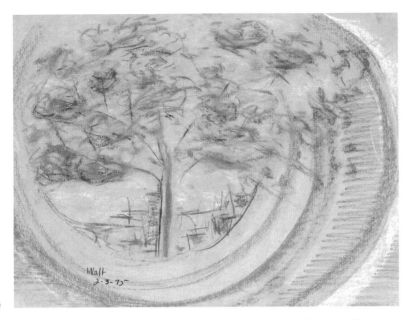

Plate III
(see p. 124)

"Walter . . . spoke at some length about the role of the leaders and his desire for their protection."

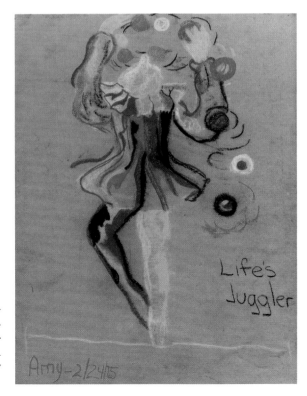

Plate IV
(see p. 126)

"Amy . . . was representing a situation of some precariousness. The juggler is balanced on a thin, wavering horizontal line. . . ."

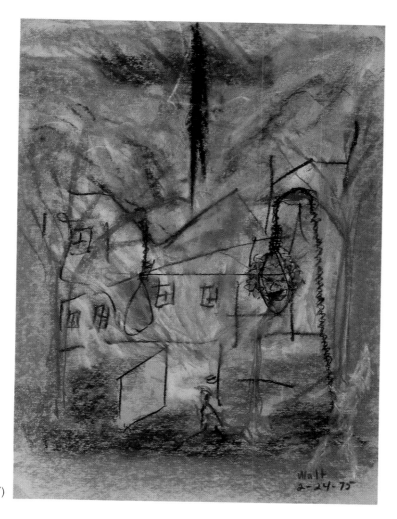

Plate V
(see p. 127)

"I lived with the constant fear that I would one day be . . . lynched.

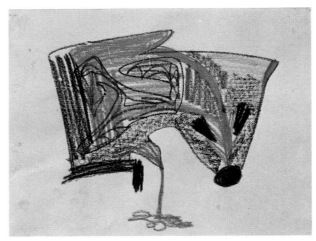

Plate VI
(see p. 145)

"A year later she said, 'It's functioning, peeing . . . it could be me.'"

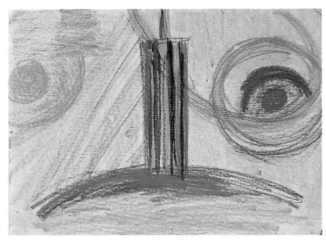

Plate VII
(see p. 149)

"I stepped *through* a door . . . I pulled it shut behind me and am in a world of hills."

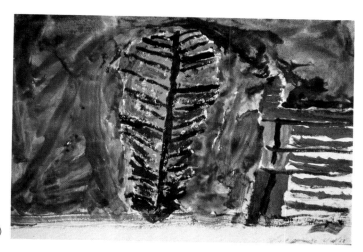

Plate VIII
(see p. 178)

"'You got me doing things I never did before.'"

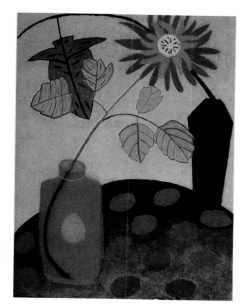

Plate IX
(see p. 180)

"The red jar pregnant
with a yellow egg shape
is woman; the blue table,
earth."

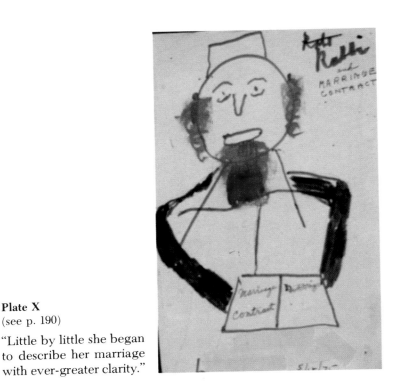

Plate X
(see p. 190)

"Little by little she began to describe her marriage with ever-greater clarity."

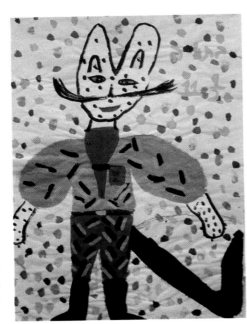

Plate XI
(see p. 221)

"Batja . . . has transformed the frightful tiger-cat into the most helpful fairytale animal—one who does away with all evil. . . ."

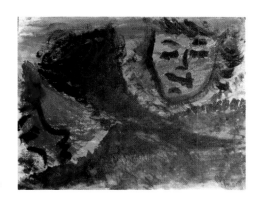

Plate XII
(see p. 275)

"Two versions of her own face are separated by a whirling black cyclone that she designated as 'destruction.'"

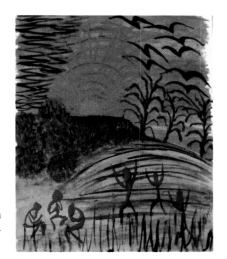

Plate XIII
(see p. 277)

"A lurid hymn to life, with flowers, trees, and gigantic birds. . . ."

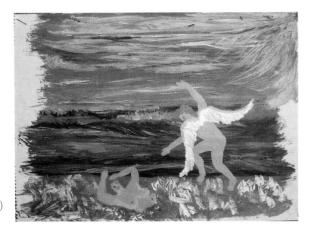

Plate XIV
(see p. 277)

". . . a girl half buried in the sand who is being rescued by an angel. A turbulent sea and sky and a hot Hawaiian sun. . . ."

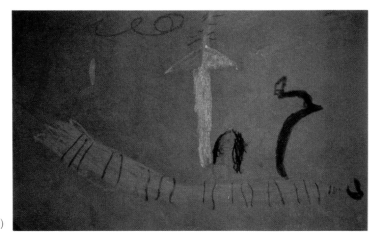

Plate XV
(see p. 286)

"Lucy . . . put in a road connecting her mother's house on the right and her father's skinny apartment house on the left."

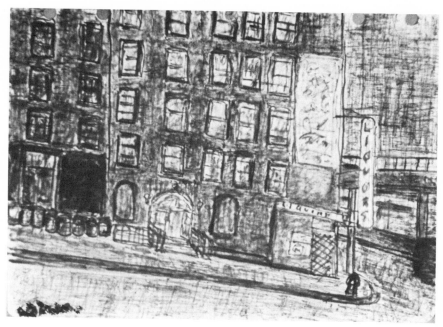

Figure 9

A Growing Interest

Louis B. is in his forties, is highly educated, and has a wide, sophisticated knowledge of art and literature. He has a lifelong history of dependency and illness.

On our first meeting he seemed deeply depressed and self-centered. He wanted attention from me but was self-deprecating and claimed that his poor vision made him unable to draw. Playing it cool, I succeeded in provoking him to start drawing anyway. He said that he had done some drawing and painting in the past, but his work was rather amateurish. From the first, however, he had a clear concept of what he wanted to create in terms of mood and poetic imagery. He responded rapidly to my teaching, and carried out my suggestion that he sketch out-of-doors and bring the results to show me at the Center. He worked up finished drawings from these sketches; Figures 8, 9, 10, and 11 are examples. Many hours of observation and drawing went into each of these richly felt, sustained studies.

He explained his intentions very clearly. Figure 8 represents deep depression. The building in Figure 9 was selected deliberately because of its wretchedness and decay, characteristic, he said, of New York City. He wanted to show a different life in each window. He told with his usual

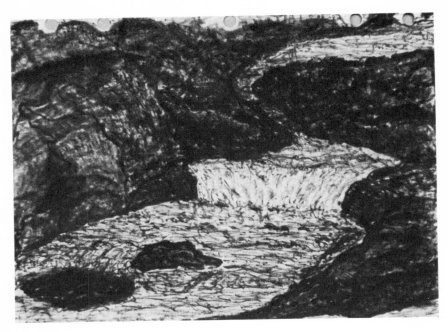

Figure 10

contempt about a passerby who wondered why anybody would bother to draw such a decrepit building.

For Figure 10 he ran back and forth searching out the hard convolutions of the rocks, the running and gurgling of the stream and waterfall. I had nothing but praise for this drawing and did not make my usual suggestions for further observation and changes. At best Louis B. accepts praise only grudgingly, and at one period he dismissed all his drawings as "finger exercises, scratchings" and accused me of being incompetent and hypocritical. Figure 11 is another passionate effort that was passionately disparaged.

In the two years that I've known Louis, although he has emerged from the extremely low state he was in, he remains uncommitted and dependent.

Conclusion

I believe this nonclinical approach has successfully stimulated many patients to produce expressive artwork or at least work that approaches that level. Among them are extremely difficult chronic cases, patients who are said to be "dedicated to their illness." One of these has responded only to art, of all the activities offered at the Center.

At the heart of my way of working is my unwillingness to accept as art a pathological work—that is, a work that evinces symptoms of illness but is otherwise inexpressive. I demand clarity of form even if a patient's painting

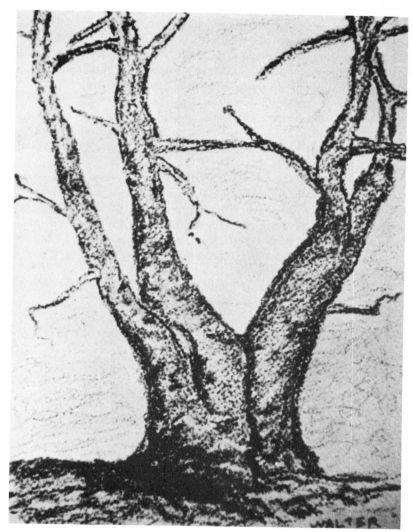

Figure 11

is *about* his illness or his miserable condition. Thus I am really demanding a healthy form of nonverbal expression.

Interpretation, that is, translating a picture into words, should be handled with care. Many levels of feeling enter into a picture, and interpretations are as likely to reflect the character of the interpreter as that of the artist. For example, a woman I know well commented that the phallic forms in Harry D.'s picture of snake plants (Figure 5) indicate his insecurity as a man. This is an acute and pertinent observation but at the same time an attack in that it focuses on a disparaging view of the picture-maker.

Certainly interpretation has its place, but it should be based on sound psychoanalytic training, and often it should not be offered to the patient. Even without such background, however, a knowledge of the language of art assists understanding of a picture's rich implications, an understanding that can be used for the patient's benefit.

As part of my teaching, I have tried to do some of my own drawing, painting, and sculpture at the Center. It is not easy to do this and at the same time be responsive to the needs of others, but my working among them has inspired many patients.

It is hard to know how long the psychological effect of this kind of art teaching lasts; probably the same may be said of many forms of psychiatric treatment. Certainly we have evidence that the combined therapeutic activities of the Center reinforce self-confidence. Some patients are helped to graduate to regular jobs by their successful work not only in art but also in the Center's activity groups of quite different kinds. This shows once again that all forms of treatment should be regarded with respect and should be thoughtfully coordinated if a rehabilitation program is to have maximum effect.

Life Review in Art Therapy with the Aged

Betty L. Zeiger

> . . . *Mem'ry's pointing wand,*
> *That calls the past to our exact review.*[1]

Art therapy with the aged needs special methods. We must do more than imitate techniques of benefit to other groups but which have little value for old people. I started working with the aged as a beginning student of art therapy, and at that time I was struck by the work of Robert Butler— particularly his theory of life review. For the past two years I have been supervising art therapist in the Hebrew Home for the Aged, a geriatric nursing home in the Washington, D.C., area. My work there has convinced me that art therapy, geared to Butler's life-review process, can be of significant value to the aged individual.

Butler sees life review as occurring naturally and arising out of the aged person's need to reexamine and resolve past conflicts in order to restructure present experience in the face of impending death. Butler writes:

> The life review [is] a . . . universal mental process characterized by the progressive return to consciousness of past experience, and particularly, the resurgence of unresolved conflicts.
>
> . . . Presumably this process is prompted by the realization of approaching dissolution and death. . . . The life review, as a looking-back process that has been set in motion by looking forward to death, potentially proceeds toward personality reorganization.[2]

If this process is successfully completed and past conflicts are resolved, then, Butler contends, "wisdom" or "serenity" may be attained. If the process is not completed, then "despair" or psychopathological symptoms may result.

---

1. Cowper, *Task* (1784), as quoted in R. N. Butler, "The Life Review: An Interpretation of Reminiscence in the Aged," *Psychiatry*, Vol. 26, 1963, pp. 65–76.
2. R. N. Butler, "The Life Review: An Interpretation of Reminiscence in the Aged," *Psychiatry*, Vol. 26, 1963, pp. 65–76.

Most (but not all) old people seem to enjoy reminiscing about past experience and need no persuasion to do so. The heightened tendency toward reminiscence on the part of the aged is not negative, says Butler, not merely a sign of increased introversion; life review activity represents a normal and positive adaptational response to impending death.

It appears that the aged, often infirm, individual attaches himself to memory and begins to talk more of his past precisely because in the present objects of pleasure become fewer and more distant. Pleasure comes to be identified more and more with the past. However, at its most active the life-review process involves consideration of not only pleasurable memories, but, more important, *painful* memories of still unresolved conflicts—in the effort to finally resolve them and find inner peace. Gorney[3] points out the heightening affect—whether anguish or joy—characteristic of various phases of active life review.

Since active life review is often painful, some old people resist it, and they suffer the toll that repression inevitably takes: a diminished ability to enjoy what pleasures life can still offer them. These people, as well as those whose memory is impaired because of physical deterioration of the brain, can profit from measures designed to encourage the recall of memories vital to the life-review process.

Irene Dewdney, writing in the *American Journal of Art Therapy,* also noted the value of "assignments that might help the patient retain his memories as long as possible" and reported that she found it wise to introduce such exercises "slowly, interspersing them among less threatening assignments." She does not explain her findings in terms of psychological dynamics, but observes that she has found that the old function better when they are in touch with memories of their younger, better functioning selves.[4]

Recall Through Art Therapy

At the Hebrew Home the seventy-five residents who have participated in art therapy have been divided into the following groups: the alert, the mentally impaired, the visually handicapped, and the depressed. This grouping is somewhat arbitrary. With rare exceptions, all residents of this particular nursing home suffer from some visual disability, some depression, and so forth. I have used a simplified life-review approach in working with residents with severe mental impairment. "Let's talk about our families," I might suggest and then, in the course of discussing our mothers and fathers and

3. James Gorney, "Experiencing and Age Patterns of Reminiscence Among the Elderly," Dissertation, University of Chicago, 1968.

4. Irene Dewdney, "An Art Therapy Program for Geriatric Patients," *American Journal of Art Therapy,* Vol. 12, July 1973, pp. 249–54.

earliest recollections of childhood homes, I encourage a few, brief attempts at putting these memories on paper with pastels.

I usually turn next to marriage as another source of significant memories. With severely impaired patients—those who are seriously confused, forgetful, and only occasionally aware of their place in time and space—the probing must be delicate. The therapist, while searching for detail capable of being translated into visual form, must always be on guard for cues that indicate stress.

I will illustrate with a brief account of my work with two very old women whose memories of long-ago events were sparked through recall of the details of Jewish marriage ritual.

Mrs. Miller, eighty-five years old, was born in Russia, has been widowed for twenty years, and was characterized by a staff psychiatrist as completely disoriented, suffering from cerebral arteriosclerosis and severe brain syndrome. She has been a resident of the Home for two years. Before our first meeting sixteen months ago, she would usually go back to her room after breakfast and lie motionless most of the day, blocking herself off from visitors by wearing an eyeshade.

During a series of sessions attended by Mrs. Miller and members of the severely impaired group, we decided that each member would draw various aspects of an orthodox Jewish marriage ceremony. Mrs. Miller drew quickly and her work has a certain dashing quality. Figure 1 shows her drawing of

Figure 1

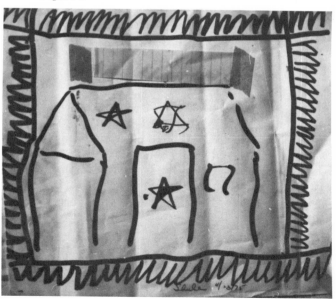

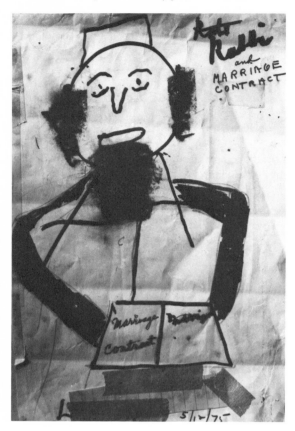

Figure 2

the synagogue. In Figure 2 (Plate X), we see the officiating rabbi holding the marriage contract. Figure 3 shows Mrs. Miller's drawing of the Bible surrounded by flowers.

These drawings were done over a period of three months. They seemed to make more vivid the pictures that were appearing in Mrs. Miller's mind as, little by little, she began to describe her marriage with ever-greater clarity as time wore on. She is still mentally impaired, but now she is boisterous, even occasionally bawdy, in her exchanges with other members of the group. Instead of staying in her room all day, she is in a hurry to go out and play miniature golf when the weather permits. She tells people she is "looking for a man," and she seems to have a somewhat clearer perception of what is going on around her.

Mrs. Croft, eighty-two years old, is much more unsure of herself than is Mrs. Miller. She walks slowly, is very forgetful, and her way of drawing reflected her hesitancy. She held the chalk poised above the paper for a long time, as if in doubt.

In Figure 4 we see Mrs. Croft's rather meagre representation of the

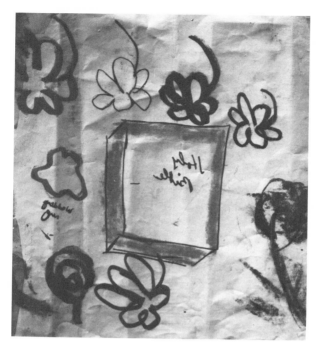

Figure 3

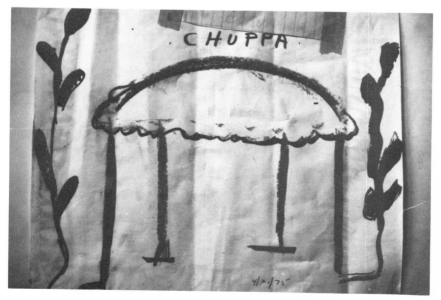

Figure 4

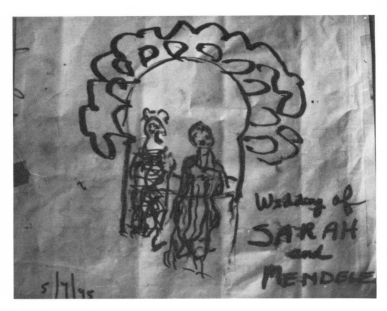

Figure 5

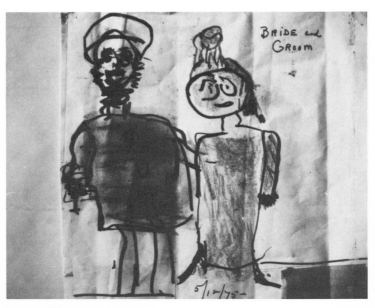

Figure 6

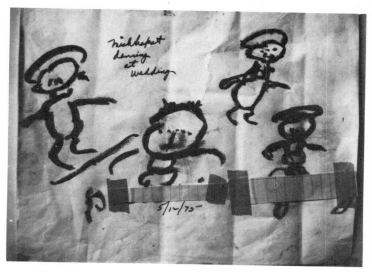

Figure 7

wedding canopy (or *chuppa*). A couple of weeks later I brought in dolls representing a bride and a groom and we decided to give them names and then draw them. Someone suggested the names "Sarah" and "Mendele," and at this point Mrs. Croft's quavering voice could be heard: "Mendele, Mendele. . . . Oh no, Mendele." One could see the poignance of agonizing memory in her eyes. Only later did I learn that her son, named Mendele, together with her husband had been killed in a terrible accident years ago, an event she had been trying to blot from memory. In blocking out recollection of her son's and husband's deaths, Mrs. Croft had inadvertently begun to block out, and thus forget, her entire past.

Figure 5 is Mrs. Croft's drawing of the dolls Sarah and Mendele under the wedding canopy. It was not possible for me to learn if Mendele, the son, had married before his death in his early twenties. Unquestionably Figure 5 is a richer and more lively work than is Figure 4, no doubt because Mrs. Croft could invest in her picture of the *Wedding of Sarah and Mendele* her memories of an important person in her life.

Two pictures that Mrs. Croft made five days later show that her work has become even more vigorous, detailed, and lively. Figure 6 shows a bride and groom and Figure 7 represents the wedding party dancing.

Mrs. Croft now is less reticent, and although her approach to reminiscence is still guarded, she has opened up more and talks about the hopes and fears of her past which had for so long been bottled up inside her.

Discussion

What does our experience at the Hebrew Home suggest? First, that, as Butler asserts, it is normal for old people to talk about their past and such talk is to be encouraged. Second, that the therapist needs to be a sympathetic listener. Third, that the sensitive use of art activities can stimulate the recall of forgotten or repressed material and thereby further the personality reorganization of the life-review process.

Life review, of course, is not a panacea for all the problems of the aged, but I believe it is worthy of the consideration of all who work with the old. Happier tomorrows for the elderly may well lie in a therapeutic searching of their past.

PART THREE

PRACTICE OF ART THERAPY WITH CHILDREN

Art for Children with Minimal Brain Dysfunction

Susan E. Gonick-Barris

When I applied for a position as art teacher in a private school for children with minimal brain dysfunction, I had had considerable experience in teaching and in working as an art therapist. However, I had never worked with children impaired in this way, and I was completely unprepared for the varied and complex disturbances they exhibited.

They ranged in age from six to seventeen and had been diagnosed as suffering from specific dyslexia, minimal brain dysfunction, and a mild to moderate degree of emotional impairment. Some children had emotional problems in addition to dyslexia or brain dysfunction; others were in the school solely on the basis of emotional impairment. All of them had experienced difficulties in learning, although their intelligence was average or above. The overwhelming majority of the students came to the school after experiencing academic failure, social failure, or both in the public schools and were referred by these schools and by social agencies, clinics, or private practitioners. Most of the students were kept on medication because it was thought that without it they could not maintain enough self-control and attention so that they could profit from instruction.

With a view to providing some continuity I observed the outgoing art teacher's last few classes. In spite of the teacher's good intentions and fairly good rapport with the students, the art lessons seemed boring and sterile. The same lesson was offered to each of ten different classes, with no regard for the ten-year range of the students' ages. It was explained to me that these children needed a great deal of structure and could not be left on their own, as children usually are in art classes. Cutouts, stencils, and forms were traced and colored or cut out and glued. The children did nothing but follow the teacher's instructions, and the lesson was as routine as reciting multiplication tables.

When I spoke to the director of the school, he defended this sterile kind of art lesson because structure and sequential learning are essential for these children. "They need to be told exactly what to do or they get lost, feel frustrated, and become depressed or enraged. The openness of creative art experience is too threatening."

I found that most of the literature supported this view. I read many very impressive studies regarding educational problems and teaching approaches for children with minimal brain dysfunction. In practically none, however, was there any mention of ways to offer such children the satisfactions and pleasures traditionally associated with creative and expressive art experience in childhood.

For the most part, works dealing with the education of brain-dysfunctioning children describe expressive art experiences as not only beyond the capacity of these children but also as something to be scrupulously avoided. Art for pleasure, for release, for joy, or for therapy is not to be included in programs designed for children of this kind. However, what the authors of such works choose to call "art" does have a place as handmaiden in the service of other goals. The following quote is representative:

Although art is usually thought of as free expression, in this program for children with learning disabilities it will be considered as one more way to practice skills and develop understandings. The goals are: to develop visual perception, to develop motor control, to aid in the teaching of writing, reading, and arithmetic, to establish spatial relationships, and to help the child in his socialization with the group.[1]

I think this is an unfortunate view. For just such handicapped children, so often disconnected both from themselves and from the world outside, living in chaos so much of the time, expressive art would be most beneficial. Here is their opportunity to extend their world and to achieve some degree of mastery over it.

Despite our different viewpoints, I came to an understanding with the school's director and began teaching ten classes a week in forty-minute periods, with about twelve children to a class. I had many failures, but I learned from my mistakes and also from the children, who were always teaching me new ways to teach. I worked out methods that I believe offered the impaired children of this school the satisfactions traditionally associated with creative art exploration by normal children. I will explain my experience below—what worked and what didn't, and why—in the hope

---

1. William J. Cruickshank *et al.*, *A Teaching Method for Brain-Injured and Hyperactive Children*, Syracuse University Special Education and Rehabilitation Monograph Series 6, Syracuse, N.Y., Syracuse University Press, 1961, pp. 249–50.

that my efforts to offer a genuine creative arts program for brain-dysfunctioning children may be of use to others working with such children. First, however, I will describe briefly the nature of the dysfunctioning child's problems.

The Learning Problems of Minimal Brain Dysfunction

Bert Kruger Smith, in an excellent and compassionately written book,[2] describes children with minimal brain dysfunction as having underdeveloped or undeveloped brain pathways—a dysfunction often difficult to detect and frequently recognized only through the behavior it seems to cause. Impairment may affect motor or psychomotor functioning, or it may become evident in one or more of the following areas: perception, conception, language, memory, and emotional control. There is no one entity. There are as many combinations of learning problems as there are children. Therefore, each child must be approached as an individual. Smith cautions us against remembering the label and forgetting the child.

Afflicted children have difficulty in getting visual and auditory messages; they see and hear the world differently from the way normally functioning people do. It is characteristic of normal perception that the whole is recognized at once. We see the total picture before the detail. Only when the whole is not immediately recognized do we take it apart, searching for clues in its components. Not so the brain-dysfunctioning child, who often does not accurately perceive the whole but instead sees one of the parts as a lesser whole.

This causes not only immediate perceptual distortion but also confusion in perception of the relationship of an entity to its background—of figure to ground. Normally, there exists a clear differentiation between the two. With little conscious effort most of us sort out shadow from substance, but the brain-dysfunctioning child who suffers from perceptual disturbance is often unable to do this. He frequently becomes transfixed by one of the parts, which leaps into the foreground as a seeming whole, thereby relegating everything else to background. Obviously the child who perceives a different image from that perceived by his normal counterpart as a result of the same stimuli is constantly building up a distorted view of reality. This cannot fail to make learning difficult or to have an effect on his total behavior.

This perceptual characteristic explains one of the most distressing learning problems of brain-dysfunctioning children: their distractability or tendency to respond to seemingly insignificant and often barely noticeable details in scenes or situations rather than to the broad and inclusive whole. Not surprisingly they often have difficulty organizing perceptual stimuli into

2. Bert Kruger Smith, *Your Nonlearning Child: His World of Upside-Down*, Boston, Beacon Press, 1968.

meaningful patterns in order to form concepts. (Since art media offer infinite stimuli, work with art can indeed pose problems, but not, I found, insurmountable ones.)

It is easy to understand how an early inability to structure the stimuli which he perceives leads to a maze of confusion at more sophisticated levels as the child matures. This explains why a brain-dysfunctioning child is often unable to relate cause and effect or to make predictions. An unfortunate snowball effect operates whereby new and misperceived stimuli must be fitted into already faulty structures. Deviation tends, therefore, to perpetuate itself, and the whole unfortunate experience of brain dysfunction results in a very poor self-image. Emotional disturbance is an all too common side effect.

The teacher of brain-dysfunctioning children must simplify conceptual tasks so that the children can understand the lesson. To summarize, when planning lessons thought must be given to ways of getting around the following weaknesses which the children may be subject to:

1. Figure–ground confusion
2. Distractability
3. Disturbance of spatial relationships
4. Insufficiently established directional orientation
5. Impaired auditory perception
6. Overlays of emotional disturbance

It is equally important to understand that no two children will have exactly the same degree or kind of handicap. In a group, the range of ability is apt to be as broad as in any group of normal children. As mentioned earlier, the approach to each child must be individual and should be based on what strengths the child does have.

Materials and Approaches: What Worked and What Did Not

Consistent and clearly understood procedures are crucial to the success of any program with brain-dysfunctioning children, especially when stimulating materials are used. I arrived at my procedures through a process of trial and error.

Working with Clay

In our work with clay I started out by giving the children too much clay—a ball about the size of a grapefruit. I worked my way down from grapefruit to tangerine size, which seemed about right. The larger amount was overwhelming for these children whose ideas leap ahead of their ability to carry them out. Another imperative was to make sure everyone had a ball of clay of exactly the same size, thereby preventing both arguments about someone being treated preferentially and "clay snatching" to correct unequal distribution.

We used wet clay, not Plasticine. I had wedged it earlier to a very soft consistency—something like mashed potatoes—so that it was responsive to the slightest pressure. Earlier experience showed that clay too hard for the children to manipulate easily frustrated them and made them angry. They lost patience and would not work the clay to make it more plastic. Giving them water to experiment with was a disaster. Mud was everywhere—on faces, hair, floor. I learned that preparing the clay in advance paved the way for quick satisfaction and more sustained interest.

The clay was worked directly on the surface of the desk. Usually one works on newspapers, clay tiles, or plaster bats and uses wet sponges and modeling tools. I deliberately refrained from distributing any materials other than clay in order to reduce distractions. From bitter experience I had learned that for these children clay tiles, normally a convenience for turning the work so it can be looked at from all sides, were just one more thing that might slip off the desk. Thus, each child had a ball of clay that fit neatly into the palm of one hand on which to focus. We started out with a very structured group experience. My instructions were simple:

1. "Here is a ball of very soft clay. One for each person."
2. "Put your empty hand behind your back. Now squeeze the ball as hard as you can." The children notice that squeezing the clay has produced interesting shapes between their fingers.
3. "Now, use both hands to put it back into a ball." We repeated this procedure several times because I saw that some children were having trouble with even so simple a task as putting the clay back into a ball shape. I rolled the clay on the desk to demonstrate how it might be done. When all the children were able to do this, I proceeded to the next instruction.
4. "Take your ball of clay and press it as flat as you can on your desk, like a big cookie." Once again I told them to roll the clay back into a ball.
5. "Make one long skinny snake [a coil] using the whole ball." Again, they formed it back into a ball.
6. "Now make two balls from the one ball." Then: "Make two more from each one." Then: "Make as many balls as you can." At the end of the lesson collecting the clay was a simple matter. "Roll all the little balls into one ball just as you had before."

When all of the clay had been returned to the crock where it is stored, and only then, I gave each child a small, damp sponge. (All the sponges are of the same color and size.) They washed the surface of their desks quickly and returned the sponges to an empty basin. This initial lesson lasted about twenty-five minutes. In subsequent and longer sessions we followed the same distribution, collection, and clean-up routines.

Anyone who has worked with clay in a free way will deplore such a carefully controlled exercise. However, with these children I have found it best to hold back initially and to move slowly. Clay can be the most threatening of media for many children, from a conceptual as well as a tactile and expressive point of view. From earlier failures I have learned that children with minimal brain dysfunction will want to make very complicated and realistic productions without understanding the limits of either their skill or the medium. I have seen many children give way to tantrums over clay legs that collapse and clay heads that fall off. My idea was slowly to build skills so that, when finally on their own, the children would know how to make what they wanted.

The children's work with clay proceeded in certain phases. The first six or seven sessions were devoted (at the children's choice) to pounding the clay—building up a mound and smashing it down—often accompanied by the sound effects appropriate to annihilation. In an earlier teaching venture, I cut off the pounding phase in my zeal to get on with the lesson. My later training as an art therapist taught me my error. Now, more aware of the importance of timing and inner needs, I respected the children's urge to pound. I learned to wait for their enthusiasm to ebb. Then and only then would they be ready to move on. As a predominantly destructive way of using the clay seemed to lose momentum, some students started to scratch lines in it with their fingernails. This signaled to me their readiness to use tools. The next clay session was almost soundless. Instead of the boisterous activity of punching clay with up-and-down arm and body movements, all the children crouched intently over their material, silently engrossed in etching the clay with toothpicks and nails. Later, we added more tools: bolts, screws, and other objects that could make an impression in the clay. Initially, the tools were distributed one to each child. As the newness of the tools wore off, they were placed in a box and passed around so that each child could select a few.

In the early sessions the class returned the clay to the crock at the end of each session. My idea was for the children to use the clay primarily for play as long as they wanted. A time did come, however, when they asked to keep what they had made. This marked the move from investigation to creation. We used shoeboxes for storage. Providing safe storage and the chance to come back to where one left off are important to the child as a sign of respect for his work.

After weeks of pounding, the flattened clay seemed to bring out a great interest in foods and masks. For a time the children acted out a variety of feeding relationships: menacing mothers shoving food into reluctant mouths, infantile protests, infantile greed. They took great delight in making endless pizza pies, gooey layer cakes, and foods of all kinds. The mask making centered around and afforded a chance for identification with the monsters of movies and television. I was struck with the way many ordinarily shy children made contact with other children through such role-playing. In a sense, their clay creations served as a costume to slip into and out of.

After a while a number of students seemed quite ready to move on to tasks which demanded more in the way of skill: making such things as animals, vases, small pots. After months of slapping and pounding, folding and squeezing, cutting and etching, many wanted to learn how to join pieces of clay together for sculptural purposes. At this point, the class seemed very like any class of normal children. Each student was able to work in the way best suited to his needs. For some, pounding was still all they wanted to do, and they continued to pound. Others kept on making masks but they were more refined and sophisticated. Some made guns, knives, and bullets. But many children wanted to learn the coil-and-slab method of building, how to make pinch pots, and how to shape increasingly complex figures such as animals and people.

After two months or so, I increased the amount of clay with which we began each session to grapefruit size. Soon the children were cutting off chunks of clay by themselves with a wire from twenty-five-pound blocks right out of the manufacturer's carton. At this point, they were quite able to decide for themselves how much they needed. The last thing I introduced was individual one-ounce paper cups of water for smoothing over cracks and making slip to make pieces stick together.

From a tightly controlled beginning, and after continuing to operate in this way as long as necessary, it was possible for the class to move into a much freer, more flexible way of working which allowed for genuine personal expression. Several children had significant experiences during our work with clay, and I will discuss two such events below.

David, in a class of seven-year-olds, refused to participate in any artwork from the outset. His teacher said it was difficult to engage him in anything. He always said "I can't." David is very short and chubby for his age. He is of normal intelligence, although he functions at least a year behind his chronological age. His head seems too large for his body, but he is otherwise not remarkable in appearance. He is a twin; his brother attends a normal public school. David is considered a show-off by his classmates, but after much boasting he seldom delivers. He pouts a good deal in a corner and generally draws as much attention to himself as possible.

When all the other children were working at their desks, I sat down next to David with a ball of clay in my hand. I had his permission to sit near him. Without speaking I started playing with the clay myself. He watched sullenly, chin resting on his hand, lips tightly pressed together. We sat in silence. After a few moments, he said to no one in particular and with some disgust in his voice, "I can't do anything."

"I know," I replied, still working on my own clay.

"How do you know?" he asked.

"Because you say so," I answered.

I continued exploring the clay, stretching and compressing it. A few moments later David said, "I want to make a man but I can't."

I said, "You want to make a man and you don't know how."

"Yeah." His voice was flat.

"I'm getting tired of fooling around," I said. "Think I'd like to make a man too. Should we do it together?" I said this inquiringly, with no special enthusiasm.

"O.K., but I don't know how. . . ."

"Well, let's do one part at a time. What's the first part you want him to have?"

"A head."

I offered him my clay, a small ball resting in the palm of my hand, and suggested he pull off a piece the size he wanted. He did so and started rolling a small piece very cautiously on the desk. When it was smooth he said, "Now what?"

"Well, feel your own head. What is it connected to?"

He looked very seriously at me, eyes bright and alert now. He ran his fingers through his hair, felt his skull, moved down to his neck, patted it gently, and enclosed it with both hands.

"My neck!" He showed excitement for the first time and pulled off another piece of clay and stuck it underneath the head. We worked together in this way to make the rest of the figure. Only through repeated reference to his own body could David slowly build a figure that had all the parts. When we finished, David beamed and clapped his hands.

"I made a man!" Other children came over to look and seemed impressed.

"What's his name?" someone asked.

David hesitated awhile, then said "Alex" clearly as he looked at me and smiled. "His name is Alex." (I discovered later that his father is named Alex.)

In the afternoon, David's teacher told me that David had become more willing to try other things. He began to draw on his own, something he had never done in school before. He drew a human figure, touching himself as a model, and named the parts. He seemed suddenly to notice things.

Certainly for this child a simple experience with clay had fostered growth. If it had been thought appropriate, we could have explored David's relationship with his father through his projection onto the clay figure of his father's identity. However, if we concern ourselves here only with David's delight at discovery, his joy in play and peer recognition, we have ample demonstration of the value of creative experiences for brain-dysfunctioning children.

In another class for nine-year-olds, clay coffins were for a time in fashion. Clearly death was of considerable concern, and we used the coffin-making as a springboard to informal exchanges about illness, death, and dying. One cannot help but feel moved by the burden imposed on many young children by the amalgam of fantasy, myth, and half-truths stored in their minds.

Carmine continued to fashion coffins long after that fad had been replaced by others. His coffins were assembled meticulously, and he pretended they were of different materials: stone, metal, and so forth. All had lids and were empty. We saved them in a shoebox. One day he opened a new coffin and showed me a small clay figure inside.

"Who is it?" I asked.

"Me."

"Oh. How come?"

"I'm dead."

"When did you die?"

"When I came home from school."

Carmine, who had hardly talked at all until this exchange, began to talk. He made a series of coffins and dead babies. All were stored in his shoebox. One day he got them all out. He was going to bury them. I asked whether there would be guests at the funeral, and he thought about it. Yes, his mother and father. He selected two class members to act as stand-ins for his parents. I left the room with them and we went to a more private place. One of the children asked Carmine who was in the coffin.

"My grandmother," he said, and looked sheepishly at me.

After the burial—we covered the box with shredded newspaper—Carmine and I talked a little bit. I told him I was glad he was still alive and not in that coffin after all.

"Well," he explained, "my grandmother really did die last year."

I learned later from his records that his grandmother had lived with his family, and that he had been especially close to her. He had been greatly affected by her sudden death. School authorities were concerned because Carmine became withdrawn, depressed, and very silent after his grandmother died. His work suffered, and he often made sudden violent attacks on other children.

Although Carmine's grandmother had died a year earlier, he was still bound up in his grief and unexpressed pain. In his work with clay he gave these emotions expression, and this time he brought in witnesses. What had been too difficult to talk about earlier became close to an obsession.

After several weeks of coffins, dead babies, and then the burial followed by drawings of black figures, Carmine was at last able to let go of the subject. Very gradually he started to turn his coffins into small racing cars by adding wheels and arching the lids into roofs. He became less moody and was more friendly. Carmine offers another example of how impaired children not only *can* use art experiences for creative expression but often also have an even greater *need* than normal children for such experiences.

I feel that my stress on routines and simplification helped bring David and Carmine (as well as the other children) to the point where they could be genuinely creative. I have come to respect the place of controls and limits in any program offering instruction and, in particular, creative experiences to children who are lost when on their own. If confusion arises when there are too many choices, it seems wisest to reduce choice for the time being—the better to extend at a later time the range of alternatives with which the children *are* comfortable.

Working with Paint

Compared with other media, paint is hard to control; it demands better hand–eye coordination. Some of the errors I made in our early painting lessons were similar to my errors in working with clay. The children could not handle their excitement over the variety of color and the far too large paper at the beginning. A large empty space of newsprint was too much uncharted space to be responsible for. Yet interestingly enough, many of the children were no longer overwhelmed by that same size paper when it had a black dot at the center. The dot seemed to serve as an island from which the brush could wander off into uncharted seas and return for refuge before taking off again.

Because I worked with ten classes a week I was able to modify my approach continuously and refine procedures until I worked out what I considered the most rewarding. I learned that the best consistency for the paint is far thicker than one would use ordinarily—almost as thick as buttermilk. Thinner, runny paint requires far more control. After the children get used to working with the paint, it can gradually be thinned. In the long run, thinner paint is more desirable, because the newsprint will crack and tear under the weight of heavy paint. As in our work with clay, we established simple routines for distribution of materials and cleaning up.

Because of the excitement that color brings to a lesson, the best colors to start with are the blander ones: green first, then yellow. For some time the children used a palette limited to green, yellow, and white. When they were familiar and at ease with the paint, the paper, the brushes, and the mixing process, we added blue to the palette. After about six lessons it was expanded to include black and red.

I had learned from earlier work that red paint could create havoc and destroy a lesson, as can black and brown (to a lesser degree). Red is a very evocative color and gives rise to "blood and guts" play. When I made the mistake of introducing red too soon, the children made a mess and acted out all kinds of wild scenes. They seemed seized by the color and could not get past their psychic arousal long enough to use the paint for a graphic experience. When I held off and added red to the palette only after the students had devoted a great deal of time to painting, the chaos and wildness were put on the paper; the action became graphically contained. Instead of painting their fingers and hands red and threatening each other with "dripping blood," they painted bloody scenes and compared catastrophes and nightmares in pictorial terms.

In our first lesson each child took a turn coming up to the blackboard, dipping a half-inch brush (the same size brush they would use later) into a container of water, and painting on the blackboard. I asked some to paint lines from top to bottom, others to paint geometric shapes (triangles, squares, circles) over chalk. In the second lesson I gave each child a blank sheet of eight- by eleven-inch paper (smaller than the surface of their desks), a small metal container about the diameter of a cupcake tin but shallower, and one brush. Last was the paint itself. I had prepared the paint thoroughly before the lesson so that it was smooth and of the right consistency. I poured about three tablespoons per person from a one-quart milk container. (The milk container made it easy for me to distribute the paint, and the children took great delight in the "green milk.") This time I told them to "Dip your brush into the paint and paint your whole paper. Use up all the paint with your brush. Cover as many papers as you wish."

Some children worked slowly and deliberately for the entire period and covered only one sheet. Others worked very quickly and used three or four sheets. When everyone had used up all his paint, I walked around with two pails of water. In one the children put their brushes, in the other their little pans. I gave each student a toothpick to scratch his name and the date in the still and thick paint of his painting(s). Some children used the toothpicks to scratch designs in the wet surface. We put the paintings on the newspaper-covered floor to dry. Then they were stored in the students' individual folders.

In the next lesson we used similar procedures and green paint again. Now, however, instead of asking them to cover the entire surface, I asked them to try to discover what they could do with their brushes by using the flat, broad side or just the tip, by pressing at different angles, and so forth. This brush lesson intrigued most of the children, and they used many sheets of paper experimenting in this way.

After I was satisfied that distribution and cleanup routines were firmly established, that everyone could control a brush, and that the size of the paper was right, I introduced white paint in addition to the green. Each student now had two cups—each containing a small quantity of paint—but still only one brush. I gave each person paper towels for wiping his brush. I asked them to use the white to create as many different tints of green as they could. The thickness of the paint kept drips to a minimum, and the blandness of the color did not distract from free experimentation with a variety of brushwork and tints.

As usual all papers were carefully dried and saved. If a paper was torn accidentally, I repaired it by taping from the underside very carefully. All this taping, labeling, and storing contributed to each child's sense that what he was doing was important and of value. It was apparent in many small ways that the children came to share this view. As time wore on they collected things and passed them to each other much more carefully. There were fewer accidents and far fewer papers thrown away. The children even commented on one another's work less harshly and became more accepting of differences in style.

When the children started demanding another color, I added yellow. For several weeks, they contentedly explored the possibilities of combining green, white, and yellow. Next I added blue. At about this time I brought in small muffin pans (six muffin spaces to a tin) and invited the children to mix colors in them. There was room on their desks for this palette and the small papers we continued to use.

After about two months of working this way with a palette of white, yellow, green and blue; one brush; and as many small papers as they needed—I felt that they were ready for larger sheets of paper. Since these sheets were larger than their desk tops and no easels were available, we worked on the floor. (The cooperation of the home room teacher was essential. She rearranged the furniture before the lesson to free as much floor space as possible.) Each child's space was covered with a layer of newspaper, and his paper for painting went on top of that. Alongside was his muffin-tin palette and brush. In the center of the room was a large pail of water and a box of small absorbent rags (facecloth size, all of the same size and material).

When we had firmly established the procedure of painting on the floor with large paper I approached the introduction of the color red by providing pale pink paint. In each succeeding session the pink became redder until eventually the children were working with pure red.

By now, the color mixing was as sophisticated as can be found in any normal art class. At the same time subject matter became more important to many children as they began to be able to take color and technique more or less for granted. They came to use painting materials and themselves as freely as any group of children of the same age.

Once again I must stress the importance of laying the groundwork in as unpressured, simple, and satisfying a way as possible, always mindful of the variety of handicaps these children face. There must be a willingness to experience each child on his own terms, to let go of expectations that may be unspoken but nonetheless are communicated to the student and felt as inhibiting. The unqualified respect for the student-as-artist must permeate the atmosphere. These children are the first to disparage their own efforts and ideas, despite frequent demonstrations of a bravado which is actually defensive. Not only do they often project their own negative judgments but they are also remarkably sensitive to unspoken ones on the part of others.

Three-Dimensional Design and Collage

Working with three-dimensional design and collage poses specific problems for brain-dysfunctioning children and their teacher. This kind of work demands a certain degree of skill in cutting, folding, and fastening things together. Ordinarily, children would be given the broadest range of materials from which to choose—assorted shapes in vibrant colors, a variety of textures. A single sketch or demonstration of a three-dimensional arrangement would be expected to be enough to set the children off on their own.

With impaired children, however, a lengthy period of gradually built-up experience must precede genuine creative expression. Once the basic skills are understood and mastered, however, there is no reason why impaired children cannot exercise ingenuity and craftsmanship to express a mood or the essence of a form or to create a startlingly dramatic effect.

We began, as usual, by limiting our materials. Each child was given a six-inch square of cardboard. In the center of each square was a small dot. I distributed smaller squares of paper and asked the children to glue them on the dot in the center of the cardboard. Then they were asked to glue a prepared circle of paper to the smaller square. (Needless to say each child's materials were the same size and color as everyone else's.) All along I watched to see who was having difficulty using glue or locating the middle.

When all was progressing satisfactorily, each child was given three narrow strips of paper six inches long with which to stripe the cardboard as he liked. So far the work had been in only one plane. The most important skill had been to apply just the right amount of paste so that papers did not slip and slide off each other.

In the next lesson each child worked with his original cardboard square and was given in addition a one-ounce cup half full of glue and a strip of construction paper about three-fourths of an inch wide. I told them to paste one end of this strip anywhere they chose. When this was dry enough to stay (about two minutes), I showed them how to turn the other end of the strip so that there was a twist in the center and then glue that end to the cardboard. The instant three-dimensional effect gave great delight. As soon as they had caught on to this technique, they used as many strips as they wished, choosing from a range of colors.

After the paper-twisting skill was established, I gave each child a small scissors and several narrow strips of paper. I taught them how to curl paper by holding it at an angle against one blade of the scissors and pulling it up. At each lesson I demonstrated a different way of shaping paper. One time it was cutting round and round in a smaller and smaller concentric curve until a spiral was formed. This was glued at one end to make a bouncy spring. Another time paper was folded in accordion style and cut into strips of steps that were glued to the cardboard.

After several lessons the children had acquired a number of shaping and construction skills. When they were all able to cut, paste, roll, and fasten paper, it was supplied in a full range of colors and shapes. It is important that the ground (the cardboard base onto which everything is attached) be small. Many different kinds of material can be used: straws, tin foil, and so forth.

Although these three-dimensional constructions started out uniform in order to reduce stimuli and confusion, nearly all turned into unique examples of individual work, reflecting the students' preferences in their color, shape, texture, and overall effect.

In making a collage with natural materials—stones, sand, twigs, dried flowers, seed pods, and so forth—the ground is again kept small. As before, we started with cardboard squares not larger than six inches on a side.

Because some of the natural materials are unfamiliar, the children, who have an unusually high need for tactile experience, had to be free to examine the objects very closely. They took great delight in the dried pod of a wisteria, for example. Its outside feels and looks like olive-green plush velvet. The irregular bumps indicate something is inside. What could it be? I allowed them to open the pods, to feel the soft, satin lining inside and admire the beautiful chestnut-colored seeds. The seeds are about the size of a penny and are often prized for their hard and richly textured surface. Stone chips about the size of a nickel (so that gluing them would be no problem) were tasted, smelled, squeezed, scraped, and so forth. Stones with imbedded layers of mica were turned to catch and reflect light. To impress the children with the delicacy (and the need for careful handling) of small, dried flowerets from a snowball bush, I used tweezers to place several on each child's desk. Finally I gave them a piece of common bark. They found it hard to believe that material like this was all around them in great abundance.

In the first lesson, after the children had examined the materials at length, I asked them to try to arrange all their materials on the cardboard square like food on a dish. After they had done this they were to come up to a row of boxes labeled "rocks," "tree bark," "dried pods," etc., and carefully return all their materials to the proper boxes.

In the second lesson, the children started with a cardboard square and a green craypas on their desks. I asked them to draw a line with the craypas dividing the cardboard into sky and ground. When all the children had done that (and a number of them needed a great deal of time), I collected the green craypas and gave each child a blue one to fill in the sky. Then I collected the blue craypas and offered them a choice between brown, black, or green craypas for the earth or ground section. When the latter had been completed and all the craypas collected, one at a time the children came up to the desk and chose from among the natural materials (the same ones they had handled in the first lesson) to create gardens or forests on their cards. After they had done so I offered them glue to make the arrangement permanent. These small collages were exquisite, and were further enhanced when we mounted them on mats of various colors.

This experience gave rise to a great interest in both collage and the environment. For the rest of the winter members of the group brought in all kinds of materials, often with a comment such as, "The school yard is full of this stuff, and I only noticed it today!" Familiar things became exciting. The children worked on collages by themselves, and many abandoned the arbitrary division between earth and sky to do freer, more abstract arrangements.

For variety I brought in many different kinds of seashells. Each child drew a figure of the creature who could be comfortably housed in the shell of his choice. He made up a history for this creature, which included its family. The brief "shell" biographies were touchingly close to each child's real or fantasy life. The children took turns reading them aloud. Some, however, would not do so, but many of these who were reluctant to read to the group were eager to read their stories to me as an audience of one.

The shell experience resulted in a mural—an enormous cardboard beach scene. The children continued to add such things as angelfish and menacing sharks to the scene long after we had gone on from collage to other working methods. A revealing and expressive dialogue between the "sharks" and the "angels" of the class grew out of the experience. The following is an excerpt from a taped exchange:

> *Shark* (First does a lot of flailing on the floor and makes eerie noises): Get the hell out of my way or I'll eat you the hell up!
> *Angelfish:* Yeah . . . you think you're so great you fat-assed pigfish. You're a fat-assed bully because you're so big. You should go on a diet. Well, I won't let you get away with it. My spit is magic; as soon as it gets in the water you shrink to smaller than me! Haaaa. . . . (Makes a spitting sound.)
> *Shark:* Help! Help! I'm shrinking.
> *Angelfish:* If you promise not to bug me no more I'll help you.
> *Shark:* O.K., O.K. (His voice is very faint now.)
> *Angelfish:* Spit, Spit, Spit!

These two boys, although often friends, had been fighting and sometimes hurting each other for some time before the above exchange. In their guise as shark and angelfish they swapped accusations and counteraccusations that reflected the ambivalence of their real-life relationship. Clearly they were not merely fish. Sometime later the homeroom teacher reported that the two boys were getting along with each other much better.

Using Felt-Tipped Pens to Make Murals

Some materials help and some hinder the student. For example, hard crayons can create muscular tensions incompatible with the production of free-flowing lines, whereas soft crayons (such as craypas) or felt-tipped pens lend themselves to a relaxed line. Children should not have to fight the medium they are using.

After the children had built up basic individual experiences with clay, paint, three-dimensional design, and collage, I felt they were ready to work together, providing I kept the material uncomplicated and easy to manage. First, the children chose partners with whom to work. The theme of their first mural was "Friends." Each set of partners was given a specific space along the wall of the room, with no more than two couples per wall. The point was to allow them enough room to work without bumping into each other and also to ensure as far as possible that partners spoke only to each other and didn't disturb others. Very large pieces of paper were taped to the wall. Each child chose one felt-tipped pen—green, yellow, or brown—and outlined his partner's body while the partner leaned against the paper on the wall. When both outlines were completed the children clothed and decorated their figures, using felt-tipped pens in a variety of colors.

The next lesson continued from where the first left off. We retaped the completed figures to the wall, and I asked the children to write something personal about themselves, mentioning perhaps their favorite food, book, or television show; or describing a hobby or a place they had enjoyed visiting. As each child finished writing his personal statement on desk-size paper, I stapled it to his figure. (I had shown them an enlarged sample of a comic-book page to remind them of the way the characters are represented as talking to each other.) Then the children read the printed statements aloud to each other. From this, a master list was made of foods loved, places enjoyed, colors preferred, and so forth, which I taped on the floor. I hoped to use it as a source for themes in subsequent small-group murals.

We continued to use the large paper figures in the following way. Two or three children would work together on environments for the figures—beach scenes, picnics, parties—and then cut out their figures and tack them on as foreground. This device was abandoned several murals later as the children spontaneously drew new figures into their murals with an increased feeling for background–foreground presentation. It was common to see from two to four children at work on one large scene, each child with his own complete set of felt-tipped markers. The large paper cutouts had served as a bridge to more spontaneous and complex behavior—both in terms of the children's attitude toward each other and their sense of spatial relationships.

Around this time, I started allowing the children to choose their own media. Since they had become familiar with a range of materials, I believed they were ready for a more individual art experience. That is, in any one art period, clay, paint, Cray-pas, felt-tipped pens, collage, and mural materials were available, and each child was free to make his own choice. This freedom, which had been earned little by little, allowed each student to go his own way, absorbed in his own work, which might be very different from that of the others around him. Thus individuality was fostered and competition was reduced. Such freedom of choice would have been out of the question had it not been preceded by months of carefully planned experiences, each building on what had gone before.

Within the limits of their handicaps, the children working at their chosen activities with a variety of media resembled any art class for normal children of the same age.

Conclusion

My experience with these handicapped young people has led me to believe that under properly structured conditions they are as able as any other group to use art as it has been used through the ages: for exploration and play, to create and to express. Traditional art programs for children with brain dysfunction—offering them stereotyped adult symbols to copy, trace, or otherwise duplicate—doubly deprive them: they are misled about the meaning of art and robbed of an opportunity for art expression.

I believe, further, that children with learning disabilities and problems in social or emotional adjustment are in even greater need of creative art experiences than are children who do not have such disabilities. Precisely because they are so often unable to make themselves understood in more usual ways, these handicapped children need alternative modes for expressing the same emotional impulses and attitudes they share with all children.

There can be no doubt that David, the child who discovered his own physical organization in his work with clay, experienced real growth. From a characteristic focus on his dysfunctional self he grew into an appreciation of his whole self. Thus his self-image became less distorted and he began to gain a more realistic view of himself.

I hope that my experience and methods will be helpful to others concerned with children who are neurologically impaired, and that art in all its forms will be recognized for its power and be accorded its rightful place in the lives of those in all our educational and rehabilitative institutions.

Art as Therapy in a Group Setting: The Stories of Batja and Rina

Hilde Meyerhoff

Before I came to Israel I always worked individually with patients; therefore, painting in a group setting was a new experience for me. I soon found that children (like adults) are usually quite lost when you tell them, "Go ahead, paint whatever you like." They keep on asking, "What shall we paint today?" and want you to give them a subject.

Then I learned something that surprised me: namely, in a group setting, even when a subject is given and the art therapist does not interpret, the child unconsciously portrays his own problem, works on his own problem, and often solves his own problem. He tries to paint himself well, so to speak. What happens, apparently, is that insights are gained not on a *cognitive* but rather on a *symbolic* level.

When I work individually with a patient, be he a child or an adult, I interpret his painting or sculpture directly to him much as if it were a dream. (A dream may be looked on as a series of inner pictures, paintings and sculptures as inner pictures projected outward.) Working with groups in a hospital setting, however, I pass on my findings to the members of the staff, who then use these insights in their individual work with each patient. Of course, it is well known that working with paints and clay is therapeutic; in hospitals the activity is, after all, called *art therapy* and not *art lessons*. But it was a revelation to me that in the unconscious the healing process is at work in an absolutely *individual* manner, according to each patient's need, even in the framework of a group. This wondrous experience I would like to share with you by telling you the stories of Batja and Rina.

The two girls were hospitalized at the Government Rehabilitation Hospital of Nes Ziona in Israel. They painted with me one morning a week. The paintings reproduced in this chapter[1] were selected from their work over a period of six months. Batja was not at all amenable to psychotherapy, while Rina received psychotherapy during the same period with excellent results.

1. The photographs are by Nechemia Ross.

Batja

Batja came to the hospital at the age of eleven. She was born in Tunis of working-class parents. When she was two years old her parents came to Israel. In succession three more children were born: a boy, a girl, and a boy.

It soon became apparent that Batja's mother was very disturbed. One day she was good to the children, the next day she treated them cruelly. By the time the last child was born, her illness had reached dangerous proportions. Once the mother took the baby boy and threw him out of a window. Miraculously nothing happened to the child. Only Batja, then five years old, witnessed the scene. Surely it is hard to imagine the terror she must have felt at that moment.

Immediately afterward, the mother was hospitalized and diagnosed as schizophrenic. She is in the hospital to date. The children were sent to a foster home. All got along well except Batja, who was so seriously traumatized that she could not get along with her foster mother. Apparently any mother figure spelled threat and danger to her. She quarreled with everybody, would not eat, would not go to school, and was bossy and cruel to her siblings and to other small children.

Batja was sent from one foster home to another but could not get along anywhere. When she was eight years old, she did a fearsome thing. She burned a cat alive, then cut the dead animal open with a knife to see what was in its belly. After this, her foster parents would not dare to keep her, and Batja was sent to the hospital in Nes Ziona.

At Nes Ziona she was given a battery of tests. The findings were summarized as follows:

I.Q. excellent, but her thoughts circle mostly about the ambivalent hate–love feelings for her mother. When she is supposed to see a woman in the Rorschach test, she always sees a cat. She is afraid of death and bodily disintegration. She can make contact but she tries to adapt the surroundings to herself. She feels like a girl—a woman— because she thoroughly identifies with the mother. Diagnosis: Character disorder with underlying psychotic traits.

Different psychologists tried to work with her to no avail. She opened up to no one. When questioned, she said, "What goes on inside of me is nobody's business."

In class she had to be the best, and she was. She had to lead, and she led. While she was painting, I never saw her take an idea from anyone else. The others always tried to copy her. If she could not make a painting exactly to her taste or if it looked as if another child was making a better painting that day or if my suggestion was not to her liking, she tore up her work, threw it in the wastebasket, and left the room. She was extremely moody, stubborn, and quick to anger. She knew what she wanted, and everything had to go her way. Batja was the undisputed queen—she excelled in absolutely everything: painting, singing, dancing, reading, writing, acting. To my mind, she was the most brilliant, most gifted, most complex, and, in her psyche, the most endangered child in the group.

Shortly before I came to Nes Ziona, a new psychologist tried her luck with Batja, who was then eleven. "What is treatment?" Batja asked. "Do you want to make me forget things?"

"No," the psychologist said, "I want you to remember things and make you able to live with them."

"That is not possible," said Batja.

"We can try, can't we?"

Batja thought it over. The approach seemed right, so she opened up enough to tell a dream:

> I was in my foster home with my brothers. The home was under the earth. We were playing outside. Suddenly a frightful, huge, green, two-legged monster came toward us. My brothers ran into the house. I had an elastic stick in my hand which I quickly tied around my waist and I jumped into the air. From high up I saw the monster slowly shrink. Then my brothers came out and killed it. They wanted to pull me down but could not. So they left me in the air.
>
> Then came an airplane which looked like a guitar. I tried to catch it, but the pilot became very angry, flew faster, and cut off my head. I could speak only with my hands. He returned and cut off my breast and my legs and feet. My feet fell down and I became very light. When my feet touched the ground, I gradually grew back—slowly, slowly—until I was whole again.

This dream shows only too clearly Batja's nightmarish imagery and her terrible fear of insanity and physical disintegration. The cut-off head may be taken to mean the loss of thinking; the cut-off breast, loss of feeling; the cut-off feet, loss of the ground, of reality.

In her paintings Batja wrestled with *one* problem only: her mother, the cause of her fears, the core of her illness. In Figure 1 Batja responds to the assigned topic, *Happy Memory*, by recalling a sunny spring day when she climbed a hill and picked a beautiful blossom from a blooming tree.

It is apparent at once what a gifted child Batja is. But what else do we see? Batja does not stand solidly with her feet on the ground; as in her dream she floats in the air without the orienting, anchoring support of the earth.

She paints herself with black hair, while in truth she has light-brown hair. (Later the reason will become apparent.) The tree stands high on a hill, alone, indicating Batja's feeling of isolation and at the same time her need to stand out and attract attention. And most important, the tree has been cut off. Its branches do not grow organically into a crown but wondrously have

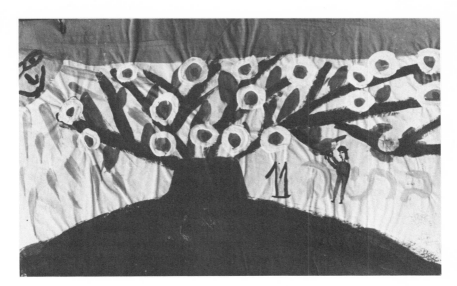

Figure 1

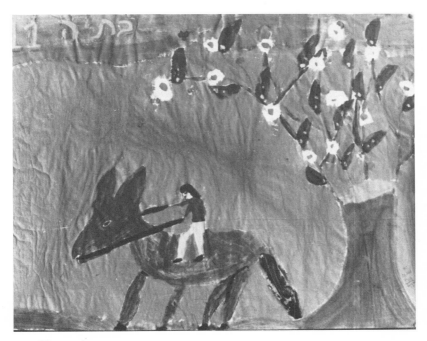

Figure 2

grown back after the cut and blossom. Exactly four branches—the four children. The unconscious makes no mistakes. This cut-off tree symbolizes Batja's family, cut off at the outbreak of the mother's illness.

Figure 2, *My Favorite Animal and I,* is again a response to a group assignment. To me it is one of the most beautiful paintings of the lot, with its perfect composition, sensitive division of space, and daring color choice (of course not visible in this black-and-white reproduction). And notice, at the upper left, how decoratively Batja has painted her name.

Again she draws the cut-off family tree, and this time even more distinctly. The tree is literally sawn off, and yet nature does not allow it to die. Again four branches spring to new life.

Batja rides a donkey. She is very small, the donkey very big. Probably the choice is no accident. Her unconscious has chosen an animal with whom she

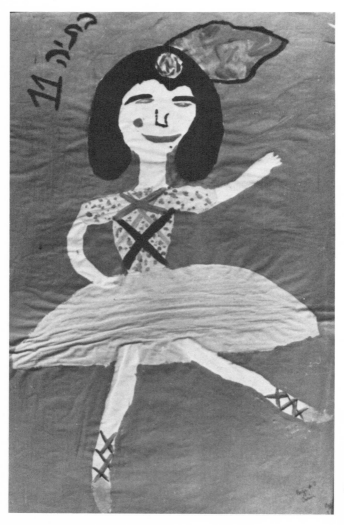

Figure 3

feels a kinship. In this painting, I believe, Batja is trying to harness that big, stubborn mule inside herself.

In Figure 3, *What I Want to Be on Purim,* a topic suggested during the Purim week when children typically dress up in costumes, Batja wants to be a ballet dancer. In this charming picture Batja's skill as a painter is again apparent. It is significant that she has given herself green eyes and once again black hair and black eyebrows. In reality she has hazel-brown eyes and, as mentioned earlier, light-brown hair and eyebrows. Notice, too, the circular flower in Batja's hair. We will see this again. The three emphatic crosses—in brown, blue, and black—may pass as an element of costume. Or may they be seen as crossing out the upper part of Batja's body, expressing the loss of feeling as did the cut-off breast in her dream?

In Figure 4, *Self-Portrait,* Batja must have asked herself quite consciously

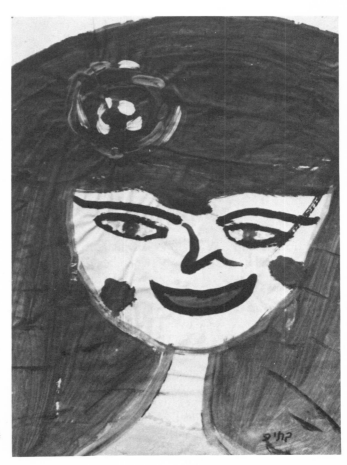

Figure 4

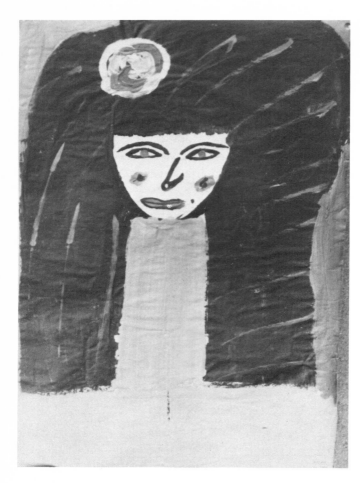

Figure 5

before starting to paint, "What do I really look like?" Here she gives her hair its true brown color, and in it she again puts the round flower. Yet two untruths have crept in after all. Batja gives herself a mass of long hair, while in reality her hair is short. And she again gives herself green eyes.

Figure 5, *Portrait of Batja's Mother*, explains everything. Batja painted it after her mother, on a day's pass, with the permission of the hospital, visited Batja together with Batja's father. This was a very upsetting experience for Batja, and apparently she found her peace of mind again only after having projected the experience outside of herself. The picture is a terrifying representation of the mother frozen in her illness. Here we find the mass of long black hair, the black eyebrows, the immobile eyes—green like the monster of Batja's dream—and the round flower. Batja's mother is a great beauty and often does wear a flower in her long black hair.

Quite unmistakably, Batja has demonstrated here how deeply and totally she identifies with her ill mother.

Batja's next painting, Figure 6, deals with the mother–child relationship in the animal world. Here she wants to show a *Chicken Feeding Her Young*. But this is not a chicken; it is a rooster. The care Batja received as a small child probably came from her father, not her mother. As a result, she gets along much better with men than with women.

The rooster has a sharp beak, made for pecking rather than feeding, and he looks mean, not gentle and motherly. He, too, has green eyes. Again there are four offspring, two still in the egg. And again, on the extreme left and not entirely distinguishable in reproduction is the cut-off tree that blooms.

In Figure 7 Batja dares to touch her sickest spot, her mother/cat identification. She paints a cruel *Cat Catching a Mouse*. The cat has the markings of a tiger and is about to seize and devour a little mouse. Predictably, this tiger-cat-killer has green eyes, like Batja's mother. Batja probably is not aware how much she still feels like that trapped little mouse, but by portraying the problem she has moved it closer to consciousness.

By the time Batja, now eleven and a half years old, painted Figure 8 (Plate XI), her cat had become a friendly *Tom Cat—Puss in Boots*. He wears a lovely suit, and he actually smiles. There is little that is frightening or

Figure 6

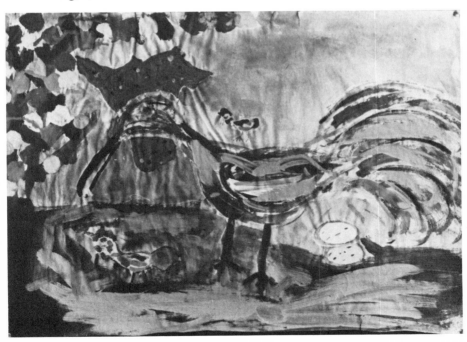

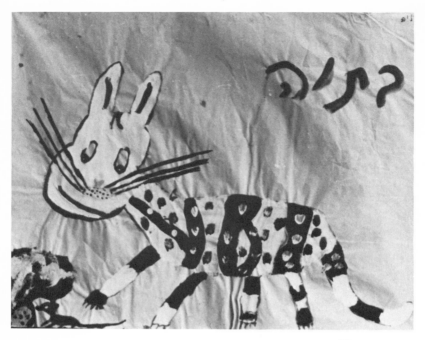

Figure 7

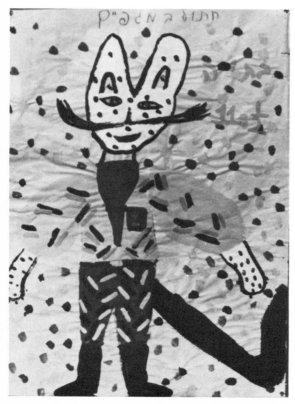

Figure 8

dangerous about this cat anymore, aside perhaps from the veiled threat suggested by the enormous, long, black tail.

In the story "Puss in Boots" the cat goes to the castle of the powerful magician. Upright, in his boots, he bows and asks, "Is it true that you can change yourself into *any* animal?" "True," the magician says and turns into a big elephant. "That is, indeed, marvelous," the cat replies. "But can you make yourself into a very small animal, too—as small as a mouse?" "Naturally," says the magician and—one, two, three—he becomes a mouse. Puss in Boots quickly pounces on him and eats him, and that is the end of the wicked man. The cat gives the beautiful castle to the poor miller's son who then marries the princess, and they live happily ever after.

What has Batja done? She has transformed the frightful tiger-cat into the most helpful fairytale animal—one who does away with all evil and may one day bring her the same happiness he brought the miller's son. The demonic green eyes have disappeared. Puss in Boots, this wonderful cat, actually has smiling blue eyes.

Figures 1–8 are representative of Batja's work over six months, painting once a week. And these eight pictures are only the milestones. I believe that Batja's unconscious accomplished a great deal of work during this time. Due to the combined efforts of the staff, the love and care she received, and last but not least, Batja's own efforts, she made enormous progress on her long road to health.

At present Batja is living in a good foster home, where she has adjusted well. She made two close friends in the hospital and is one of the best scholars in the municipal school.

Rina

Rina is a girl with a beautiful soul, but when she arrived in Nes Ziona she was an unmanageable wild animal.

Rina's parents came from Persia. Her father, a laborer and a rather primitive man, has been married three times. He had several children with the first wife and several with the second, who became mentally ill and committed suicide shortly after Rina's birth. Her father then married his third wife, but she did not want any of the children from the two former marriages. Thus the children were split up and sent to different institutions. Rina was placed in a home for orphaned or homeless children.

Rina's physical development proceeded normally, but she became hyperactive and nervous—undoubtedly because of her lack of one stable mother figure. When she was five years old, she was sent to a foster home. Her foster parents loved Rina very much and slowly she began to blossom. Rina stayed in this foster home for two and a half years, at which time her foster mother fell ill and could no longer keep the child. Thus Rina lost her second mother—but this time, at age seven and a half, the trauma was a conscious one. Rina reacted violently to the loss, becoming very aggressive, naughty, loud, and unruly. She was then sent to Nes Ziona.

The child felt so deeply unhappy that she did not even want to be a human being anymore. She called herself "Kofiko"—little monkey—and exhibited all the bad animal sides of herself: not sitting still for a moment, running about, making faces, climbing walls and trees, and being terribly noisy. She really behaved like a wild monkey. After a while, she attached herself to one of the cooks, who gave her much warmth and affection. Rina improved a little. But then the woman got pregnant and had to stop working. For a third time Rina lost her mother and regressed to her former wild-animal stage.

Then Mira, a new occupational therapist, came. Mira loved and understood the child and gave her a great deal of freedom. For instance, one day Rina wanted to paint one of the small playrooms black, and Mira courageously let her do it—ceiling, walls, doors, and all. It was ghastly. Again Rina improved. But she still called herself Kofiko.

After one year, Mira went to America for further training and Rina lost her fourth mother. The child was desperate.

At this point, Ruth, a young and gifted psychotherapist, began to work with her and—in time—became Rina's fifth mother. Rina was nine years old and back where she had started: an unmanageable, wildly unhappy child with no one to cling to—Kofiko, the monkey. For the first time, Rina received proper therapy now, one hour every day.

Ruth's treatment at first consisted in letting Rina do whatever she wanted. She let her be a monkey, she let her climb trees and run wild. Rina, wanting to destroy the whole world that had treated her so badly, tried to light fires in the room. Ruth let her light fires, but outdoors; and together they roasted potatoes in the fire and ate them.

In the beginning Rina did not want to talk to Ruth—no more opening up, no more loving, only to lose again. Instead of answering Ruth's questions, Rina simply repeated what Ruth said. Echolalia was the beginning of contact.

Ruth walked in the country with Rina, played with her, talked with her, and slowly—probably against her will—Rina grew to love Ruth. She said, "Come let's go to the black room; it's warm and good there. Come let us die there together." Now we understand more explicitly the meaning of the black room to Rina. She had made her grave. And if Ruth were to die with her, Rina could never lose her.

Rina now called Ruth "Doctor Kofiko," uniting herself and Ruth in the name. She scratched "Ruth and Rina" into tables and trees, the way one does when in love.

One day Ruth brought her a toy dog. Rina immediately ruined it by tearing off an ear; she could not stand owning anything anymore. "It's easier to have nothing," she said. "But now you won't love me anymore."

"Of course I love you," Ruth said, "and your hour will always be your hour."

Around the time Rina began painting with me—she was ten and a half years old then—she found a yellow bird on the ground. It was perhaps the first thing she really wanted to own again—something living that would belong only to her. And lovingly she took care of the bird. However, the bird had been injured internally and soon died. Rina was heartbroken but pretended to be indifferent. Ruth was worried.

In response to the first topic assigned, *My Favorite Animal and I,* Rina chose to paint her bird (Figure 9). She shows herself bringing it food. Ruth was greatly relieved. She felt that this picture, painted two weeks after the death of the bird, signified Rina's reconciliation to her loss.

Since Rina did not know how to draw herself in a bent position, she ingeniously lowered the ground to put herself on a level with the bird. Flowers are spread all over the ground in a decorative pattern. And *every* bare branch on *every* bare tree sprouts a bud. Nothing has died during the barren, loveless years; earth and trees have come back to blooming life.

In her picture, *What I Want to Be on Purim,* Figure 10, Rina chooses to be a clown, a silly clown who makes faces; yet we know the clown is sad inside. The clown is an evolution of Kofiko raised to the level of a human being. Rina wears pants and stands with legs far apart, even on stilts. You will see her in

Figure 9

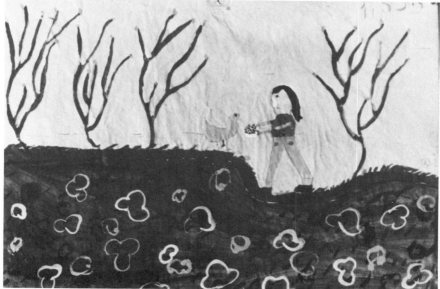

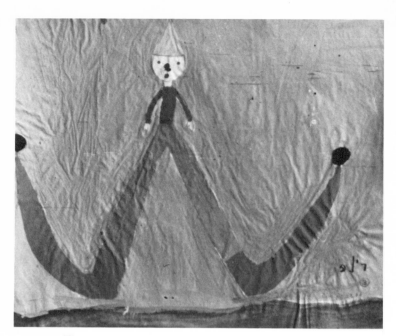

Figure 10

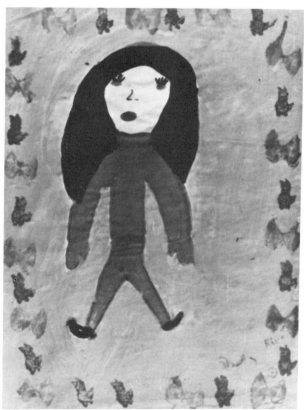

Figure 11

this posture—her typical defiant stance—and in pants in every picture but one. I believe that Rina would have perished if she did not have this stubborn strength in her.

In Figure 11, she paints an idealized *Self-Portrait*. Again we see her stubborn stance. And, as always, she wears pants. I do not know why she drew her legs so short this time, for her legs are actually very long, perfectly in proportion to her slender body. In reality Rina has short curly hair, olive-colored skin, and deep brown eyes. In her self-portrait she gives herself white skin, blue eyes with glamorous long lashes, and a mass of long black hair. The frame of butterflies and cats, made by means of potato prints, was my suggestion.

When I saw that Rina *always* painted herself in pants, I wondered whether in her unconscious she wanted to be a boy; but with that hair and those lips and eyelashes, my speculations vanished. Rina most certainly wanted to be a girl—if for the time being a wild one. Apparently, her tomboy pants and posture symbolize her stubborn wish to remain a child. She wants to be Peter Pan, the fairytale figure who never grew up. For if she grows up, Rina must face the sad reality that she is all alone in the world.

In Figure 12, *A Horse Eating the Fruit of a Sabre Cactus*, Rina uses a marvelous color scheme. She dares to put orange next to red. And she gives the horse a yellow face and blue eyes—blue eyes like Ruth's and mine, the blue eyes Rina would so much like to have herself.

Figure 12

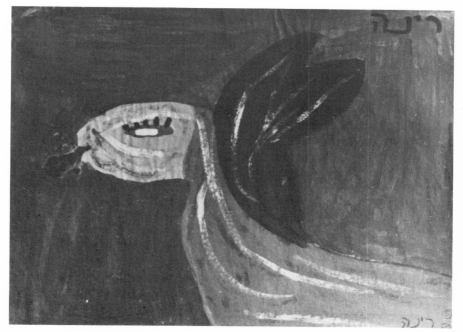

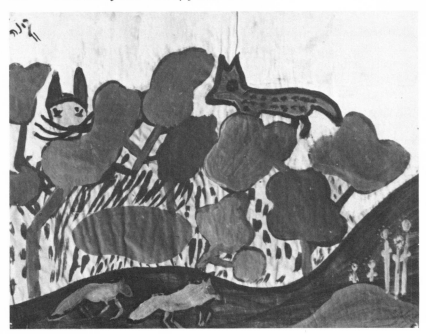

Figure 13

Figure 13, *Animals Coming to an Oasis to Drink,* shows Rina's good sense of composition. The pond, the most important thing to the animals, is the focal point of the picture. It is a desert scene with cacti growing at the lower right. Notice the funny tiger at the upper left. Rina's clowning sense of humor is coming more and more to the fore.

In Figure 14, we see *Rina Driving with Ruth* in Ruth's blue car—a happy scene. They drive along a river lined with trees, and all the trees are in bloom and have huge crowns. Rina-Kofiko, in the back seat, copies Ruth's driving, learning by imitation. Her yellow bird perches on the hood of the car, and in the air fly two big, beautiful butterflies—the symbols of transformation. It is significant that the road goes uphill.

Figure 15 is Rina's version of *What I Want to Be When I Grow Up.* She wants to be a cook, perhaps in grateful memory of the cook who mothered her. But also, she is a deprived child, and to deprived children even more than to others food and drink are love. Being fed is being loved. Indeed, many of Rina's pictures portray eating and drinking: *Feeding the Yellow Bird, A Horse Eating the Fruit of a Sabre Cactus, Animals Coming to an Oasis to Drink.* In these pictures it is Rina—in the form of her beloved animals—who is fed, while in Figure 15, it is *she* who is doing the feeding. In spite of all that has happened to her, stubborn, defiant Rina, always in pants and with legs apart and firmly planted on the ground, little Rina has enough love left in her to want to feed others.

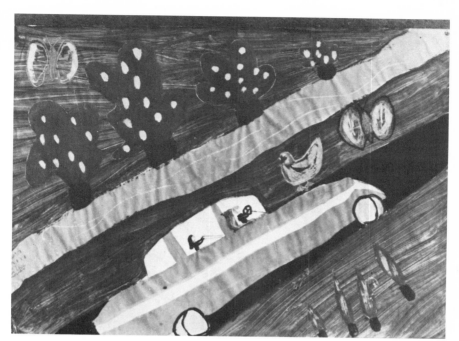

Figure 14

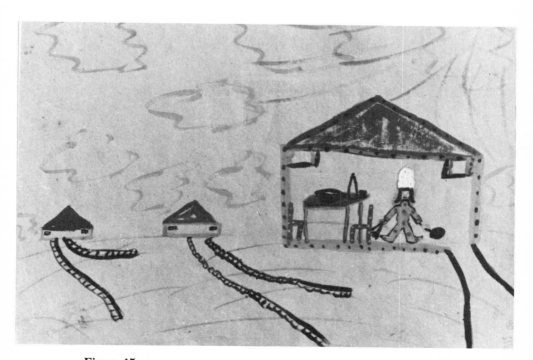

Figure 15

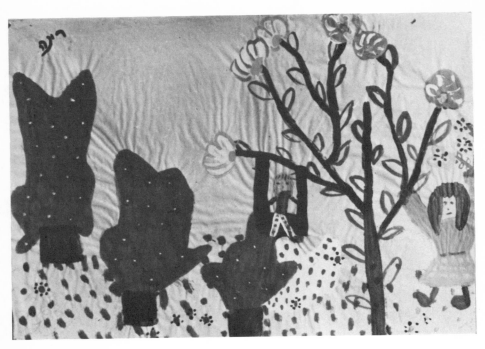

Figure 16

In Rina's last picture, Figure 16, *My Favorite Friend and I*, the whole world is in bloom. Rina's typical trees with the big crowns are laden with fruit. Fruit is food, and food is life-sustaining. We say, the tree *bears* fruit. And we speak in a general sense of *fruitfulness*. Fruit is thus a fertility symbol, and Rina's fruit-laden trees are a most glorious affirmation of life.

In the tree with the children's swing, the main stem—symbolizing the parents—is cut off, but *all* the branches—symbolizing the children, the offspring—are flowering. Rina's friend in the swing is much smaller than Rina and is perhaps someone Rina can mother. And now look at Rina herself. Rina has undergone a transformation: she wears her first dress!

During this period, Rina was transferred from the Nes Ziona school to the municipal school in the village. Children and teachers like her; she learns well and excels in painting, acting, and sports.

Ruth became pregnant and temporarily stopped working. But Rina, now convinced that Ruth loves her, accepted the separation with grace. When at last Rina was allowed to visit Ruth at her home, she greeted her shyly with a kiss. It was the first time Rina had ever dared to show Ruth her love.

I think that Rina has made the grade.

Conclusion

I began this paper by noting that even when I work with patients in groups, give them general subjects, and do *not* interpret, each patient unconsciously states his own problem, works on his own problem, and often solves his own problem. He tries to paint himself well, so to speak. What happens, apparently, is that insight is gained, not on a cognitive level but on a symbolic level.

We may draw a parallel with findings of research on the the phenomenon of sleep. It has been demonstrated that man can be deprived of sleep for some time without damage to his mental health; but he cannot be deprived of dreaming for any length of time without such damage.[2] Thus the dream has a health-promoting function; it affects our mental household even if we don't remember it.

It seems to me that the same is true for the arts. We paint or sculpt ourselves well—even if we don't know what we are doing and why, even though intellectually we do not understand our product or its message.

In a dream and on paper the unconscious seems to work toward insight in the language of pictures, a language of symbols.

A long, half-conscious thought process such as "Mothers have green eyes. Mothers have babies in their bellies. Mothers are cruel. . . . Cats have green eyes. Cats have babies in their bellies. Cats are cruel. . . . But perhaps there are some good mothers, for there are some good cats," can be expressed in one picture as Batja did in *Puss in Boots*, her portrayal of the good fairytale cat with smiling blue eyes, inspiring *trust*, not fear. This is powerful symbolic language, comprehended in a flash.

Of course, in a hospital many influences are at work. One cannot isolate the effect of art work but must consider it in conjunction with other therapeutic interventions and the whole protective environment. Nevertheless, seeing the healing process at work in Batja's and Rina's paintings was such a rewarding experience for me that I present it to you with the hope that you will share some of my satisfaction.

2. Ramon Greenberg, Chester A. Pearlman, and Dorothy Gampel, "War Neuroses and the Adaptive Function of REM Sleep," *British Journal of Medical Psychology*, Vol. 45, 1972;. Caroline Grieser, Ramon Greenberg, and Robert H. Harrison, "The Adaptive Function of Sleep: The Differential Effects of Sleep and Dreaming on Recall," *Journal of Abnormal Psychology*, Vol. 80, No. 3, 1972, pp. 280–86; and Ramon Greenberg and Chester A. Pearlman, "Cutting the REM Nerve: An Approach to the Adaptive Role of REM Sleep," Chicago, University of Chicago Press, *Perspectives in Biology and Medicine*, Vol. 17, No. 4, Summer 1974.

Art in a Class for Mentally Retarded Children

Lena L. Gitter

A special class for mentally retarded children in a regular public elementary school has important advantages but poses particular problems. While those whose intelligence is far below average cannot learn at the pace expected in the ordinary classroom, separate schools wall them off from the contemporaries among whom they will have to find their place as adults. In my experience, art provided the best means to help overcome the stigma of the special class. Largely through their art work, the retarded children won the acceptance, even the respect, of their more intelligent schoolmates. But this was perhaps the culmination of values developed within each child and among the children in the special classroom itself. Art played a paramount role in alleviating emotional stress and enabling the pupils to master basic school subjects to the limit of their ability.

The program I shall discuss was developed according to Montessori principles for a special class established at the request of the principal of the Greendale Elementary School, Seat Pleasant, Maryland. Most of the children referred to the class had been unable to handle regular school work. The age of these seven boys and four girls was from seven years one month to ten years nine months; and their intelligence quotients ranged from sixty-two to seventy. Their mental handicap had, of course, been compounded by the frustration of being unable to grasp what was being taught. In addition, many of them had physical problems such as speech defects and poor vision, which were the more difficult to correct since the parents seldom carried out the recommendations of the public health nurse.

The pupil personnel worker found it difficult to persuade the parents to accept the special placement. The fathers are laborers with unsteady employment, and a number of the mothers have jobs. These families, most of which are large, move frequently from one makeshift home to another.

Greendale School is a modern, one-story building with private exits from the primary rooms leading to the playground and a nearby wooded area. Each classroom has hot and cold water, drinking fountains, and lavatories—important luxuries that obviate many problems. There is a well-equipped cafeteria in the school. The special class is at one end of the building, a good location for the peculiar needs of this group. As teacher of the new class, I was determined to make it an integral part of the school community.

Art and Personal Identity

Art, in its broadest sense, played a stellar role in the early days when "Getting to know you" is so necessary, and "Getting to know myself" is possibly even more urgent.

Each child's physical outline was drawn by the teacher as he lay on a large piece of paper. The child cut out the silhouette, then filled in the details of his own likeness in color—eyes, skin, hair, and the clothes he was wearing at the time. Each life-size figure was put on display, and one could almost see learning take place.

Each pupil seemed overwhelmed at the realization that this was truly his own image. He was amazed at his own size, his proportions, the placement of his legs and arms, his individuality. Distinguishing himself from his classmates involved new awareness first of his own self. This set off the first spark of pride in his appearance.

The next step followed naturally: the comparison of himself with his classmates. The concepts of size—of small and large—and of pairs, the counting of the digits, limbs, and other parts of the body, and the recognition of the clothing that covers the body, grew out of this experience.

Sometimes consciousness of self seemed to dawn suddenly. On a sunny day a child suddenly observed and then sought for his shadow—his own shadow—and found it was distinct, different, his very own. The concepts of an image, a shadow, the self, took on a meaning that would have been almost impossible to achieve by any other method than the creation of the individual cut-out likenesses.

The children began to recognize their own reflections in the puddles left on the playground after the rain, and to fully comprehend the similarity as well as the difference between reflection, image, shadow. The beginning spark of curiosity about the world around them, the wonder about how the reflection got into the puddle, a new awareness outside of self, came to life. They ran after the shadow of a low-flying plane and marveled that the dog and cat cast shadows too. They took great pride in learning new words that signify ideas whose meanings they had grasped. That words need not be the names of persons, places, or things was something they had not understood before this awakening through the use of art.

Soon the children were trying to draw pictures of themselves. At first these drawings were all out of proportion, but gradually they discovered how the limbs fitted on the body, and observed relationships of size more accurately. Later we acquired a full-length mirror, and by studying themselves in various positions the children continued to develop the sense of their own identity that had begun with the cut-out figures.

They had seldom heard Mother Goose rhymes and children's stories, and so in class we did much reading and exclaiming over the pictures in the books. When they were familiar with a tale, they drew—each child's image of the part of the story he liked best. Or they drew pictures suggested by music; favorite records were *Sleepy Family*, *Peter and the Wolf*, *Swan Lake*, and *Sleeping Beauty*, the last three augmented by filmstrips. The children were very proud of these pictures which showed their own personal reactions to rhymes and stories.

This led to questions about the mechanics of art: "How do I color it? How do I draw it? How do I paint it? How? How? How?"

To help answer this bombardment, a number of excellent filmstrips are available, which explain color, line, and form, and stimulate imagination. We discussed fully what was shown, sometimes using only part of a filmstrip on a single day. Some of the older children showed that they had grasped what colors can do in the creation of a foreground or a background. There was even a slight hint that it might become possible for them to understand perspective.

Painting and Writing

Some children who had never been able to master the alphabet learned to make letters through music, dancing, and painting. First they danced with sheer abandon to the compelling rhythm, then recorded sweeping gestures on the paper with colored chalk as they continued to stand and sway to the music. Then we developed exercises delineating the shape of letters. This rhythmic movement forming each letter seemed to enable the pupils to write correctly after the exercises had been repeated and repeated and repeated.

A brush and a jar of paint helped enlarge vocabularies. The brush was used like a big, fat pencil to draw the pictures that words like "smoke," "sunshine," and "wind" conjure up. Or the process was reversed, and pictures or designs were developed out of the letters of a child's name. Each was eager to have his name used. This not only helped the children remember the alphabet, but was a source of much pride to the child selected. He was delighted by this use of what was so very much his and his alone—his name! Some very inhibited children, who thought they could never make any kind of picture, were drawn into painting almost without knowing it by playing this sort of game with letters and numbers.

Sometimes during the art period we played a phonograph record called *The Nonsense Alphabet*, where the letters stand for silly characters or unusual animals that become involved in dramatic situations. This inspired the children to use the alphabet as a base for cartoon-style characters. For instance, one child drew a large "A," then added eyes, ears, and mouth, and from this developed a funny animal. Meantime alphabet cards were on display, and between the rhythmic exercises, the nonsense record, and the cartooning, the sequence of the alphabet, so vital to their academic work, was grasped by some children who had never been able to learn it by rote.

The children loved making the funny pictures, and what started as a writing exercise resulted in another important, good, new experience. Looking at each other's work and laughing at each other, they discovered that they not only could enjoy laughing, but they didn't mind being laughed at. Being laughed at when making a caricature meant success—the more laughter, the more success. They were used to the kind of laughing at another's work which brought on anger, tears, and blows, and usually ended with the ridiculed child destroying his own picture. Now they learned for the first time that one doesn't always laugh at people to hurt them, but sometimes with warm, friendly feeling.

Children spontaneously sought from each other the help they sometimes needed to complete a picture. By working together in this way they learned the value of cooperation, without the teacher's intervention. The helper gained through the realization that he could help; the one helped surmounted a problem through the extension of this hand of friendship by his classmate. However, we did not attempt murals, as I did not think the children were ready for sustained work in organized groups.

Children often understand each other's expressive needs, so that spontaneous joint effort does not destroy the personal character of the drawing. It is quite unlike the well-meaning adult's drawing on a child's picture in an alien style that leaves the child bewildered, with a work no longer his own. And when children choose to imitate a classmate's work, it is usually because something about it suits their inner demands. They take from it what they wish, and are free to transform it or depart from it. This kind of copying therefore has an entirely different effect from the teacher's setting up things to copy, and insisting that they be copied accurately.

The Angry Drum

Sometimes the children could work off violent feelings through movement, sound, and eventually through painting. We made a big drum out of an empty barrel, and decorated it with Indian designs and musical notes in bright colors. It came to be known as "The Angry Drum," so often was it beaten on by an infuriated child, who formerly would have slammed doors, smashed equipment, and attacked his classmates.

For Kevin, the drum was not always enough. Sometimes beating on it seemed to intensify his anger, and he would turn from it to knock over furniture and strike out at other children. Whether or not they hit back, after a while he would burst into tears, then calm down.

On one occasion he was able to tell me the cause of his distress: it was his eighth birthday and his mother said he was now too old for playthings, so she was going to throw out all his toys. Kevin asked again and again whether I too was going to forbid him to play. Despite all my assurances he was still very upset. This time, instead of banging on the Angry Drum, he seized paint and brushes, and with violent, slashing strokes made a big picture of it (Figure 1). The jagged design was Kevin's own contribution; the decorations on the actual drum are much more static.

For once, instead of letting his rage drive him to destructive acts that left him sore and exhausted, or just dissipating it in harmless banging, Kevin had managed to harness all this wild energy. Everybody admired his vivid picture, and the principal asked to have it hung in her office. She told Kevin how much she liked it, and for many months I found opportunities to send him to her office so he could see that his drum was still hanging there.

It is sometimes difficult to maintain discipline with children such as these. Sandra, who painted Figure 2, explained that the long, menacing arm showed it was a portrait of me scolding her. The other children naturally

Figure 1   The Angry Drum

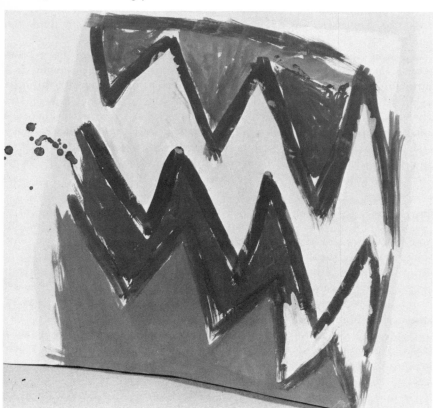

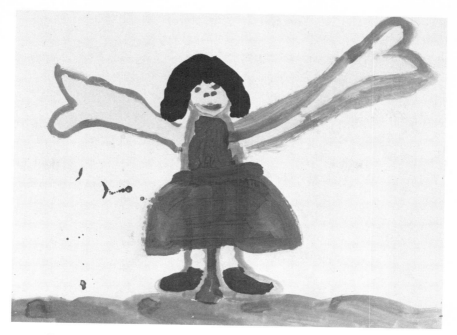

Figure 2 The Angry Teacher

appreciated her caricature, and I could join in their laughter at the teacher with the long, long arm. Before we introduced painting, and had the materials available so that the children could turn quickly to them in a moment of stress, Sandra met my reprimands with curses, and sometimes even hit me, inevitably generating more bad feeling in me and herself. Her picture, on the other hand, evoked a good response, and remained as a source of pride, since it was displayed for a long time on the classroom bulletin board.

The Angry Drum figured in other paintings too. One of them seemed to mark a turning point for ten-year-old Jimmy, one of our most disturbed boys. He is the oldest of eight children, and they live in a sordid, *Tobacco Road* sort of neighborhood. Jimmy's instability had been noticed ever since the time, five years before, when he saw his twin brother struck and killed by an automobile. Their mother, who was carrying her youngest child and leading a toddler by the hand, held Jimmy responsible for the tragic accident. "See what you've done," she screeched at him.

Jimmy was always covered with bruises and cuts, some of them self-inflicted. He had frequent infections, and once he had stuck something in his ears, piercing both drums and inducing a chronic trouble that became worse from time to time. He was frequently hospitalized, losing a lot of school time, so that it was hard for him to keep up even in the special class. He was another child for whom beating on the drum sometimes was not enough to stave off a violent temper tantrum.

Before Easter I asked the children to bring in hard-boiled eggs to paint.

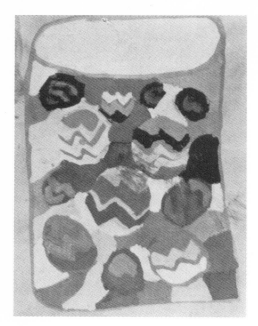

Figure 3   The Easter Drum

Jimmy's father had work only occasionally, and the big family was very poor. Perhaps Jimmy's mother would have liked to give him the eggs but could not. All she said to him was, "You're too big now to color Easter eggs. That's for babies." So Jimmy was angry not only at his mother but at me, because I had asked for something that his mother considered "baby stuff."

Here were the beautiful colors and hard-boiled eggs laid out, and everybody went to work—everybody except Jimmy. After a while he pulled out a big roll of manila wrapping paper, knocked it down on the floor with a loud bang, unrolled a large piece and cut it off angrily with a long shears. With black paint he outlined a huge drum, as big as the real one (about three feet tall and one and a half feet wide). Then he decorated it with notes similar to the musical notes on the original drum—but each note looked like an Easter egg (Figure 3).

The other children took time out from painting their eggs to admire Jimmy's very pleasing picture. We could see the joy in his face over this creation—a joy that overcame his jealousy of the beautifully colored eggs of the rest of the class.

Jimmy had not only dealt with a difficult situation, but he had shown for the first time a talent for handling color and form. When his interest in painting continued, I displayed some of his artwork. With this recognition, his self-confidence increased and he began to have some success in academic learning. His tantrums became less frequent, and he did not even have to resort so often to violent beating on the drum.

Effects of Poverty

Possibly holiday pictures mean more to children from poor homes than they do to those who are better off materially. We discuss the meaning of the holidays, and by painting pictures of related themes (Figure 4) the children seem to feel that they have a part in the celebration even though their parents cannot afford fancy dinners or elaborate gifts.

The school provides special holiday food because some children might not otherwise get any, making a nominal charge so that they will not appear to others or to themselves as objects of charity. Before Thanksgiving, Danny's mother sent a note asking permission to pay later for his turkey dinner, since she could not spare even thirty cents that week out of her meagre relief payments. Danny, in turn, painted a turkey (Figure 5) to take to his mother and the other children at home.

When families like Danny's get a real turkey, it comes from a charitable organization, and the uncertainty and suspense surrounding the donation, plus mixed feelings about accepting it, make the approaching holiday a source of anxiety. Danny's turkey picture not only helped ease the holiday tension, but represented another kind of triumph. He was a very timid boy who came from a broken home; for a long time he couldn't learn to write, and was unable to draw without using a ruler or the Montessori geometric insets.

It seemed as if he started to write all of a sudden, and at about the same time he gave up these supports of his own free will. His pictures, however,

Figure 4   Thanksgiving Theme

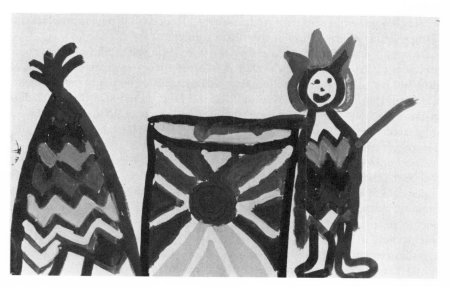

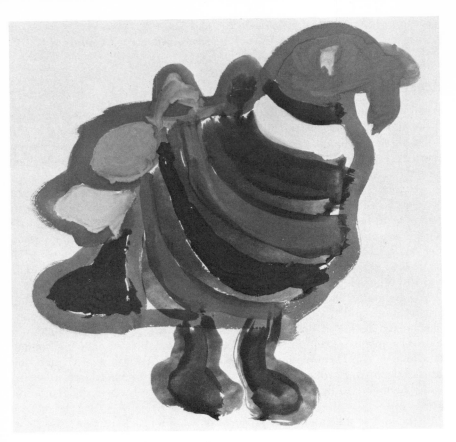

Figure 5   Thanksgiving Turkey

still tended to be wishy-washy. The turkey was the first one where he achieved a powerful effect through contrast, using dark browns and blacks to bring out the bright colors of the bird's plumage.

I have observed that for some children with little self-confidence the ruler serves as a sort of temporary crutch. I tolerate their use of such mechanical aids, but try to be alert to the moment when they may be ready for a change, and to find some positive suggestion that will help them make the break. For instance, when Danny had one day stated his plan to draw a boat, I suggested that it should be a great *big* one, and I must have hit it right, because from then on he stopped asking for the ruler.

The houses where the children live are likely to be condemned, and for this and other reasons, the families move frequently. Nancy showed her concern over an impending move by first portraying the entire family around their rural home (Figure 6). Although usually mother is the most important person in these children's lives, Nancy's father is the strongest member of this particular household. The mother, who drinks to excess, is the small, pale figure at the top center. Next, Nancy seemed to derive a good deal of comfort from trying to visualize the apartment house (Figure 7) which she

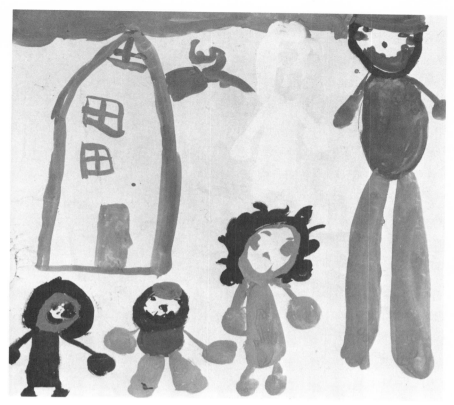

Figure 6   House and Family

Figure 7   Apartment House with Lots of Lights

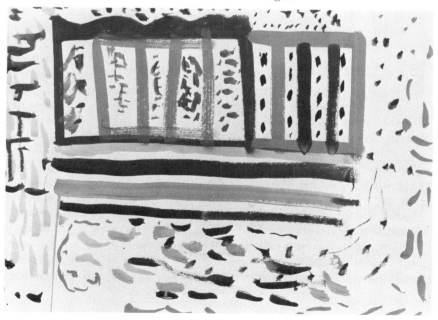

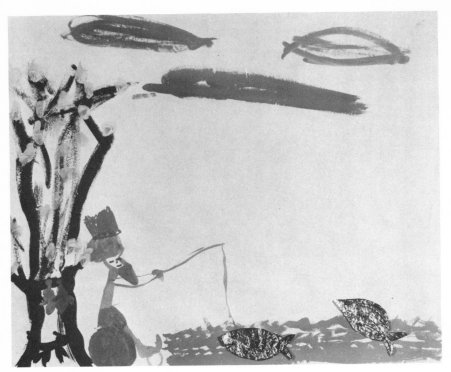

Figure 8   The Royal Fisherman

had heard described as her future home but which she had never seen.

Betty was able to seize on a fairytale, "The King's Fisherman," to illustrate (Figure 8) at a time when a parallel theme was a source of real consternation to her and her family. All the children adored their handsome, unreliable father, who had just lost his job because he was AWOL once too often in order to go fishing. The king in the story had plenty of troubles; Betty wanted to think of her father, despite all *his* problems, as something of a regal figure too. Concentrating on her picture, she apparently could contemplate the real situation with a little detachment; certainly she appeared somewhat relieved. It was near the end of the school year, and we displayed Betty's picture in the main corridor with a sign wishing everybody a "King-Size Vacation." Many people expressed their admiration.

The fish in this illustration were carefully shaded and decorated with colored pencils, then cut out and pasted onto the more freely brushed-in background. This kind of small, highly finished drawing, where a ruler can even sometimes be used appropriately, used to be common in European schools. Attractive effects are possible, and children like the feeling of reality and solidity they can achieve by working in this way.

Unfortunately, artwork that meets the children's emotional needs does not always appeal to their parents. Sometimes I have to help the pupils make something usable, which may not be very original but will help the child gain stature in the eyes of his family. One Christmas I got some inexpensive fabric we could cut into doilies and napkins, and with alphabet stamps and green, red, and black stamp pads we were able to make up attractive designs which were easy to execute with almost machine-like perfection. The parents admired these gifts and it helped them accept art as something useful and beautiful. Too often they tended to look upon it as a waste of class time. These applied art or craft projects were important in maintaining a good feeling between child, home, and teacher.

Later, when the children had become bolder in making experiments, they took scrap plywood and followed the grain to draw abstract shapes, which they painted in various colors. These decorative pieces were shellacked and made into trays or scrapbook covers. Almost all the children, from the sloppiest to the most inhibited, could produce something reasonably attractive by this method. Not only were the products popular at home, but the discovery was taken up by the children in the regular classes, making the retarded children feel even more proud of their invention.

The Special Class and the Regular Classes

Through art much of the curiosity about the designation of our class as "special" was dispelled, and a healthy exchange with children from the regular classes became possible.

To bring the special class into closer contact with other pupils, two films were shown to them together with all the primary grades. One film gives a simple explanation of artistic principles; the other was *Make Way for Ducklings*, a beloved story whose situations and language are close to these children's experience. The children made their own illustrations of the story, and we held a contest. Each class selected its own winner; these pictures were displayed together, and a faculty committee awarded the final prize.

Some people disapprove, I know, of art contests in schools. I felt that the children had to learn that people do compete with each other, and I wanted to help them realize that not everybody can win, and nobody can win all the time. That is one reason why I chose *Make Way for Ducklings*. Author-illustrator Robert McCloskey won an American Library Association award for the illustrations of this book. The children also knew and loved several of his other stories. I could point out to them that McCloskey kept right on making books and pictures for us to enjoy even though only *one* of his books won a prize. The children were eager to select the "best" picture in the class, and were exceedingly proud of their classmate whose picture hung in the main corridor with the other winners. Comparing the retarded children's drawings with the others, we observed that at best their pictures were on the level of work by normal first-graders. Yet somehow they managed to become the leaders of the whole school in esthetic matters.

Returning from a trip to Europe, I brought back some children's paintings and recordings, as well as slides of great pictures that I thought would appeal to the children at Greendale School. My class helped prepare displays, and invited other classes to hear the recordings and see the slides. All the children were excited to discover that they could "read" the pictures by foreign children even when the words on the recordings were quite incomprehensible. But they were most enthusiastic about the Dutch master, Jan Steen, because he depicted everyday life, including a lot of disorder—animals in the house and water spilling on the floor. It wasn't very different from their own home surroundings. If they had understood only one artist, I would have been pleased, but that was not all. I was amazed to be bombarded with questions when I showed some Rembrandts: "How does the light get into his pictures? Where does it come from?" So the slides led to still greater interest in techniques of painting, and we secured children's art books which explained and illustrated ways of using different art media.

By this time there were two special classes in the school, mine having the younger students. The teacher of the older group and I discussed ways in which our pupils could earn money for the March of Dimes, and concluded that shining shoes would be practical.

The children designed posters to advertise their shoe-shine shop to the school; a lot of language and art work went into these. There was quite a bit of competition between the two special classes. My class compensated for the handicap of being younger by setting up an interesting shoe display—shoes of different colors, sizes, and materials; shoes for various sports or to go with certain uniforms. It was later moved from our classroom to the public display case in the center hall, and drew contributions from all the pupils in the school.

The shoe display stimulated picture-making; they wanted to draw the strange-looking shoes brought in by other children, shoes that their fathers had collected while overseas with the armed forces. But beyond inspiring the children's art productions, the shoes became the stepping-stone from which they stepped into the whole world. Suddenly they were interested in geography and the people who inhabited the many places from which the shoes came, and they wanted to draw these different people. We were able to find a few appropriate slides on art, such as Van Gogh's painting *The Old Shoes*. They were amazed that a famous painter would concern himself with such a common subject as shoes—battered, work-worn shoes just like those they often saw at home.

But perhaps most important of all, the shared display of shoes brought the other children of the school into the world of the retarded child, making for all of these children a piece of common ground where they could share the same interest. This atmosphere of goodwill was reflected in a beautiful poster my class created: the old woman who lived in a shoe. Some of them thought it represented me, but they said it was no longer the old woman who "didn't know what to do." All of them had found their place in the school and in the community, and so it was now the "old woman who knew what to do." For the sake of the children and this wonderful experience they had had, for once I didn't mind being called an old woman.

PART FOUR

CASE STUDIES

Do You Know What Is a Djobbeh?

Sondra K. Geller

Rose Klein, a seventy-eight-year-old resident of the Hebrew Home of the Greater Washington (D.C.) Area, had never worked with clay. "I don't know how to do this thing," she said. "I never learned."

I brought the clay to the table. When she saw it her face twisted into a grimace. "Ich!" she said with disgust, nodding disapproval. I cajoled her into handling it, even in its sticky, clammy state. "Martha, Gussie, Hyman, Gertrude, Fanny—they have all worked with the clay. You're a sissy! Have you ever made a matzo ball?" I queried. "Yes, of course," she boomed. "Well then," as I handed her a mass of clay, "make a matzo ball!"

She made contact . . . her hands held the brown lump and then she started to roll it. "A *groise* or a *clainike*?" (a big one or a little one) she asked. "Whatever you like," I replied. Soon she was busily rolling out clay matzo balls. "I like this," she said. At that point, my attention moved to someone else for a few mintues. When I came back to Rose, I saw the shape represented in Figure 1. I started to ask what it was, but I checked myself. Sometimes an interruption stops the creative flow, making the client/artist self-conscious.

Some twenty to thirty minutes later Rose announced that she had completed her work (Figure 2). She asked, "Do you know what it is? How do you say in English—this small animal that lives near the water?" She began to make jumping movements with her hands and a croaking sound emerged from her throat. Her eyes twinkled with delight. "A frog," the reply was chorused by the group. "That's right. You see his legs and his big eyes? Who knows this word 'frog' in Yiddish?" she asked. "Frog?" "Frog?" the group strained to remember. "I know this word," said Rose. "It is a *djobbeh*." "Djobbeh." "Yes, *djobbeh*." The others nodded their heads. Very pleased with her experience with clay, Rose lifted herself from her chair, took her walker, and slowly made her way from the room.

I was captivated by her spontaneous creation—pleased with her pleasure.

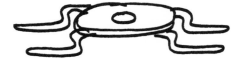

Figure 1

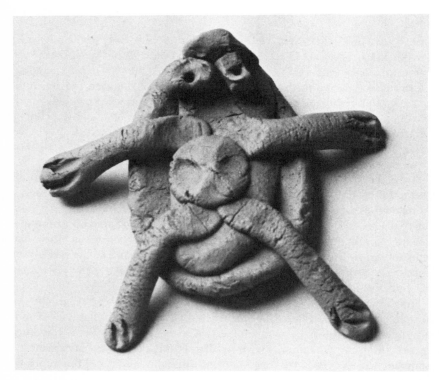

Figure 2

The following day I passed Rose on my way into the Home. She was sitting outdoors, knitting. I stopped and we chatted. "You know," she said, "I've been thinking about that frog. I remember now . . . it was during the war. We were in a place that had many trees. What do you call that?" "A forest," I offered. "Yes, a forest. We were in a forest, hiding . . . and there was this water and we could see the eyes of many frogs along the edge." She paused.

"Ach! the war! You know, we had no water to drink. People here don't know what it was like . . . we had no water and we went to that little water, with the frogs." She cupped her hands and dipped them into the water of her memory, then put them carefully to her mouth. "We drank that dirty water . . . it was terrible . . . the war. People here don't appreciate, they think it is this way. I appreciate. Always, I say, thanks God, even for a little water."

The day after Rose's story to me about the frogs, I saw her again in the second of her group's twice-weekly art therapy sessions. I was excited about her experience and hoped she would share it with the group. How surprised I was when Rose looked at the little frog in my outstretched hand and made the gesture of spitting over her shoulder! She shuddered as she said, "Take it away! I don't want to look at it!" But she responded to the silent questioning of the group. "It's about the war . . . it was . . ." She proceeded to tell them the story in spite of herself.

I remembered then one of the first things Rose had said to me five months before. "I will try Art, but I have already tried Poetry, News Discussions, and other events. I will not go to these. They talk of things that make me remember the war. I can't . . . I can't talk about it." I respected her obvious determination.

Rose had entered the Home seeking refuge from thirteen years of virtual imprisonment alone in her small apartment in a rough section of town where old people were mugged regularly and drunks slept on her doorstep. She had known only four years of happiness in the United States when her husband died.

The war-scarred couple came to the Washington area to be near a niece and nephew. Precious few members of their large families had survived the Holocaust. Both Rose and her husband eagerly attended Americanization School. She proudly displays their graduation certificates in her room at the Home. They began to settle down to what they hoped would be a secure, quiet life.

Thus it was with great hesitation that I followed my instincts some days after her refusal to look at the frog and took the Djobbeh story to show Rose. She reacted as I hoped she might. The words, typewritten on the pages I handed her, told the story of the spontaneous production of a frog and some poignant associations to it. The story provided Rose distance from her pain. We sat together on her bed as she read aloud. She chuckled with delight, nodding her approval and saying, "That's right, that's it exactly! Exactly!" Then her voice began to crack as she read her own description of the war. Her eyes filled with tears. "I do appreciate." She reached out and gave me a bear hug.

In the weeks and months that have followed, Rose has not shut herself off as much from her memories of the war. She has told me of the horror of her separation from her husband, neither knowing where the other had been taken after they were dragged from their home, or, indeed, if the other was still alive. It was nothing short of miraculous, she says, that they found each other after the war through newspaper advertisements in the European press. Recently, she has pulled out dozens of dog-eared snapshots which she has pasted up all over her room. She introduces them lovingly; "Mama, Papa, my brothers, my sister, my two uncles, my cousins . . . fifty members of my family . . . all killed in the war." She pauses, taking her head in her hands. "Hitler" . . . her voice fades. I feel the pain in her silence, but can only guess at the agonies she carries in her heart.

Autobiography of a Ten-Year-Old

"Introduction" and "Comment" by Edith Kramer
"Self-Biography" by Angel

Introduction

I have described work in art therapy with Angel, an unusually talented disturbed child, in two articles which appeared earlier in the *Bulletin of Art Therapy*.[1] The experiences that form the basis of these discussions occurred when Angel was between the ages of six and eight. I have continued seeing him for two more years and now present his own account of his life as he wrote and illustrated it in his art therapy sessions at the age of ten.

For readers who do not recall the previous material, I recapitulate briefly. Angel was the first child of an unmarried Puerto Rican woman who, shortly after his birth, married a man who was not Angel's father. The family moved to New York when Angel was between two and three years old and there his two half-siblings were born.

At the age of four years and three months, Angel was brought to Jacobi Hospital. He had stopped speaking, watched television incessantly, and seemed to believe that he was Superman, climbing onto window sills and acting as if he were about to fly off. Also he had become dangerously aggressive toward his younger siblings.

As a patient in the children's ward, Angel soon emerged from his withdrawal. He began to speak and formed good relationships with staff members and other children. His preoccupation with Superman, whom he impersonated in a homemade cape, persisted.

1. "Art Therapy and the Severely Disturbed Gifted Child, Part 1," Vol. 5, No. 1, October 1965; "The Problem of Quality in Art, II: Stereotypes," Vol. 6, No. 4, July 1967.

At the age of five, Angel began drawing pictures of Superman and thereupon ceased wearing the cape. In addition, he drew other heroic figures, such as Hercules, and later Batman and Robin. This became his major preoccupation. The precocious skills developed in the service of his delusional fantasies attained a certain degree of autonomy, so that he could also draw excellent pictures of subjects not related to his need for omnipotence.

Angel's treatment at the hospital included intensive psychotherapy, occupational therapy, and, from the age of six on, art therapy. When he was seven and a half years old, he had improved considerably and was placed in a Catholic children's home for normal dependent children where he remained for the next three years. Placement was necessary because Angel's parents had separated, and his two half-siblings had been left by the mother in the care of their paternal grandmother. The resulting situation in the home of Angel's stepfather and stepgrandmother was too insecure and chaotic to risk as an environment for the still-vulnerable child. Since the institution where Angel lived was not far from Jacobi Hospital, it was possible for hospital staff members to continue treating him for the next three years.

During the first two years, art therapy sessions were held at the Kennedy Home. In the third year, feeling that Angel needed to broaden his horizon, I took him out on sketching trips, or held art sessions at my studio.

The production of Angel's autobiography extended over three sessions. In the first, he dictated the story of his past and drew most of the pictures for it. He also insisted that I add my recollections of him to his own account. This led us to look at his old drawings and choose two of them to illustrate his early style of work.

In the following session Angel added the passage on his hopes and worries about the future and drew the picture of his future home.

Angel had now produced all the material needed for his book. He could not, however, have completed it without some technical help from me. His original drawings were made on sheets of paper of different sizes, some of them too large. I therefore photographed them all and had eight- by ten-inch prints made. I also typed the story, which had been taken down in longhand. Since both narrative and illustrations were well conceived and entirely his own, and the whole undertaking was an important step in Angel's development, it seemed worthwhile indeed to help him succeed in completing his book.

At last Angel composed the dummy, working with scissors and paste to put photographs and text together. He added some new illustrations as he went along. A number of Xerox copies were made for him from this dummy.

As Angel dictated his story he remarked, "Isn't it marvelous how much I remember of my past!" His account, which is indeed essentially correct and coherent, will be followed by the art therapist's further comments.

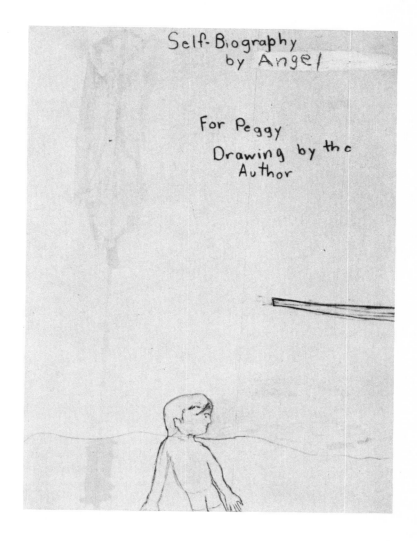

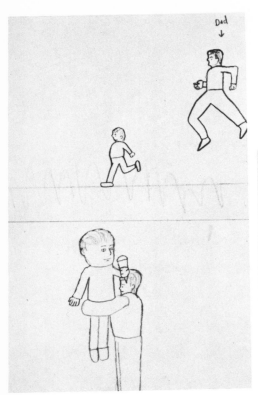

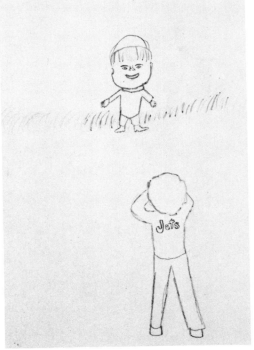

I was born on March 18, 1957, in San Juan, Puerto Rico. Nothing really happened until I was two years old, and then it all began. I ran away, and then when my father found me he gave me an ice cream cone.

My father was playing baseball with other people one day. One guy hit the ball too far and it came to me. I thought it was something to eat and tried to lick it. My father came and took it away. After the game I had my picture taken with a baseball cap.

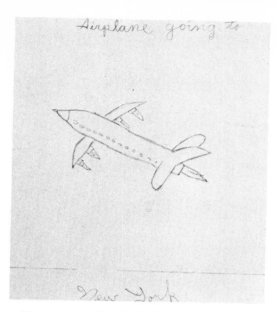

We moved to New York when I was three years old I think.

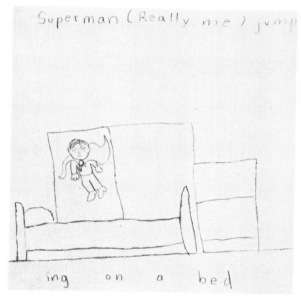

When I was three my brother was born and I was mad because I wanted to be the only child in the family.

When my brother grew older I began to hit him. I pretended I was Superman and that he was the bad guy, and I hit him real hard when we had fights, like Superman does. I said I hate a little brother, because he always bugs me!

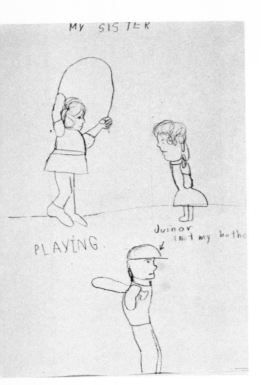

MY SISTER

PLAYING.

Junior not my brother

A sister was born two years after, but she was alright for she played with other girls instead of bothering me.

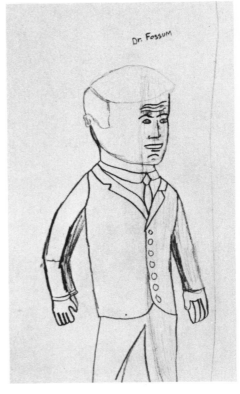

Dr. Fossum

When I was four years old I came to Jacobi Hospital because of what I did to my brother. I met Doctor Fossum, a nice man over there just like a social worker. He is a talking doctor; he helps you with your problems. When I wrote this book at the age of ten, I was in Kennedy Home at the Bronx, and Dr. Fossum comes to see me every week on Friday, in case we have something to talk in private.

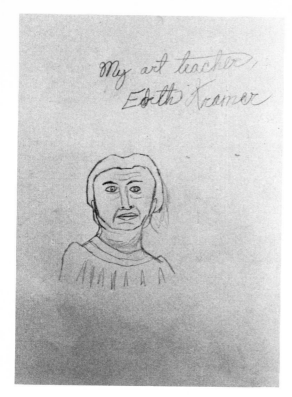

My art teacher, Edith Kramer

And then I met Miss Kramer when I was six years old. I already could draw. I am a very good drawer, and reading is one of my hobbies too, but I did not read until I was in Kennedy Home.

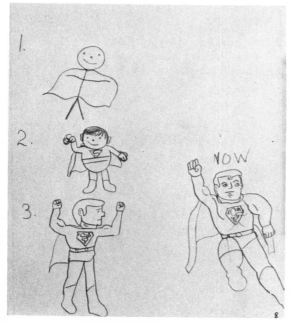

1.

2.

3.

NOW

When I started drawing I first drew stick men, and then I drew circle men and then men that looked like the cartoon of Dick Tracy. Here are samples:

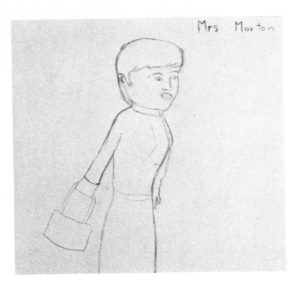

Every time there was no art lessons and I was
not in school the nurse would take some drawing
paper and crayons and coloring books, and I would
do some of both of them. And then when four
years passed, I went to Kennedy Home. And then
when I got there Miss Kramer came on Wednes-
days but now it's changed to Saturday. And Mrs.
Morton comes on Tuesday and Dr. Fossum comes
on Friday.

And then when I was nine I got into the seven
feet swimming pool and when I got on the diving
board I got scared and I overcame the scaredness.

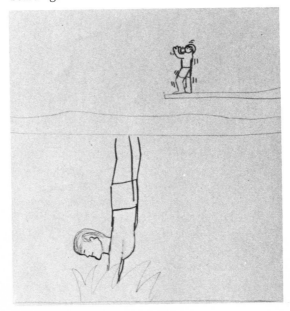

And then at ten I made up a song. Here it goes in the tune of "The Whole Wide World in His Hand."

> I got a big family, oh yes (repeat two more times)
> And they do something all day
> I got a little brother, oh yes (repeat twice)
> And he keeps bugging me all day
> I got a tiny tiny sister, oh yes (repeat twice)
> And she plays house all day
> I got a big father, oh yes (repeat twice)
> And he complains all day
> I got a little mother, oh yes (repeat twice)
> And she keeps house all day

Miss Kramer's Story

I am Angel's art teacher. I am helping him write his self-biography. He asked me to write my impressions of him when I first met him when he was six years old.

At this time Angel could already draw very well, and he was proud of it. On the walls of the hospital I saw many pictures of Superman which Angel had drawn.

When I told Angel that I was an artist he asked me to draw something for him, and so I drew his portrait. He took it and added a long black necktie to the drawing and then he drew a picture of his father beside it and gave him a long black tie too. He explained that his daddy would let him wear his tie next time he came for a visit. I thought this little boy likes his father very much and thinks a lot about him.

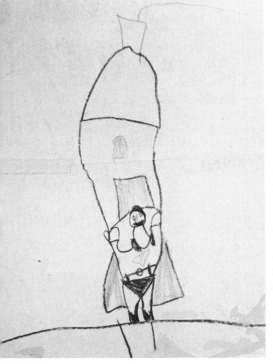

Next Angel drew a picture of Superman picking up a house. I wondered in my mind what house this was, but I did not at this time ask Angel about it. Now, as we were talking about the story, Angel explained that the house was Jacobi Hospital, and that Superman would throw the house, but that he would run fast, and catch it again, and put it where it belongs.

Next Angel drew Clark Kent taking off his coat and his glasses and turning into Superman. Now, Angel explained that he thought when he was six years old, that his father made Clark Kent's glasses. He got the idea, because his father was at this time working in a factory where frames for eyeglasses were made.

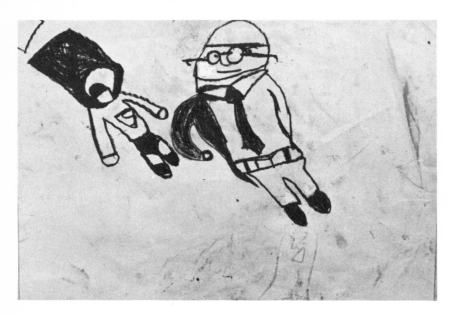

Angel continues:

Next I am anxious about my nearby future. About when I am going home for good and when I am becoming a real artist.

When I do go home I will wait until I am about eighteen and then I am going away. I will move to the country. I will move to a lake where I can swim and fish. And I plan to get married. And have two children, a boy and a girl, one of them named after me. I can build a little shack to be my studio.

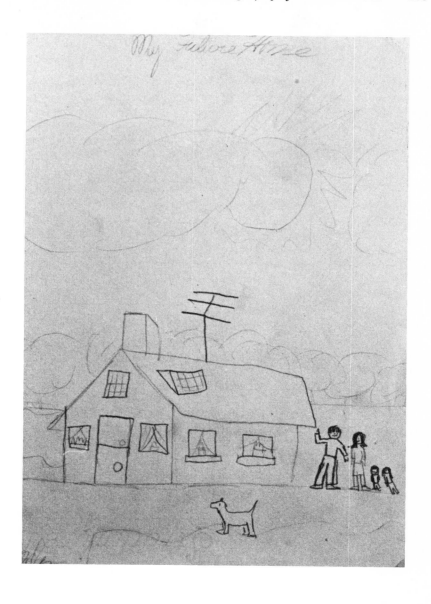

Comment

Angel's story of his infancy, where father protects and feeds him and mother is not mentioned, reflects real experiences. Mother seems never to have been able to give her children much care and warmth. Angel's stepfather, who has known him since he was a baby, always treated him as if he were his own child and has been, insofar as he was able, a kind and faithful parent to him.

It is interesting that in his account of the etiology of his superman fantasy Angel stresses jealousy of his younger brother, an element to which, in my earlier account, I gave relatively little weight. On the other hand, Angel says nothing about his need for omnipotence, a motive which I had stressed. It seems likely that Angel is unconscious of the latter aspect of his disturbance because the need for omnipotence persists, while he can admit to the sibling rivalry because it has been successfully worked through in psychotherapy. At ten years of age Angel still maintains a stream of fantasies about the heroes of television, and in times of stress he withdraws into this fantasy world.

Angel's presentation of his development as an artist and of the three people who worked with him for so many years needs no comment. The likenesses of his doctor and of the art and occupational therapists are excellent.

In his song about his family, Angel permits himself to express negative feelings in a jocular form, but he also improves on the real situation by bringing back his mother and thus restoring the family's unity. At the time the song was written mother did not keep house for her husband and children, but lived apart from them. On home visits Angel stayed with his paternal stepgrandmother who kept house for his stepfather and Angel's two half-siblings.

Angel's conquest of the water is the major success story of the book. On the title page we see him coming up after a high dive, and the whole book is dedicated to his swimming teacher. When Angel learned to swim and dive, his early fantasies of possessing the power of levitation were to some extent fulfilled. The transformation on page 260 of the shivering little figure on the diving board into the victorious diver recalls his earlier drawings of the transformation of Clark Kent into Superman. Thus Angel accurately portrays his present state, poised between fantasy and reality but moving toward the conquest of the real world.

Angel has not much to say about his future, which is indeed uncertain. It is encouraging that his aspirations are realistic rather than megalomaniac. After the story was written Angel was placed in a foster home, and he and his foster family seem to be pleased with each other. After six years of institutional existence, Angel will, if all goes well, experience a few years of family life before his childhood ends.

Conclusion

Angel's autobiography is not merely an interesting postscript to my articles. It is presented because the child's own words and drawings are the most eloquent testimonial that could be found for the value of continued treatment geared to a child's special needs. It testifies to the importance of continuity in the therapeutic relationship, to the need for teamwork, and last but not least it shows how art therapy can help the feeling of identity to crystallize and the sense of past, present, and future to develop.

Children who live for a long time in institutions suffer from changes of personnel. Counselors, social workers, teachers, therapists come and go. The child can draw little sustenance from an endless succession of personalities even though each of them may be well-meaning and competent. If he allows himself to be drawn into strong relationships he finds that his attachments inevitably end with loss. After a while he learns to hold himself aloof. He keeps his relationships shallow, and so it comes to pass that a great many children who live in institutions grow up to be empty people even when the adults who took care of them were kind and well trained. Ultimately these conditions also erode the child-care worker's and therapist's professional zeal and capacity for empathy so that they also are in danger of becoming hollow shells.

An encounter such as this one with Angel is, therefore, a sustaining experience also for therapists, who must as a rule face tragedy and can seldom contribute to the good outcome of a situation which is not without hope. It remains tragic that Angel's story is exceptional not only because of his rare gifts but because the kind of help which he received is unusual in our public institutions.

Postscript: Twelve Years Later

Angel is now twenty-two years old, and art continues to be an important stabilizing factor in his life.

The foster home where he was placed at age ten proved unsuitable, and Angel again lived in a group home until he went away to an out-of-town college. Meantime he had won a place in the High School of Music and Art in New York City where he readily learned commercial art skills. He did well in college, earning his way by means of restaurant jobs. It was in the middle of his junior year that I wrote asking his permission to reprint the "Self-Biography" in this collection. Angel's reply to my letter was in part as follows:

It was very interesting and very revealing to read about my past in detail. . . . It came at a very opportune time and I needed to read that in order for me to open some doors in my head that were closed at the time. . . .

College and I will be parting our ways after this semester. . . . I need something more than school at the moment. . . . After I made dean's list, the challenge of a liberal arts education suddenly disappeared. . . .

I do have a job as a commercial artist starting this summer . . . but I can't see doing this the rest of my life. Of course I would still like to go overseas and study art. . . . I just couldn't go to school, work at McDonald's, study, and concentrate on my artistic progress, so for now I think I will work and draw at the same time. . . . I plan to take a year off from school.

He also enclosed the following poem, apparently inspired by the look into his past afforded by reading my comments and his own story about his early years:

Nothing but the Light

By the time he could kick he was constant motion
legs pumping piston-fast accelerating over all obstacles—
in fact he was so fast he could outrun the wind

No matter what he would go his way oblivious to all
*   that was captured inside that little head of his*

But when he sat down to recollect himself,
visions of his past pleasure floated by so quickly all he could
*   see was the tail-end of his future running toward a star at the*
*   end of the sky*

Before he could think
he was up chasing what he would hope to find ahead

Calling upon that little extra he thought he must've used years ago,
he pumped—pumped so hard he was nothing more than a blur and
when
*   he was a grasp away . . .*

He just plain fizzled out

Angel's present plans include learning a skilled trade other than commercial art. He hopes to complete his college studies someday, to travel, and to pursue a career as an artist.

Art Therapy with Three Patients at Hawaii State Hospital

Anna Wagner

Art therapy at Hawaii State Hospital, Kaneohe, has been conducted by volunteers since 1956. At the time of writing, there is reason to hope that the State Department of Mental Health is coming to view such a program as worth expanding and paying for. Years of demonstration with patients and efforts to educate the public and the hospital staff may soon bear fruit.

The Art Therapy Program

From the beginning, hospital authorities have encouraged the volunteer art therapists and have given them valuable training. A few fine artists have worked in the program, but most volunteers came without art training. Therefore education in art is offered, and trainees are urged to use the medical library freely to gain understanding of psychodynamics. Continuous training sessions follow the weekly two-hour art therapy conference. An effort is made to acquaint the new therapists with the world of symbolism; the development shown in sequences of paintings is studied, and the artists' comments are considered. The trainees are encouraged to ask patients about their intentions and their interpretations of their own work, and to invite their attention to what they may have expressed unconsciously. We emphasize respect for the patient, for the medium, and for the psychiatric team effort.

At present, four volunteers offer three weekly programs. Community organizations and the hospital auxiliary make it possible to provide a wide variety of art materials, ranging from charcoal to acrylics. (Acrylic paint dries fast, and this is important in our humid climate.) One session is for adolescents and takes place during school hours. These younger patients are encouraged simply to enjoy the experience of art rather than to discuss its meaning, yet their pictures often give the staff glimpses into the less obvious aspects of individual personalities. Those who must be overly exact are drawn into freer expression, while the explosive ones are encouraged toward organization.

In addition to the volunteer art therapy program there is an art class initiated and run by an especially sensitive ward aide. His patients are geriatric cases, many of whom cannot speak coherently. Using thick acrylic paint, despite physical awkwardness they show strong and consistent individual styles. Color would seem to be the key to communication here, and a study is being made to correlate color choice with behavior. Pictures by these patients are displayed throughout the light and gaily decorated geriatric ward.

Recently, the volunteers have undertaken art therapy with alcoholics, who are no longer arrested in Hawaii but are referred to the state hospital. We have found that patients in this category tend to take a rigid view of art. Talent is often evident, and the gifted alcoholics almost always work at realistic landscapes. Freer approaches are used only after much coaxing, and often at the cost of a severe breakdown of defenses.[1] Our drug addicts tend to be younger, and fond of a more expressive kind of art. We hope to learn more about the therapeutic possibilities of art for these groups of patients. Meantime we count as success anything from the discovery of a real gift for original work to the selling of pleasant pastel mountain views for a dollar apiece.

In our efforts to win the sympathetic understanding of the entire professional staff, we learned to be aggressive about taking part in meetings and knocking on office doors, pictures in hand. We also set up a small gallery in a central location, with an exhibit of patients' paintings that was changed each week. This was as good for the morale of the patients as it was enlightening for hospital personnel, and we began to hang works by patients in the canteen and the cafeterias as well. Then, with permission of the hospital and the patients, we took pictures to the marketplace, hoping to help break down the barrier that separates the mentally ill from the community at large. Sponsored by the Mental Health Association of Hawaii, our first annual exhibit was held in 1969 at a large shopping center. Pictures were titled mainly with remarks made about them by the artists, and were priced from twenty-five dollars down, one dollar going to the art therapy program and the rest to the artists. Over 10,000 programs were handed out, many appreciative comments were recorded, and most of the paintings were sold, with a total of about $1,000 taken in.

In keeping with current trends, Hawaii's mental hospital population has been halved while the total population has grown dramatically. Most patients are only in the hospital for a few weeks or months, and art therapists must try to engage their interest quickly. Yet despite modern treatment

1. These observations are strikingly similar to those reported by Diane K. Devine ("A Preliminary Investigation of Paintings by Alcoholic Men," *American Journal of Art Therapy*, Vol. 9, No. 3, April 1970). Our closely coinciding impressions had already been recorded before the appearance of Miss Devine's article.

methods there will always be some patients who resist all efforts. The entrenched schizophrenic can easily be lost sight of in a group that includes a few demanding young people. Nevertheless we observe that the loud, witty exchanges do penetrate the silence barrier, and even arouse an amused interest. A long-term patient sometimes develops his first relationship in many years with an art therapist, their mutual interest in art serving to establish a bond. This may lead to friendly exchanges with other patients, and finally to a new alliance with members of the ward staff. The slow process is clearly charted by the increasingly integrated character of the patient's art. For some the experience is complete when the picture is finished; they are not interested in discussing it. For others, painting is the beginning of an objective look at themselves.

In the following instance, art played a major role in the relationships of three patients with each other, the art therapist, and regular members of the hospital staff.

Emil, Rose, and Robert

This study is concerned with a triangular relationship whose development can be traced through art productions. While our main focus will be on Emil, Rose provides the connecting link, and the story begins with Robert, an artistically gifted young Japanese. Rose was the first woman to give herself to him, and he expressed his happiness and gratitude in Figure 1, showing himself handing her a bouquet of roses, with the hospital building in the background.

After he was discharged, Robert became absorbed in writing a novel, and neglected to visit Rose. Then his sister read his manuscript, declared he used too many dirty words, and destroyed the work it had taken him six months to produce. Bitter and angry, Robert returned to the hospital, only to find Rose in love with Emil.

Emil, part Puerto Rican and part Portuguese, had grown up in the slums of Honolulu in a poor family marked by emotional instability. Mother, uncles, sister—all had a history of hospitalization at Kaneohe, known to Hawaiians as the "pupule [i.e., crazy] house." Religion, cruelty, and a belief in ghosts and magic shaped the world he came from.

Emil's mother was his father's third wife, and the small boy witnessed the many beatings he gave her. When his mother died of cancer, thirteen-year-old Emil went to live with an aunt. He grew up shy, lonely, worried, and ultimately haunted by feelings of guilt. He graduated from high school, then served in the army. After discharge, he returned to the golf courses on Oahu where he had caddied and played as a growing boy. The peaceful, beautiful lawns and graceful shade trees spread out under green cliffs were his comfort, and he enjoyed the simple, easy way of life still possible in Hawaii.

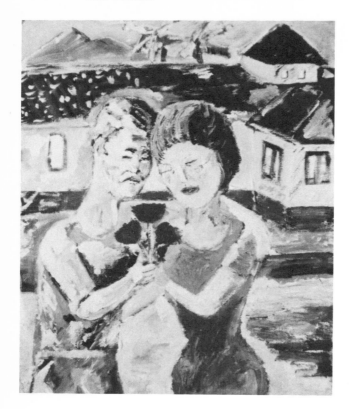

Figure 1

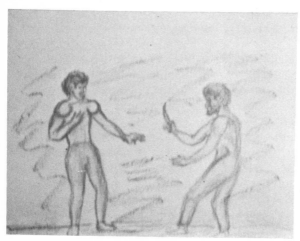

Figure 2

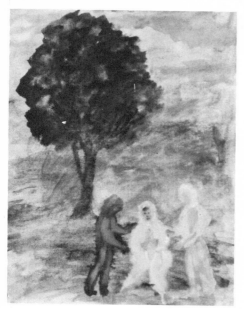

Figure 3

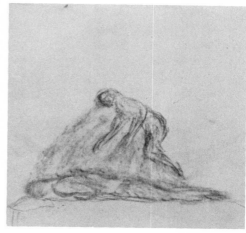

Figure 4

At thirty he began to experience hallucinations and a compelling fear that he would be killed by a jealous brother (see Figure 2), and was admitted to the state hospital in Kaneohe. He had been sleeping very little and ate hardly at all. His emaciation, coupled with the black beard he grew at this time, gave him an ascetic look; we noted some ambiguity in the aggressive "brother" figure.

Shortly after admission, Emil entered art therapy, where his natural talent was immediately apparent. His pictures illustrate his dreams and fears, his love, and his discoveries, all translated into his own poetic mode of expression. In the course of his hospital stay, his life became more complex, and today he wrestles with new problems.

At first inarticulate, he would respond to questions about his paintings in a few vague words or with a shrug. Nevertheless, the pictures spoke for him. First, he chose soft pastels to depict a dream of his "good and bad conscience" (Figure 3), each tugging at him as he sits in the moonlight. In another dream (Figure 4) he felt himself rise from his bed, only to look down and see himself asleep. The drawing suggests a disguised homosexual fantasy, as does Figure 2. Later came a series of "cosmic" themes in vivid colors.

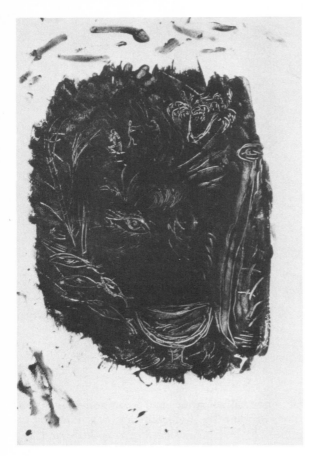

Figure 5

Feeling somewhat better, Emil left the hospital and went on a grand drunk with friends. When he returned, he abandoned the pastels for crayon resist. After scratching out a graceful hummingbird, he experienced a moment of truth, and using a chopstick he conveyed his self-disgust in Figure 5, a frightening, one-eyed face. He said the fighting stick-figures on the forehead stood for the other eye, "the mind's eye," and the seated figure was himself thinking of joining the fight; he was worried about a recent urge to strike out. The mouth of this face is a wineglass and a large bottle stands alongside. The smearing and messiness fit with the cathartic purpose the picture appeared to serve.

Emil turned to paint and introduced a theme that continued to appear whenever he was at peace—a beautiful but rather distant green landscape, as bright as he could make it. The paintings, together with his comments on them, eloquently revealed a simple man of sorrowful nature and history.

The landscapes of Emil's mind at first were empty, but later there grew in them plum trees, frail but graceful and resilient, that, he said, represented himself. Then one day Emil met Rose and fell deeply in love with her.

He was very happy for the first time in his life. He tended a flower garden he had planted behind his ward, and painted pictures of its colorful blossoms and lush leaves.

Rose is a Japanese girl whose childhood was as cruel as Emil's. She had the reputation of being promiscuous; she once said ruefully that she was good only for bush therapy. Nevertheless, Emil saw her as resembling his mother and sisters, as many of his portraits of her show (Figure 6 is one of them). He found that their relationship gave him a new sense of manhood, and he began to improve rapidly. His sexual experience was reflected in explosive designs.

Like Emil, Rose had a family history of schizophrenia and she lived a miserable life of highs and lows that left her groggy. Intelligent, witty, and given to rapid shifts of thought and frequent punning, she was often misunderstood and had become reluctant to confide in anyone. Although Emil had never known how to converse very well, he and Rose began to spend much time together, talking and planning. When he went on home visits he took Rose to visit his sister.

Robert, meantime, returned to the hospital and discovered that Rose was absorbed in her love affair with Emil. He tried to figure out his feelings toward her in a series of pastel drawings; he was almost deaf, and art was his major means of communication. In Figure 7 he portrayed himself holding a stalk of bananas, scowling at a seductive Rose. He colored over the end of

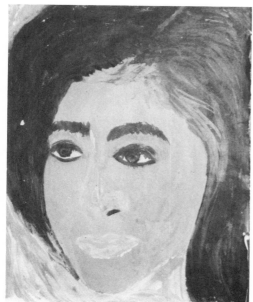

Figure 6

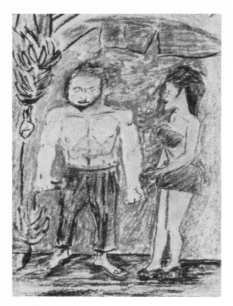

Figure 7

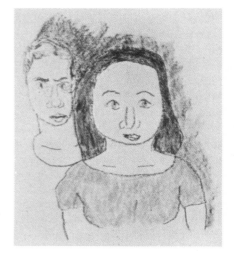

Figure 8

the banana stalk, suggesting symbolically the denial of any more sexual favors. Soon after this he did a pastel drawing expressing the idea of a violent death for Rose. Her head is shown as if suspended from a yardarm or a gallows and flanked on two sides by crosses. In the foreground, he and Emil stand, Robert laughing, Emil sad. Next came pictures of himself and Rose in varying moods, beginning with Robert very angry and Rose with a worried stare (Figure 8). In the last picture of this series, Robert looks sad and lost while Rose appears confident. In both of these double portraits Robert drew himself slightly behind Rose.

Soon after, he attempted suicide by swallowing a caustic poison, with the result that his vocal cords were injured. Now not only was he partially deaf, but also he could not speak. More than ever frustrated, angry, and bitter, he retreated to an infantile state, referring to himself as "baby Bobby." In this condition, he ran away into the mountains, where he somehow survived wet days and nights on the cliffs, keeping himself alive on a diet of guavas and bananas. He finally went to his home, and his mother refused to return him to the hospital. There seems to be some hope for him, since his family now appears to have become more understanding and ready to try to help him begin again from the beginning.

When Emil was discharged, Rose continued to visit him, leaving the grounds without permission. The staff became resentful and made accusations and threats. Emil was no longer welcome at the hospital, and efforts were made to separate him and Rose on the ground that the sexual relationship was bad for her because it revived the guilt attached to damaging childhood experiences. One of her paintings (Figure 9, Plate XII) seemed to confirm this idea. Two versions of her own face are separated by a whirling black cyclone that she designated as "destruction." The closed eyes look downward, she said, in shame. Yet we may also interpret the painting as showing her reluctance to face truths that she nonetheless instinctively felt.

Gradually, a sort of silent truce evolved between Emil and the hospital staff. He was allowed to visit Rose almost daily, and often accompanied her to the weekly art therapy sessions. His landscape was no longer empty of human life. Figure 10 is a vivid painting of Rose in a billowing green dress, the color of the meadow she stands in, one arm seeming to beckon. The sky is orange, especially brilliant directly behind her.

Rose was faithful to him but he became jealous and imagined slights. In one powerful painting, his face in perfect likeness glares at the observer from amid fiery flames of anger. No longer did he always have to hide enraged reactions to frustration behind a shy, retiring manner.

But there was always a flash of laughter that relieved the tension as the three of us would study the paintings and Emil would struggle to find words to describe feelings he had easily depicted with the paint brush. He and Rose continued to show their heightened sexual awareness, he with portraits of her, now more realistic and life-size, leaving no room for anything else on the page just as his relationship with her left no room for anything else in his

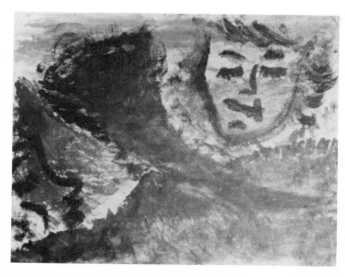

Figure 9

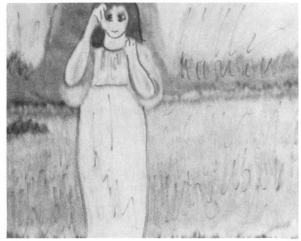

Figure 10

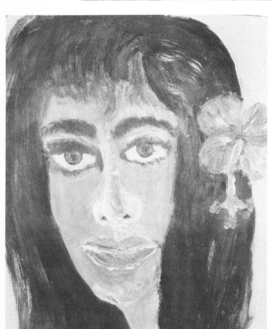

Figure 11

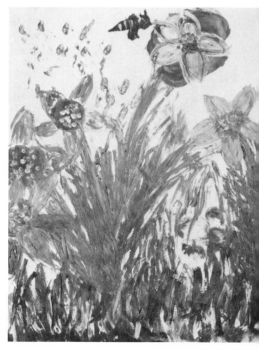

Figure 12

life. In Figure 11 he seemed to incorporate his own likeness with hers. Rose, likewise making large, emphatic paintings, showed a black bee pollinating a hibiscus in a wild garden (Figure 12).

Emil's confidence grew; he painted pictures to show "stages of learning." In one of these (Figure 13; Plate XIII) he called the figures sitting slumped on the bright-green grass "people who think they know everything," and the others, dancing with arms outflung, "people who think they know nothing." Behind the figures is a lurid hymn to life, with flowers, trees, and gigantic birds backed by a huge, radiating, rising red sun.

There may be an element of bravado in Emil's feeling of power, but he tells us in his sometimes florid paintings that through his successful defiance of the hospital's authority he now sees himself as the only one who can help Rose and himself; perhaps he is right. Figure 14 (Plate XIV) shows a girl half buried in the sand who is being rescued by an angel. A turbulent sea and sky, and hot Hawaiian sun contribute a feeling of intensity. Emil tended at this time to be not only minister to Rose but also preacher to the world at large, especially the hospital staff.

He urged Rose to paint painful memories, offering one of his own: a walk through a strange and hostile neighborhood at night. She responded with Figure 15, an erupting volcano, red lava spewing into the sky and flowing down the mountainside, a sight common on her native island but also aptly suggesting the frightening, sexually tinged violence of her life.

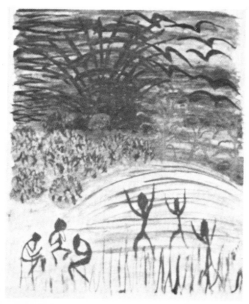

Figure 13

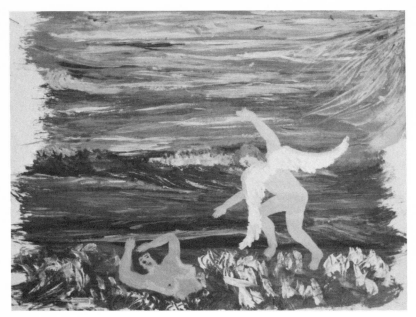

Figure 14

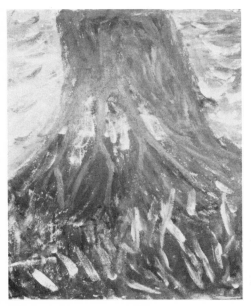

Figure 15

Often she would retreat to her moody, witty play with words and scribbled paintings. With Emil she talked about happy times, recalling the 4-H activities and parties of her childhood, while he chatted, counseled, soothed, and attended her as much as he was allowed to.

Rose also has now been discharged from the hospital, and she and Emil have been living for several months with a kindly aunt of his. With much care and help they may move toward some level of independent living. Without such investment on the part of others, they will be left like Hansel and Gretel to find their own way out of the woods. Their lives and problems are probably paralleled by thousands.

Postscript: Ten Years Later

I have not been able to track down Robert—as far as I know, he did not return to the hospital.

Emil and Rose lived together for a while in a trailer on a golf course where he caddied and served as a guard. Eventually, she left him and was referred to a rehabilitation center in Honolulu. She still works there, producing delightful stuffed animals that she contracts to sell to tourist shops. She has recently moved into an apartment with two other women and has become quite independent.

This last Christmas, when I didn't get my first card of the year from Rose, I knew she had made it on her own.

Preventive Art Therapy with a Preschool Child

Edna G. Salant

At the National Child Research Center in Washington, D.C., I conducted an art therapy program that I was asked to design for the purpose of helping preschool children with a variety of problems. Because the children are so young, I use both art therapy and play therapy.

The center, a private school, was started in 1927 as part of a research project of the Rockefeller Foundation. It has a population of about 150 normal children, ranging in age from two and a half to seven years. Many of the children in the school come from professional families, mostly middle and upper middle class. Some are black, but they are in the minority. The staff consists of ten young women and men trained in child development. These teachers are well informed, intelligent, highly sensitive to children's problems, and, in general, most cooperative with any person who, like me, is there to add to their understanding of the children they work with. The children in the school are often observed as a sample of "normal" population by psychiatrists, psychoanalysts, and students training in mental health.

After school has been in session for about a month, the director asks the teachers to observe children in their classes, looking for any presenting a problem or problems which may range from excessive aggressiveness to overpassivity and failure to join in the activities of the group. A troubled child may have great stress at home: a new baby's arrival, illness or death of a parent, separation of parents, death of grandparents, and so on. After the teachers' selections are made, I observe these children myself, selecting those who seem most in need of art therapy and likely to benefit from it. When I know which children I will be working with, I appear in their classrooms and get to know them by joining in their play. I make myself very visible to them on each visit. This is the beginning of building trust between the child and me. Next, I invite the child to come to my art therapy room alone. The children can stay as long as they wish and return to the classroom whenever they want. This gives them control of the situation, and they usually come with me quite easily. After they feel comfortable and come willingly I see them individually once or twice a week, the sessions usually lasting about forty-five minutes.

When I have seen the child in therapy a few times, I make an appointment to see the mother or father, or sometimes both parents, to get a full early history. This history covers the infant years of the child, his eating, sleeping, toilet training, and any illnesses or traumas that may have occurred before his entrance into our school. Attitudes of the parents and of the other siblings toward the child are discussed at this time. No such history is taken from the parent when he or she applies for the child's entrance to the school, and teachers rarely have the opportunity to get this information from the parents later. Therefore, there is an enormous amount of useful information to be obtained in this first meeting with the parent(s).

Before the child is accepted into the art therapy program, the parent(s) have to agree to meet periodically with me for conferences, so that I will be kept up to date on what is happening in the home. In the case of separated parents, I need to know how often the absent parent sees his child and what kind of visits they are, what emotions seem to be caused by those visits, and so on. A working relationship between art therapist and parent can be most useful to the treatment of the child. I keep in touch with the parent by telephone and also through personal meetings about once a month, or more if I think it is necessary. The parents are free to call me whenever they want to discuss some change in or problem with the child. At periodic meetings with the teachers I report on the parent conferences and bring along the child's drawings to illustrate what the child is communicating in the art therapy sessions.

I conceive of my program as both preventive and therapeutic. It is most effective in both respects when it involves both parents and teachers. There is nothing new in using a parent, usually the mother, in treating a child. In therapeutic nursery schools therapy is frequently handled by means of "treatment via the mother." Freud used a similar approach in the classic case of Little Hans, when he treated the child via his father. I use the help of the mother (or father) in therapy because parents are the most influential people in their child's life at this age and the most important instrument for effecting and sustaining change; it is natural for them to be involved in the changes going on during therapy. At the outset of treatment parents give the therapist her best picture of the early development of the child and of his environment. As therapy progresses their observations of the child at home give helpful information about how therapy is affecting the child.

The teachers are also important to the art therapist in that they can give her a view of the child's relationship with his peers and bring up current problems which in their view need further attention. In addition, they report on changes in behavior in the classroom as therapy progresses. The teachers, in turn, learn a great deal from the art therapist. In our conferences, they see in the child's drawings his fears, wishes, and other significant emotions of which they often have not been aware. My recommendations also carry weight in their planning for the child's classroom routine. For example, I may point out that an unmanageable child will probably calm down if greater intellectual demands are made upon him.

I may also recommend to the director that a child should receive tutoring or psychiatric treatment, or possibly that he ought to be transferred to a different kind of school.

Children of Separated Parents

Preschool children are particularly vulnerable to the disruption of family life which divorce or separation of the parents entails. At their young age they are often unable to verbalize how they feel about what is happening in their family. They do respond, however, with the help of an art therapist, to the use of art materials. Through drawing, painting, or clay modeling, painful feelings of aggression and anger, fear and anxiety can be expressed—as well as can feelings of love. Without help, such children frequently act out these feelings in school, which results in learning difficulties and behavior problems. Often, psychosomatic illnesses develop as a direct result of their unexpressed anger or helplessness.

Although the children whom I see for art therapy may have any of a number of stressful situations at home, I have for some time had a special interest in children of one-parent families. The case I will use to illustrate the art therapy program at the National Child Research Center is of such a child.

An Illustrative Case

Lucy illustrates some basic problems related to the experience of a child in a one-parent family. A vivacious, gifted, mature child of superior intelligence, Lucy was three and a half years old when her parents separated. Her younger brother, George, was two and a half at that time. Whereas George reacted openly to the separation with outbursts of anger, tantrums, and bowel regression, Lucy never showed her emotions about the separation in any way. She lived with her mother after the separation but didn't talk to her mother about it and in fact seemed to deny that it had happened. Her mother, a physician (as is the father), recognized that Lucy's behavior was not normal and was concerned about it. To me, it seemed obvious that, being in the oedipal phase of her life, Lucy was probably suppressing strong feelings about her parents' separation. The mother also felt considerable guilt about the effect of the separation on the children.

At school Lucy showed few outward signs of needing help. She was doing well in her class work, learning to read quickly and to write. She was well liked by her peers and dominated them most of the time. The teacher did report that Lucy was very demanding of adults and incessantly interrupted stories and conversations with questions that she insisted be answered. In her artwork, at which she was quite proficient and in which she was greatly interested, Lucy would deny any difficulty that confronted her. For example, if she began work on a drawing which was too big for the paper, instead of beginning again she would continue drawing, saying, "It's just fine; this is going to be the best picture I ever made." This seemed to parallel the denial by means of which she was defending herself against the impact of family problems.

Many of the foregoing factors made Lucy a good candidate for art therapy, which she began with me at the age of five and a half.

In my first conference with Lucy's mother, she described Lucy as having been a very easy and delightful baby. She also said Lucy was the kind of child who stands off until she is sure of you—"She doesn't give of herself quickly. She is introspective and not impulsive." During the time I was seeing Lucy in school her father moved to Florida. The mother described him as "not wanting the responsibilities of childrearing," although he seemed to be very fond of the children. The maternal grandparents are very close to the mother, Lucy, and her brother. The mother is in analysis, trying hard to keep things normal.

Figure 1

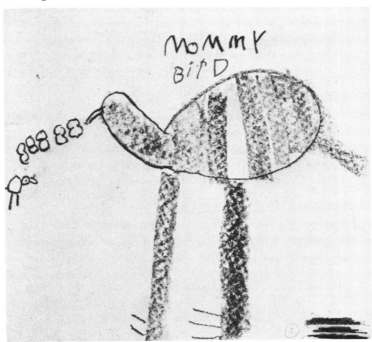

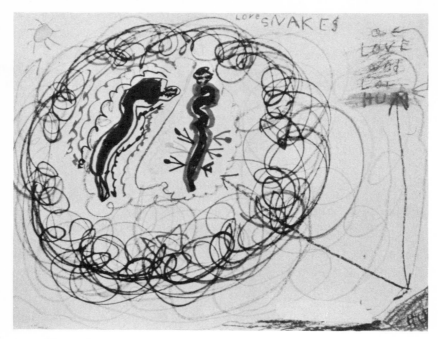

Figure 2

When Lucy came to the art therapy room for the first session, she immediately began drawing a picture of her cat. I knew she had a brother in the school and I asked about him. Then Lucy drew her brother and herself. When I asked if there were any other people in the family she said, "No," but then said slowly, "Well," and drew another picture (Figure 1) of a large bird and a much smaller bird next to it. She labeled the large bird "Mommy" and called the small bird "Poppa," and said, "He's smaller because he's far away and looks smaller in the distance." However, I later observed that Lucy habitually represented her mother as "a big girl" and her father as "a little boy."

At the next session Lucy began playing in the doll house. After putting the mother doll and father doll in the living room together she started fixing up the bedroom. "See," she said, "the mother and father have separate dressers because they are separate people." Then Lucy began drawing two snakes (Figure 2). After the picture was finished I asked her for the story of this picture. "There was a lady snake and a man snake and they were getting married; there were lots of guests around them. There was music and love all around and a big celebration of love." If one looks closely one can see that the snakes are divided from each other by a line and each is separately enclosed. This picture, coming so soon in the therapy, was a great surprise and indicated to me that Lucy had been waiting for an opportunity to open up and let out some of her thoughts and feelings about her parents' separation.

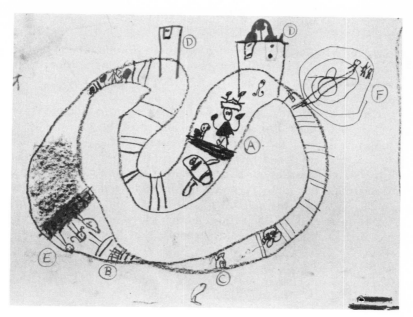

Figure 3

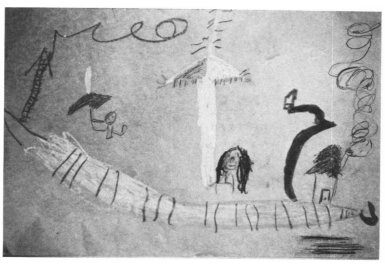

Figure 4

The next picture Lucy drew (Figure 3) expressed several losses in her life. Close friends who lived nearby had moved away (A). Most important, her father's new apartment (B) is removed from her mother's house (C). "My father can't live with my mother anymore," she said sadly. Lucy illustrated a number of memories: traffic lights (D) seen on the drive to her father's, and

walking over a bridge (E) and going to the zoo (F) on outings she and her
brother had with their father. This picture, with its emphasis on the loss of
the family who moved away, acted as a catalyst in helping Lucy to talk about
her parents' separation.

During the session that followed Lucy drew Figure 4 (Plate XV), one of
her pictures showing a "little boy" (on the left) and a "big girl" (on the right).
She began by drawing the umbrella in the center of the picture, which she
said her mother had as a girl. Note that the "little boy" (the father) also has
an umbrella, but a smaller one than the mother's. As in Figure 3, she put in a
road connecting her mother's house on the right and her father's skinny
apartment house on the left. We notice again the separation—father's
apartment on one side of the picture, mother's house on the other. "The big
girl is a doctor," Lucy explained. (Her mother, as I mentioned earlier, is a
physician).

The Necklace (Figure 5) is another in this series of separation pictures.
Lucy began by drawing an oak leaf she had seen the day before at a farm

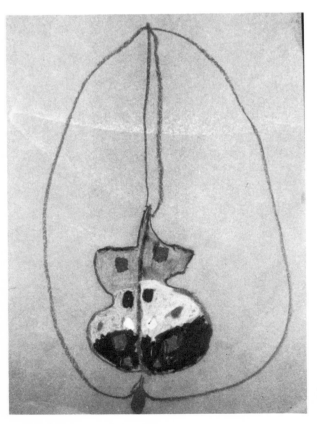

Figure 5

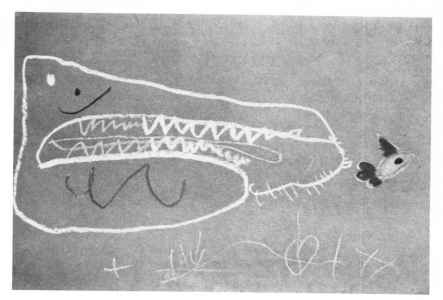

Figure 6

where she was walking with her father. After coloring the leaf very carefully, she suddenly drew a circle all around it and said, "My father gave my mother a necklace like this once."

This circle around the oak leaf is split by the line that divides it into two halves. Apparently, the oak leaf triggered a memory of happier times between her parents. Usually Lucy showed no strong emotions while drawing because of her fascination with the actual art process. However, while drawing this particular picture she looked very sad, and seemed almost to be mourning the loss of her parents' earlier closeness.

Figure 6 shows an alligator pursuing a little fish that seems to be looking back at its pursuer. The alligator is baring his teeth and looks pretty ferocious. As Lucy was finishing the picture she put whiskers on the alligator. "You know," she said, "my father has a mustache." In an earlier conference with Lucy's mother, she had talked of the father's closeness to Lucy. Was this a picture of the seductive father and the half-frightened, half-coquettish child?

Figure 7 is another illustration of Lucy's longing for the closeness of past days. It shows the house that she and her brother had lived in one summer with their father. She remarked, longingly, how happy they had been. "My mother was not with us," she said. However, on the left side of the picture is a fruit tree, a symbol Lucy often used in other drawings to stand for her mother.

About two months later Lucy did a series of pictures of a flower with a curled-up form on either side of it. Figure 8 is one of these. Lucy drew this the day after having had a happy visit with her father. In the center of each of the curled-up shapes is an eye (barely visible in reproduction). I felt Lucy

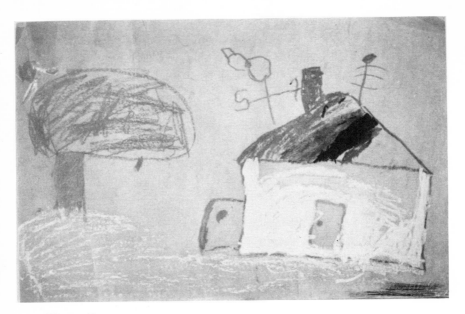

Figure 7

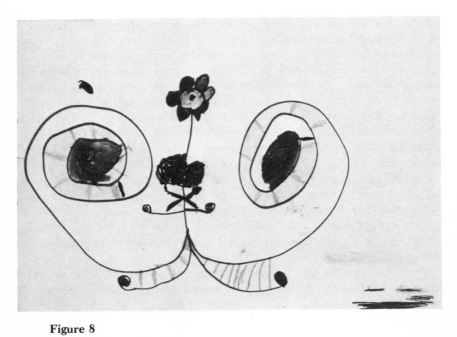

Figure 8

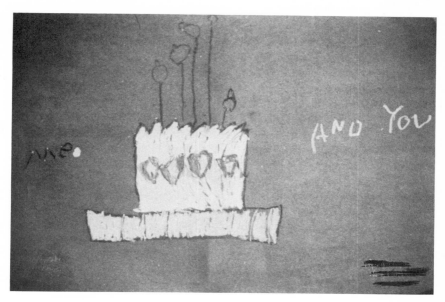

Figure 9

represented herself here as the flower in the center who seems to be supported by her two parents, one on either side. Confirmation of this state of equilibrium in Lucy's life came from her mother who said she was adjusting to her parents' separation. She has also been able to maintain a close relationship with both of her parents.

When nursery school ended in June, the therapy sessions stopped until August, when Lucy's mother called me and asked if I could see Lucy for a while before her new school began. During this period she made several pictures showing great affection for me. One of these was *The Birthday Cake*, Figure 9. Lucy's birthday was coming soon and she drew a beautiful cake with candles on it. On the left side of the picture she wrote the word "me" and on the right side "and you." When she read it off to me her eyes smiled and she nodded, saying, "You know what I mean." The last picture (unfortunately not available), entitled by Lucy *Large White Mother Cat*, was another expression of Lucy's positive feeling for me. The cat looked human, and when Lucy was drawing its mouth she turned to me and said, "What color lipstick do you wear?"

The therapy was finished for the time being. Lucy was doing very well in her new school, her mother reported. However, at spring vacation, six months later, Lucy visited her father in Florida. When she returned she began having nightmares, wanting her mother to stay with her at night, and being quite tense. One day she said, "You know the lady I made pictures with at school last year? I'd like to see her again."

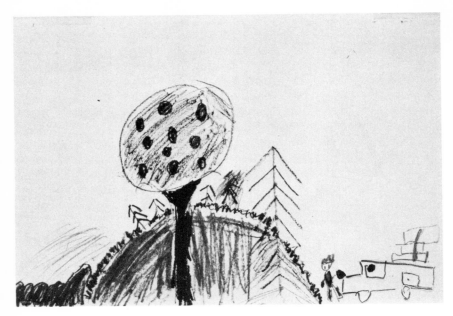

Figure 10

After a couple of sessions Lucy did a series of three pictures. Figure 10 is the first of these. It's a park and in the center there is a large apple tree bearing fruit, one of Lucy's symbols for her mother. The apple tree dominates the drawing. In the lower right corner there is a truck with a man sitting inside. You can only see his head. Lucy told me the man in the truck is being arrested by a policeman who is giving him a ticket. Handcuffs are being put on the man. "Why is he being arrested?" I asked. "Because he made a fire and stole some logs," Lucy said. The second drawing, Figure 11, shows a man making a fire in the park. He's camping and has a sleeping bag. At first, Lucy said the third drawing of the series, Figure 12, was a rocket; then she changed it to a pencil. In either case the form is obviously phallic.

These three pictures puzzled me at first until Lucy's mother told me that her new boyfriend is a lawyer. Then I was able to piece their meaning together. It seems clear that Lucy's father, who does a great deal of camping, is being arrested by a man of the law. Lucy is worried that her father, the camper, will be taken away by the policeman or lawman who may become her new father. The phallic symbol tells us she has an idea about the sexual side of love and marriage.

In a recent conference, Lucy's mother told me that Lucy had had a good year in her new school, was accepting the new man in her mother's life, and would be visiting her father for the summer. Art therapy apparently contributed to better communication and more openness between mother and daughter. Lucy talks freely about her feelings with her mother now.

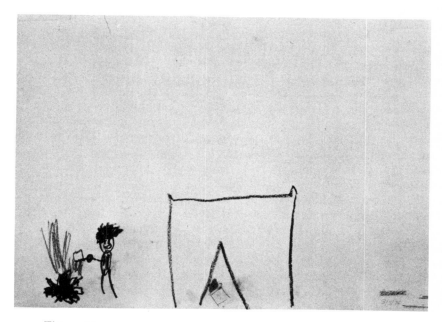

Figure 11

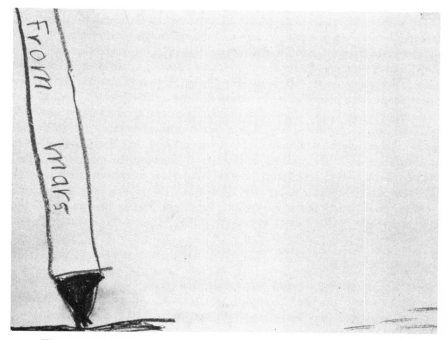

Figure 12

An important event occurred toward the end of the nursery school year at a conference with the mother. She had asked earlier that I show her Lucy's drawings made over the past months. I thought very long about doing this and considered both the confidentiality of the drawings and their possible effect on the mother. Confidentiality in the treatment of a five-year-old where a mother is already being apprised of her child's progress through conferences is quite different from the confidentiality one would respect in an adolescent's treatment. After weighing all the knowledge I had about the mother—her capacity to understand, her being in analysis, her intense desire to know more about her child in order to help her—I decided to show her the drawings.

The mother's reaction to the pictures was extremely emotional at first. She burst into tears at seeing the picture of the *Two Snakes* and said, "My God, I never knew the depth of Lucy's feelings. How she must have suffered over these past two years." However, after we talked a bit longer about this, she said, "Now I can talk with her about what's happened, knowing she does understand." The mother has been very grateful for being allowed to see her daughter's drawings and, through them, to understand her feelings about the parents' separation.

Summary

I have presented briefly a case illustrating treatment through art therapy of a preschool child of a one-parent family. The goal in working with such young children is to prevent emotional problems resulting from crises or traumas in their lives from causing the development of serious symptoms.

Lucy's reluctance to talk with her mother about the separation of her parents may have been caused by her guilt feelings about it—her feeling that in some way she was responsible for its happening. Bringing the whole problem out in the open, expressing her complicated emotions to the art therapist through the production of many significant drawings, helped her to communicate with her mother for the first time about this painful subject.

Lucy was a comparatively intact child, and even short-term therapy with children like this goes a long way. The mother's understanding of Lucy's feelings also helped make it possible for them to talk openly about the separation.

Discussion

I think a word should be said about the extraordinarily personal content of the pictures Lucy made. Although the walls of the office at the school were covered with paintings and drawings Lucy made in her class, they were completely different from those she made in the art therapy sessions. The class pictures were colorful, abstract, gay designs with no deeper meaning, but the ones done during the art therapy sessions were intimately related to what was going on in her life at home. They freely expressed the story (as it unfolded) of her parents' separation and her view of it. All the many pictures Lucy made during her work with me told a story related in some way to her problem. And yet nothing was said to Lucy at the beginning of the art therapy sessions about why she was coming to see me. The class teacher just told Lucy she would be going to Mrs. Salant's room to make pictures. At our first meeting, possibly by asking Lucy if there were anyone else in her family besides her brother and herself, I triggered thoughts of her parents' separation.

How do the very young children who come to the therapy room know what they are there for? No one tells them that because they are under stress or unhappy or having difficulties they can go and express their emotions in the therapy room once or twice a week, using the art and play materials there to do so. And yet the children intuitively understand that the therapist is different from their teacher, and that the room, which like their classroom has toys and art materials, is special and different from their classroom. For one thing, the therapist, like the room, is *exclusively* theirs while they are there for therapy, and everything is done to create an atmosphere of approval, warmth, and personal interest. Gradually—and sometimes quite soon—in the treatment the children understand that this time with the therapist is for them to use as they wish, playing out or communicating pictorially whatever seems important to them in their lives, something perhaps that is painful and not easy to tell. A nonthreatening, all-accepting environment encourages the lowering of the child's defenses and the expression of his repressed feelings.

The periodic conferences with the mothers of the children in the art therapy program help the mothers understand the impact of changes in the parental situation on the child. Thus the parents are helped both to handle the child better and to conduct their relations with each other in a way less damaging to the child.

There are in fact two phases in this program of prevention. At best it is possible to intervene in the life of a healthy child such as Lucy when the troubles are occurring and before they cause serious psychopathology. There is a second chance for prevention by means of treating a child's symptoms— for example, extreme aggressiveness—before they harden into a set behavior pattern.

As I see it, then, there is an opportunity with the very young child to help him over difficult times in his life by the use of art therapy. By engaging the help of one or both of his parents as well as his teacher one can prevent more serious problems from developing in his future.

PART FIVE

SYSTEMATIC INVESTIGATIONS IN ART THERAPY

The Use of Families' Art Productions for Psychiatric Evaluation

Hanna Yaxa Kwiatkowska

Art therapy at the Adult Psychiatry Branch of the National Institute of Mental Health is connected with a number of research projects. These projects differ from each other in their goals and techniques, but most of them include the family in treatment. One of the offspring of these families presents symptoms of psychiatric illness. He is designated by the family as the patient and in most cases is hospitalized on a small ward at the institute's Clinical Center in Bethesda, Maryland. Art therapy is an integral part of each program; the techniques we use follow and adjust to the treatment and research goals of the different projects.

The development of family art therapy has a natural history, which began in 1958 in the Section on Family Studies under Dr. Lyman C. Wynne. The hospitalized patient was at that time seen individually in art therapy as an adjunct to psychotherapy. Family members who were interested in what the patient was producing in the art therapy room were admitted only if they would join him in his work. The interaction of these family subgroups as well as the art productions themselves provided such interesting material that we eventually decided to include the whole family regularly in the art therapy program; this is how family art therapy was born. The many modifications of these sessions which occurred through the years have been described elsewhere.[1]

Gradually family art therapy spread beyond the Section on Family Studies, and was included in programs of the Personality Development Section headed by Dr. Roger Shapiro, and the Twin and Sibling Section headed by Dr. William Pollin and Dr. James Stabenau.

In addition to these projects where art is used in evaluation or as an

1. Hanna Kwiatkowska, Juliana Day, and Lyman Wynne, *The Schizophrenic Patient, His Parents and Siblings; Observations through Family Art Therapy*, Bethesda, Md., National Institute of Mental Health, U.S. Department of Health, Education and Welfare, 1962; Hanna Kwiatkowska, "Family Art Therapy: Experiments with a New Technique," *Bulletin of Art Therapy*, Vol. 1, No. 3, Spring 1962.

adjunct to psychotherapy, another project is being conducted where family art therapy is the only form of treatment. I was braced for strong opposition and resistance from the first family we saw: the son has an acute mental illness, they come for psychiatric help, and these crazy people have them draw pictures! At the first session, however, significant material was brought up through the drawings, and to my surprise, the family responded readily from then on to this form of communication even though its members are not artistically gifted or interested in art.

Dr. Gentry Harris, the cotherapist at these sessions, became interested in the potentialities of art in family therapy after having observed an art evaluation session with another family he had treated. In that case it was a final evaluation after long-term treatment. Dr. Harris found that in this session he had impressively deepened and enlarged his understanding of the family dynamics, even though he had already worked with this family intensively for a long time.

Each developmental phase of family art therapy was logically linked with another, and unfolded naturally. Family art evaluation, the subject of this paper, is a typical example of how our most significant experiences in art work with families were gathered together to evolve a method. To make comparisons possible, an identical set of procedures is repeated with each family. Each procedure is a distinct but connected step toward knowing the family; together they give us in a very short time a picture of the family, their problems, roles, transactions, and thinking processes.

Family art evaluation may be seen as a projective technique but it differs from the usual projective tests in that the families here create their own projective material. Because of this, we are shown additional aspects of personality: the family members' creative resources and how they can use them, their capacity to express abstract themes and concepts, whether they can produce appropriate material or whether on the other hand their responses are bizarre, their individual or joint abilities to focus attention on a task and proceed in an orderly fashion to complete it. These four points are among the criteria being developed for comparison of different families by means of art evaluation.[2]

When we compare family art sessions with verbal family sessions, we also find a significant difference. In the latter many things may be going on at once but only one person at a time can express himself in words and be heard. When the family works together with art materials, on the other hand, all members are engaged simultaneously in expressive activity. Without interrupting this activity they can comment spontaneously on each other's creations; they can see how they are perceived by others, or expose

---

2. The criteria are described and applied in a paper dealing with families of twins, which is co-authored by Dr. Loren Mosher, and will soon be ready for publication. The twins studied were concordant or discordant for schizophrenia or were members of normal control families.

their own perceptions of others. They move, change places, seek or give support, withdraw, lead, or dominate the other family members. Therefore the family art evaluation session gives us an unusually rich amount of information with a minimal expenditure of the family's and the therapists' time.

This single session provides an opportunity to see and understand the family at many levels. The family roles and relations as presented in the customary history-taking are inevitably exposed to possible distortions and omissions because of the bias of the family member who gives information. Family art evaluation is a new situation for the family, for which they cannot mobilize their usual defenses. They do not know by what criteria they will be judged; they are apt to be more themselves, less preoccupied as to what they should be.

The analysis of the behavioral and pictorial material has to be made by an experienced art therapist or psychotherapist, but the application of the procedures themselves is relatively simple. With the present interest in the family's role in mental illness, especially in the genesis of schizophrenia, this technique may be useful in settings such as the general hospital, where the staff often has to fulfill multiple functions and where only brief contact with the family may be possible.

Elinor Ulman in her article "A New Use of Art in Psychiatric Diagnosis"[3] describes a technique similar in some respects to ours; both emerged more or less parallel. However, they present basic differences:

1. Miss Ulman's patients were referred for individual diagnosis while our families are referred for the study of family relations.

2. Miss Ulman evaluates and describes an individual personality and through the pictorial material she draws very sensitive conclusions and speculates as to where personal characteristics spring from, while we have the advantage of actually experiencing the family process.

Method

Each family is seen during the first two weeks of treatment for a single session one and one half to two hours long. The art therapist conducts the session with a participant observer, who is a psychiatrist or social worker engaged in the treatment of the family. When the family comes to the art therapy room they are invited to use the art medium (rectangular hard pastels) as a form of communication or self-expression. The art therapist emphasizes that art ability or talent is not expected of them. There is no right or wrong—they should just do the best they can. They are invited to start right away and see for themselves what it is all about. A permissive and unintrusive attitude on the part of the art therapist helps to loosen initial

---

3. *Bulletin of Art Therapy,* Vol. 4, No. 3, April 1965.

restraint; never in our experience has a family refused to go through all the procedures. Very rarely, when a family member is acutely psychotic, he may be unable to follow the instructions; valuable material nonetheless may be obtained from his interaction with other family members and from his fragmentary art productions.

The procedures have been carefully devised and each has its own purpose. They are:

1. *A free picture, no subject assigned.*

2. *A portrait of the family:* "Draw each member of the family including yourself, not a detailed, photographic resemblance but also more than a matchstick figure."

3. *Abstract family portraits:* "No bodies or features—just the way you feel or think about each member of your family, including yourself."

4. *Individual picture from a scribble.*[4] All family members do arm-loosening exercises in preparation for making a scribble as the starting point of a picture. Each then draws his own picture inspired by any line or lines of his scribble.

5. *Joint picture started from a scribble.* Each family member does a second scribble and then, among themselves, they decide which scribble they will use to start a joint picture in which all family members collaborate.

6. *A free picture, no subject assigned* (as in procedure number one), made individually by each family member.

These procedures include free art expression (1, 6) and definite, identical assignments given to all families in order to obtain comparable data (2, 3, 4, 5).

All the sessions are tape-recorded, but notes are taken during or immediately after the session. This is important because after some time has passed it is difficult to recapture the investigators' subjective experience and their fresh impressions of the family members' interaction, motor activity, and other forms of nonverbal communication. All these add immeasurably to the pictorial and verbal material. Videotapes or movie films of these sessions would be very useful.

In the present phase of development of this technique, I try to have as little knowledge as possible about the family history and the patient's diagnosis so as to draw my tentative conclusions only from this one encounter. The participant observer, on the other hand, through his role in

---

4. Florence Cane, *The Artist in Each of Us,* New York, Pantheon Books, 1951; Margaret Naumburg, *Psychoneurotic Art: Its Function in Psychotherapy,* New York, Grune and Stratton, 1953; *idem, Schizophrenic Art: Its Meaning in Psychotherapy,* New York, Grune and Stratton, 1950; *idem, Studies of the "Free" Art Expression of Behavior Problem Children and Adolescents as a Means of Diagnosis and Therapy,* New York, Nervous & Mental Disease Monograph No. 7, 1947.

treatment, has had more contact with the family and the patient and of course knows much more about them. Nevertheless, the family art evaluation session invariably broadens his understanding of the different family members and of the family relations and dynamics, either reinforcing or raising questions about the previous diagnostic impression. In addition the pictures become available for reference in the course of psychotherapy, and, if desirable, can be reviewed with the family.

Illustrative Examples

I will illustrate the first procedure with free pictures made by two twenty-five-year-old twin sisters. Twins and their families come to the Clinical Center for a two-week period of intensive investigation. I have absolutely no earlier contact with them or the families. I don't know if one twin or both are schizophrenic or if they are normal controls.

At the family art evaluation session neither of the twins we are going to discuss exhibited psychotic behavior; they both presented a façade of good adjustment. Both drew landscapes (Figures 1 and 2) related to their homes. The first impression is of representations fairly well organized and complete, even if naively primitive. Upon scrutiny, however, one perceives that they present differences, which immediately throw light on the pathology of one of the sisters, Mary.

Mary said that Figure 1 was her own yard and that she was homesick for it.

Figure 1

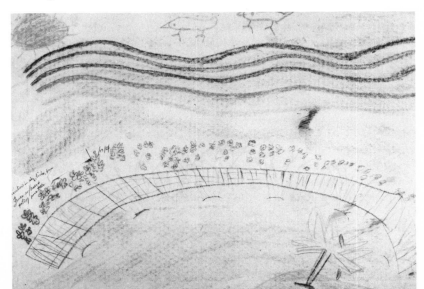

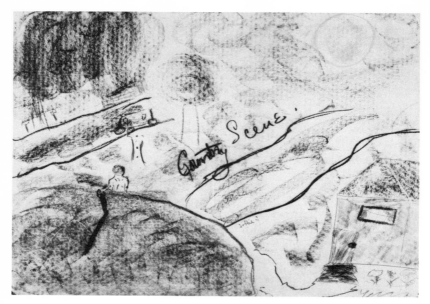

Figure 2

She called attention to the patio, the fence, the roses, and so on. She added a rainbow of a most unrealistic shape. When asked to give a title to the picture, she wrote a list of all the elements she had drawn, "rainbow in sky, birds, sun, fence, roses, patio, pine tree," but she lost the meaning of the whole picture and failed to indicate its emotional content; she reduced it to a bunch of fragments.

Her sister, on the other hand, drew a complex, somewhat incongruous landscape (Figure 2). She first called it *Farm House*. Then, with an obsessive need for exactness, she said that it did not truly represent a farm, and changed the title to *Country Scene*. She tried, through her search for an appropriate title, to relate the elements to each other, by this means seeking to attain greater coherence.

The organization of each sister's thinking processes was clearly displayed; after the first ten minutes I had some reason to believe that Mary was the schizophrenic patient. This was confirmed by the succeeding procedures and was in accordance with what I later learned of her history and preadmission diagnosis.

Examples of our second procedure, family portraits, follow. Figure 3 was drawn by a twenty-three-year-old male patient who displayed the kind of disorganized behavior that enabled me to identify him as schizophrenic. In this picture the enormous mother almost appears to be carrying the tiny father in her arms. Other family members are slightly larger than the father and like him helplessly extend their arms into space. The only exception is a sister who is drawn in profile and turned toward the patient. I later learned

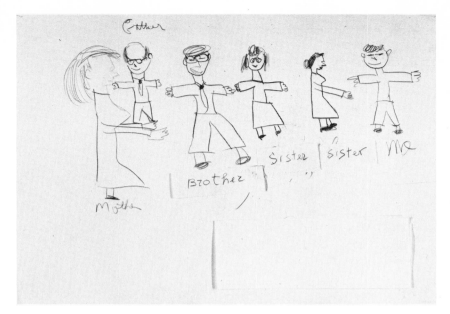

Figure 3

that even though she is much more successful and better adjusted than her brother, she shares his tendency to worry and is closer to him than is anyone else in the family. It was not difficult to infer the parental roles in this family.

Figure 4 is another family portrait. It was produced by a twenty-two-year-old male schizophrenic patient during an acute psychotic episode. In family psychotherapy sessions as well as during the family art evaluation he constantly insulted his mother.

Here we see his paranoid view of the mother's malignant influence on all family members. They are all tied to her; she directs them by means of electrodes implanted in their brains, reducing them to marionettes on strings. The patient is the one who accuses and in a mixture of French and schizophrenese designates her as the evil one.

It may look as if these two patients made distorted portraits because of their own oedipal or other problems regarding the parent depicted. In both these examples, however, the bizarre representations merely magnify the real role and personality of the mother: in each case a domineering, castrating female, as was shown more and more clearly throughout the session by her interaction with other family members and by the family's art productions.

The third procedure, the abstract family portrait, is not an easy task even for well-integrated individuals or families. I have nevertheless introduced it into family art evaluation because it gives reliable information about each person's capacity for organized abstract thinking. The samples we obtain frequently depict objects related to people's occupations or hobbies, or other concrete objects used as symbols. Less often we obtain true

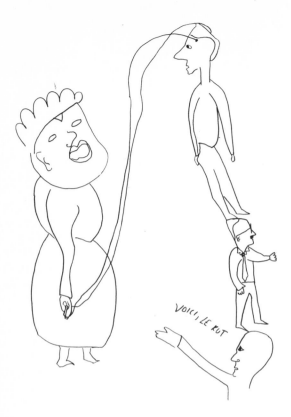

VOICI, LE KUT

Figure 4

abstractions, where colors and shapes alone convey a meaning. In the family of a schizophrenic usually not only the designated patient but most of the family members make concrete representations rather than abstract ones. In normal and less disturbed families it is more frequent that one or several family members are able to grasp and represent an abstract idea.

To illustrate this and the remaining procedures of family art evaluation, I have chosen a family where the member recognized as the patient was not as severely decompensated as the patients whose family portraits I have just shown. This family's behavior was not as chaotic and confusing as that of some other schizophrenic families. At times I leave the sessions of the more severely disturbed families not only with a feeling of extreme fatigue and discomfort but with my mind completely drained of ideas.

Evelyn Valachos, the hospitalized family member, is an eighteen-year-old girl, the oldest daughter in a middle-class family of Greek descent. About a year before her admission to the Clinical Center she left college after only three days. She had difficulty concentrating, was preoccupied with her obesity and with masturbation, and feared she might have a venereal disease. Later, after an unhappy affair, she become mute, negativistic, and withdrawn, as well as transiently suicidal. Of her four siblings only the two older ones, Vicky (aged sixteen) and George (aged thirteen), were taking part in family psychotherapy, in research interviews, and in family art evaluation. The behavior of the patient and the rest of the family was very well controlled during the family psychotherapy sessions and during the art evaluation. Laughter was their constant defense. One sensed the patient's anxiety and discomfort but the family brought enough humor into the evaluation session to make it relatively easy to bear.

Although five of the seven family members were present, I am going to concentrate on the three—mother, father, and Evelyn—around whom the conflict seemed to focus.

Figure 5, a family portrait drawn by Mrs. Valachos, is one more example of our second procedure. It is a rather immature drawing, which could easily be attributed to a child between eight and ten years of age. There are no gross distortions except the infantile appearance of all family members; mother hardly looks older than her five-year-old daughter. The father does not appear much more mature but he leads the group. The mother drew herself next to him, then crossed out her name and placed the patient's name instead under the figure next to the father.

The next three pictures are examples of procedure number three, abstract family portraits, drawn by Evelyn, Vicky and George. Figure 6 is by the patient. We see that this girl's thinking is very concrete and her symbols are overgeneralized. Women in the family are flowers, boys are toy animals, only the father is a big, strong tree. The interesting part is that Evelyn at first

Figure 5

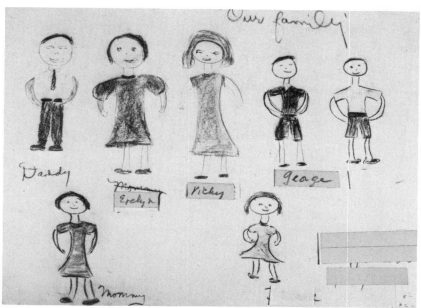

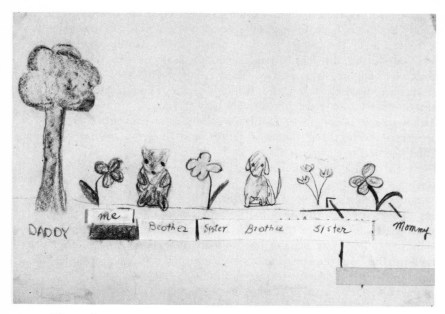

Figure 6

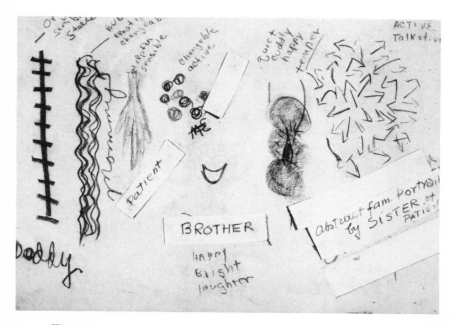

Figure 7

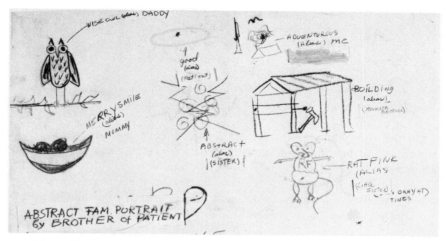

Figure 8

refused to draw herself in the family group. It was only when the session was over and the family was ready to leave that she very shyly asked, "May I add something to one of my pictures?" She then drew one red flower at the end of the row, wrote her mother's name under it, crossed out the inscription "Mommy" from under the flower next to the father and wrote her own name instead. She said she did not want to be "left out."

These substitutions, indicating confusion of identities on the part of both mother and daughter, were certainly not without meaning. Evelyn's and mother's roles were shifting: Evelyn displaced mother, mother displaced herself. Our first thought was that this might be an expression of the oedipal conflict. The later course of the session indicated that this conflict could also be viewed as preoedipal, concerned with Evelyn's wish to take the mother's place in a nurturant role.

Figure 7 is a second example of procedure number three, the abstract family portrait; the picture was made by the patient's sister Vicky. Vicky was less concrete than the patient; she used movement and color successfully to represent the different personalities.

The ladder or vertical fence-like shape on the left is inscribed "Daddy—organized, sensible, stable." Next to him the wavy, multicolor lines are "Mommy—bubbly, emotional, changeable." The patient is represented by a hand, inscribed "helpful, sensible." We are struck by the contrast between these adjectives and the character of the hand, which is blue and hangs like an empty rubber glove, lifeless and entirely lacking the helpful strength it is supposed to have.

Figure 8 is George's abstract family portrait (again, procedure number three). He pictures Daddy as a "Wise Owl," Mommy as a red mouth labeled "A Merry Smile," his sister, the patient, as a halo entitled "Good."

We see a consistent image of the father, the mother, and the patient in these three abstract family portraits:

1. The father is a pillar of strength (tree, ladder, owl).
2. The mother is the merry, changeable, unstable creature (red flower, bright wavy lines, smiling mouth).
3. The patient navigates between the parents in an indefinite role—competitive or complementary? (Her siblings represent her as a helpful hand or a halo.)

During the session, George and Vicky were constantly teasing their mother about her foolishness, nuttiness, helplessness, and lack of talent, when actually she managed well and was up to all required tasks.

We also notice that in the abstract family portraits made by the well siblings this trio—mother, father, and patient—were represented next to one another, while the patient and the mother shift their places in their own pictures.

As examples of procedure number four, individual pictures developed from a scribble, we take the two pictures done by Evelyn and her sister. Figure 9 is by Evelyn, the patient. She chose just a fragment of the scribble and made no changes in its lines. The final result shows her inability to integrate fragments into a whole. Such coloring-in of shapes formed by the lines of the scribble without using these forms as a stimulus for imagination is characteristic of fragmented or constricted schizophrenics. Evelyn's picture is not an extreme example, since she gave the colored portion of her lines a title, *Goose Head*, in an effort to achieve more than just a filling in of space. I

Figure 9

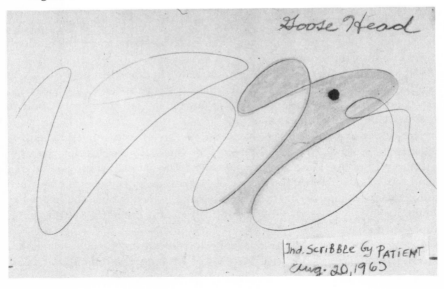

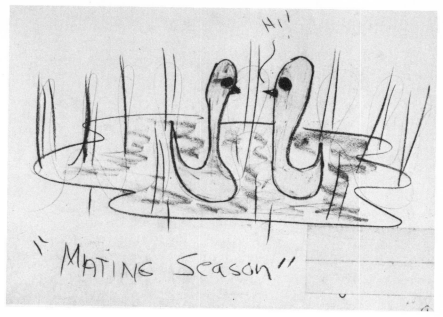

Figure 10

later found that this fitted with her diagnosis, which was constricted, schizoid personality with occasional circumscribed, frankly schizophrenic episodes.

Figure 10, *Mating Season*, is Vicky's drawing. Notice the difference between this and Figure 9, the freedom and imagination Vicky displayed. She departs from the original lines for the subject of her drawing, and then she freely adds other shapes and colors, becomes involved in the creative activity, and obtains a delightful, harmonious, and complete picture. Her title—whatever its implications may be—is again imaginative, and suggests a meaning far beyond the labeling of the obvious.

Vicky, the well sibling, has shown in all her individual pictures consistently good integration and ability for organized abstract thinking. So-called well siblings in many of our families, however, demonstrate no such capacity. Frequently we have noticed that a sibling whose behavioral and educational adjustment is adequate shows in his pictures signs of underlying thought disorder or personality problems.[5]

Let us now see how this family functioned in a joint enterprise, the family scribble (procedure number five). We recall that first each family member makes his own scribble and then they choose one to develop together into a picture. Frequently families, especially those having a schizophrenic member, decide which scribble to develop on the basis of who made it

5. Juliana Day and Hanna Kwiatkowska, "The Psychiatric Patient and His Well Sibling: A Comparison Through Their Art Productions," *Bulletin of Art Therapy*, Vol. 2, No. 2, Winter 1962.

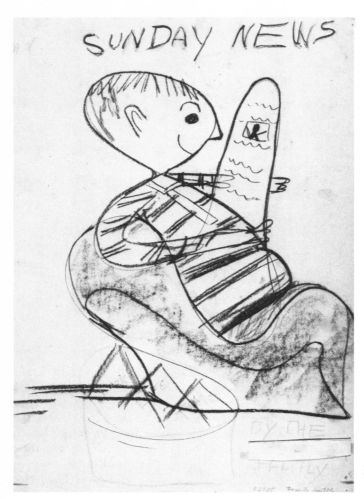

Figure 11

rather than because of what they see in it. This appeared to be the case with the Valachos family, who chose mother's scribble. There were many different associations but finally Vicky forced the decision by simply asking whether everybody agreed to father's first idea, a man reading a newspaper. They managed to produce a fairly complete picture (Figure 11) but it is limited on the whole to the original lines of the scribble just like Evelyn's, although I repeated a couple of times my initial instruction, "You can add, omit or change as many lines of the scribble as you want."

The phallic character of the newspaper in the finished picture is puzzling and adds a bizarre note to the otherwise humorous and imaginative even if somewhat limited picture. The father and the patient's brother did most of the drawing. The patient abstained completely. When I later found out about her sexual problems the thought came to me that she may have withdrawn because this phallic shape disturbed her.

The last procedure, number six, is identical with the first, "a free picture, no subject assigned." The comparison of the first and last pictures is often very revealing. The emotionally charged family portraits and the uncovering experience of the scribble rarely fail to bring out differences between the first free picture and the last one. This is why the session is started and ended with such a picture. Reactions vary. The person with a poorly integrated ego is likely to become more fragmented and disorganized. For an emotionally stable person the intervening experience has usually stimulated his creative potentialities; his last picture has a good chance of being freer and less inhibited because of the emotions stirred by the various procedures of the art evaluation. We have observed yet another kind of reaction in people who seem well adjusted but whose real ego strength is less than it appears. Their defenses have been mobilized and the last picture is frequently rigid and constricted, often a geometrical design. This is what happened with Mr. Valachos.

Figure 12, *Quiet Country Scene* (Plate XVI), is his first picture (procedure

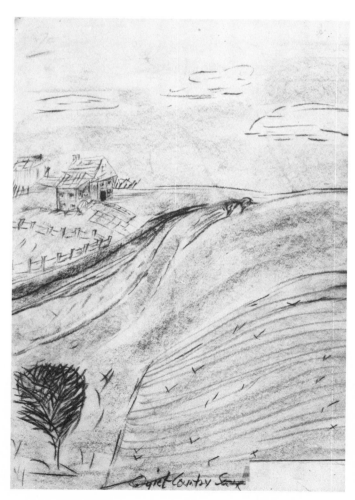

Figure 12

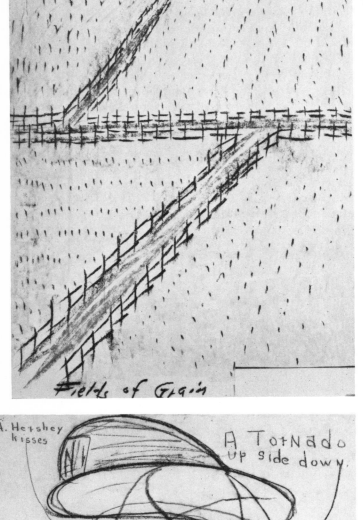

Figure 13

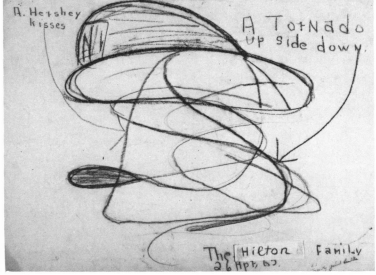

Figure 14

number one), drawn with freedom and ease. Mrs. Valachos commented, "This is what he wishes for, a farm." Let us compare it with *Fields of Grain*, his last free picture produced at the end of the session (Figure 13).

We see a complete change from the pleasant, carefree *Quiet Country Scene* to these empty and forbidding rows of fences. In the light of this change one wonders how burdensome it is for him to maintain the role, pillar of strength, assigned to him by his family. Is he really able to live up to their expectations?

He also may be responding defensively to the danger of the triangle, his wife, Evelyn, and himself. We recall the earlier pictures (Figures 5 and 6) where mother was displaced and Evelyn took her place next to him. How much is he threatened by the unclear, complicated aspects of this relationship? It appears that he has to protect himself by denying all feeling; he is expected to be "wise as an owl," "reliable, organized, sensible." He now builds fences and barriers around himself, and yet at the beginning of the session he was able to express a poetic fantasy, a cherished wish.

The diagnostic potentialities of family art evaluation will be highlighted by the contrasting result of one procedure performed by another family with an offspring having a different form of schizophrenic illness. For comparison with the Valachos's limited but well-organized effort to produce a picture together, we present the joint picture started from a scribble by the Hiltons.

The Hiltons' hospitalized seventeen-year-old daughter Rose, a chronic process schizophrenic with amorphous, disorganized, poorly differentiated forms of thinking, exercised little control over her impulses. Her brother John, aged twelve, was not overtly psychotic but his mannerisms and gesticulations were frequently infantile and bizarre, and his art productions indicated extremely low self-esteem combined with frequent impulses toward violence and destruction.

Figure 14 is called both *A Hershey Kisses* and *A Tornado Upside Down*. During its production, the Hilton family was extremely active and they showered us with associations. They switched from one scribble to another, could not settle on anything. John pointed out a "big nose" and "a boomerang," and finally outlined in red on his father's scribble what he called "A Hershey Kisses." His father accepted this title and wrote it on the sheet but they continued to work on the picture. The patient saw a "balloon," then outlined an "S" for "snake." The father brought up a childhood memory of being scared by "a snake with a wide-open mouth in a strawberry patch." The mother at first protested that the things recognized by the family in the lines of the scribble did not make sense with each other. But finally she gave in to the irrationality of the group and outlined in black what she had earlier identified as "a fireman's hat." As if encouraged by this, the rest of the family continued to make irrelevant additions to the picture. John drew a letter "A" in blue, the patient another "S," then suddenly she said she saw in the lines "a tornado." The mother again remarked on the bizarreness of the picture, found it a "little disjointed" but let her objections go and joined the others, outlining another letter "A."

The confusion in the family grew, and so probably does the reader's. This chaos is conveyed not only by the picture itself but by John's excited exclamation: "A tornado upside down! Here are the Hershey kisses, chocolate tornado upside down! An arrow pointing to it! I love chocolate tornadoes."

It is worth noting that in this family the mother does not use her potential common sense in dealing with the family's irrationality but lets herself be swayed by the mass confusion. We have observed in a variety of families that the offspring are regularly more severely ill when both parents contribute, passively or actively, to the family transactional disorder than if one takes a stand against the confusion or at least refrains from taking part in it.

Summary

A new method of evaluating family relations and dynamics through art productions has been described. It is currently used at the National Institute of Mental Health, but it presents special advantages where the program does not regularly include family psychotherapy. This method provides an opportunity to observe family members in action in circumstances new to them, in a situation that has a good chance of eliciting their habitual patterns of behavior. It is economical in time and manpower.

The standardized procedures used in family art evaluation were illustrated by examples:

1. For the first procedure we compared *free pictures* by twin sisters. In the picture of one of the twins one could easily recognize characteristics indicating schizophrenic thought disorder underlying apparent behavioral adjustment. The other twin, who is not known to have had any psychiatric difficulties, tried to integrate her picture into a meaningful whole and was relatively successful in doing so.

2. The second procedure, *family portraits*, was demonstrated by two pictures, both by acutely psychotic schizophrenic patients, both presenting magnified, paranoid views of genuinely domineering mothers.

3. A series of pictures made by one family was presented to show *abstract family portraits*, *individual* and *joint pictures from a scribble*, and the *final free picture*. Through these examples we could see how the art productions of family members bring forth unconscious material which is usually inaccessible in an equally brief, purely verbal encounter. Certain facets of family psychopathology and problems unfolded before our eyes, even though the family presented a façade of good adjustment.

4. Two families' joint scribbles were compared. Differences in the ways these families handled this task corresponded with the kind of schizophrenic disorder in their offspring.

Although this paper focuses on the use of art techniques in evaluation of families rather than as a means of therapy, the method is also being applied in the family treatment process at the National Institute of Mental Health.

Family art therapy and family art evaluation are based on the dynamic analysis of images projected from the unconscious advocated by Margaret Naumburg, the pioneer in the use of art in psychiatry. We broadened the scope of this analysis from the individual to the family. This enabled us to obtain enlightening material concerning family relations, transactions, and possible underlying thought disorder in family members. Family art evaluation provides even in one session a rapid but revealing glimpse of the psychological functioning of a family unit.

The Effect of Training on Judging Psychopathology from Paintings

Bernard I. Levy and Elinor Ulman

This paper is the fourth of a series devoted to the use of art as a representation of psychiatric disturbance. In 1967[1] and 1968[2] the authors reported the results of the first study, based on the simplest diagnosis that can be made—psychiatric patient (P)/nonpatient (N). The results of that study encouraged further work, reported in 1973.[3] In the latter study the diagnostic accuracy of art therapists was compared with that of mental health workers and that of judges without experience in dealing with psychiatric patients. A comparison of judgments by members of these three groups forced the conclusion that art therapists are not superior to others in making the P and N diagnoses. However, almost all subjects made the correct diagnosis more often than would occur by chance.

In discussing their results, the authors raised the question whether the diagnostic skill of individuals can be increased through training. Interest in that question rested on the supposition that art therapists need to cultivate such a skill to make their work as effective as possible.

By initiating a course in psychological assessment by graphic means the senior author was able to get data bearing on training for diagnostic skill. The semester course investigated the assessment of intelligence, personality, and psychopathology from the Bender-Gestalt, Human Figure Drawings, Kinetic Family Drawings, Kwiatkowska's Family Art Evaluation, the Ulman Diagnostic Series, and free paintings.

1. Bernard I. Levy and Elinor Ulman, "Judging Psychopathology from Paintings," *Journal of Abnormal Psychology*, Vol. 72, No. 2, 1967.
2. Elinor Ulman and Bernard I. Levy, "An Experimental Approach to the Judgment of Psychopathology from Paintings," *Bulletin of Art Therapy*, Vol. 8, No. 1, Oct. 1968.
3. Elinor Ulman and Bernard I. Levy, "Art Therapists as Diagnosticians," *American Journal of Art Therapy*, Vol. 13, No. 1, Oct. 1973.

Method

The members of the weekly graduate seminar exploring psychological assessment by graphic means were asked at the first meeting of the seminar to diagnose the sixty-five paintings described in the 1973 study of art therapists.[4] The students judged them again two meetings later, for reliability purposes, and then again at the close of the semester three months later. Thus, it was hoped that the effect of training upon diagnostic accuracy could be determined.

The judges were asked to view each colored slide of a painting done by either a patient or nonpatient for five seconds and immediately to note their diagnosis as either P or N. At each of the three judging sessions the same slides were presented in the same order.

The judges were graduate students, with the exception of one talented undergraduate—a senior who had been given permission to enter the course—and came from the disciplines of clinical psychology, developmental psychology, social psychology, special education, counseling, and art therapy. Several members of the seminar held graduate degrees and were working in clinical activities or in teaching. The total enrollment in the course was twenty-three. Not every member of the seminar was present for each of the three showings of the slides; therefore, the number of judges will vary to some extent for each statistical analysis.

Results

In the first study of the series,[5] the question of judge reliability was left open because of lack of repeated measurements over time. In this study, however, the judges repeated their diagnoses a week after the pretest. Data on nineteen judges were available. The correlation between first and second trials was 0.79. With an N of nineteen pairs of measures, that correlation is significantly different from zero at the $p \leq .001$ level of statistical confidence. That is to say that the judges ordered themselves in a quite constant fashion across the first two trials: the high- and low-accuracy judges tended to maintain their positions in both trials. One can infer from such data that the capacity to diagnose from paintings is a consistent characteristic and not one that fluctuates. Some are good at it and others not so good.

With respect to the central question put to the data—does improvement in diagnosis occur as an outcome of special training?—the results are encouraging. Sixteen judges were available for all three trials. They averaged 44.3 correct diagnoses at the first meeting of the class; 46.3 correct diagnoses two weeks later; and 47.4 at the close of the semester thirteen

---

4. *Ibid.*
5. Levy and Ulman, *op. cit.*, 1967.

class sessions later. Thus, there was a total gain of 3.1 correct judgments out of sixty-five opportunities to diagnose. The greatest spurt in ability occurred early in training, and improvement slowed down as time elapsed. On the average, 68 percent of the diagnoses were correct at the time of the pretrial and 73 percent at the close of the course.

The pattern of increase of accuracy is statistically significant. With *df* equal to 2/30, an analysis of variance of repeated measures yielded on *F* of 4.12, which is significant at less than the *.05* level but not quite at the *.01* level. Thus, there is good reason to believe that the increase in diagnostic competence is real.

Our conclusions are weakened by a flaw in the study—the lack of a control group; in this study each judge was his own control. A proper control group would enable serial testing of diagnostic ability without intervening training. The junior author attempted such a procedure on an informal basis with a small group of psychiatric residents. While the residents were made familiar with art therapy products for a year, they were not purposely taught to use art for diagnostic purposes. A study of their diagnostic accuracy early and late in the year did not give evidence of improvement.

In analyzing the first two sets of responses by students in the course, the overall number of correct responses attained by each subject across the two trials was used to indicate judge reliability. Judge consistency across trials was measured for each subject by calculating the percentage of agreement without regard to accuracy. Thus, changes in diagnoses, whether P or N, were determined for a judge within his own trials. The percentage of agreement between trials 1 and 2, trials 1 and 3, and trials 2 and 3 was obtained. High percentages reveal high judge consistency, while low percentages reveal that judges are operating less consistently even though their accuracy may have changed relatively little. For trials 1 and 2 the judges' consistency ranged from 63 to 92 percent, with an average percentage of 78.2; for trials 1 and 3 the range was 66 to 89 percent, with an average of 77.5; for trials 2 and 3 the range was 77 to 89 percent, with an average of 82.9. Two conclusions are apparent: accuracy of diagnosis increased over time, and consistency was greater between adjacent trials than between trials 1 and 3. With increase in both accuracy and consistency as the criteria, learning truly appears to have occurred. Could judges have improved even more with a longer training period?

A final aspect of the data was explored—the contributions of the paintings themselves to the diagnostic process. Some paintings are difficult to judge because of the major impact of the intelligence factor;[6] thus, paintings by psychiatrically normal yet mentally retarded subjects are frequently diagnosed as P by judges. Conversely, the work of highly intelligent schizo-

6. See Ulman and Levy, *op. cit.*, 1968.

phrenics tends to be seen as that of nonpatients. In both the earliest study and the present one most of the "difficult" paintings—the same in both studies—were consistently misdiagnosed. For example, in the most extreme case, a low-I.Q. normal subject was misdiagnosed by all the judges in this study on trials 1 and 2, and by fifteen out of sixteen on trial 3. Such difficult works—there are about a dozen among the sixty-five paintings used—set a real limit on judge accuracy. Without more knowledge about the clues to differential diagnosis in the paintings of retardates and schizophrenics, there can be no lifting of the accuracy ceiling in this area. In the case of the sixty-five paintings in this study, the presence of difficult paintings (primarily those by retardates) would limit accuracy levels to a maximum of about 80 percent, or fifty-two correct diagnoses. That figure was approached by several judges. At least once during the three trials, one judge scored 52, three judges received scores of 51, one judge scored 50, and three judges scored 49.

Discussion

It appears likely that one's ability to diagnose psychopathology from paintings can be improved with training. However, more knowledge is needed about the differential diagnosis between retarded and schizophrenic functioning and about the influence of high intelligence upon the art of some schizophrenics. Such knowledge could break through the ceiling that now limits accuracy of judgments. Furthermore, an attempt should be made to develop a scoring system which reflects the cues used by the most successful judges in judging the presence of psychopathology, so that assessment could be made to depend less completely on the hunches of talented judges.

One could argue that the art therapist's interpretation of patient art is an essential ingredient in his contribution to the assessment of the patient's maladjustment and its psychodynamics. We have observed that the art therapist makes unique and decisive contributions to diagnostic discussions of patients. Without skills such as are implicit even in the crude diagnosis required for this study, such contributions are likely to be pallid.

One may view psychotherapy as, in large measure, an intensive process of continuous assessment oriented to gauging the client's progress. What better gauge of current state than the products of art therapy sessions? It is by observing the client's behavior while creating and by reading the graphic language of the products that we can sometimes make pertinent and helpful responses to the client. The same process of observation and "reading" may also lead to changes in the tactics, strategy, and goals of therapy. We must always remember that the painting *is* the person who made it; it is a projection of a host of psychological processes.

If effectiveness as a healer is based, in part, on diagnostic skill, then the need to understand the meaning of our clients' art is important. One would expect that effective practitioners would also be good assessors. That prediction is an empirical matter waiting to be studied systematically. Upon the outcome of such future studies rests a decision about the relative importance of diagnostic training in the art therapist's course of study.

Graphic Perspectives on the Mother–Child Relationship

Selwyn Dewdney and Irene M. Dewdney

Introduction

In an earlier paper we pointed out that drawings of certain specific subjects could be explored by the mental patient with especially useful therapeutic results.[1] Here we propose to examine explorations of drawings that deal with a single subject: a mother and her child. Although many other subjects are likely to stimulate significant reactions in the art-centered interview, none is potentially more useful than this one. Through this study, although it will be concerned exclusively with drawings of this single subject, we hope to illustrate what rich therapeutic possibilities may be opened up by encouraging a patient to render *any* subject that promises to have a personal meaning for him.

It is important to note that this method may prove equally useful *outside the realm of art therapy* proper. For therapists who deal mainly in words, such drawings can be extremely productive at one or another stage of treatment. Neither patient nor therapist needs to have any particular background in art, and only the simplest materials—no more than a pencil and a piece of paper—are required. Drawings can remain on file to be used again and again to confirm or test insights acquired in the course of verbal exchange, or to break a therapeutic impasse. Finally, drawings of many significant subjects can serve not as substitutes for verbal expression, but to *promote* verbal responses.

The Graphic Material

Origin and Sources

In the art therapy files for the years 1955–1967 inclusive at Westminster Hospital, and 1962–1967 at the London Psychiatric (formerly Ontario) Hospital (both in London, Ontario), we found mother–child drawings in the folders of forty-nine patients. During this period some three hundred fifty patients had been referred for art therapy in the two hospitals, and we had

---

1. Selwyn Dewdney, Irene M. Dewdney, and E. V. Metcalfe, "The Art-Oriented Interview as a Tool in Psychotherapy," *Bulletin of Art Therapy*, Vol. 7, No. 1, 1967.

filed every piece of their work, regardless of whether they had attended a single session or a hundred. The total of forty-nine, therefore, includes all patients in the two hospitals who made mother–child drawings during the stated periods.

Neither interest nor ability or training in art has ever played more than a minor part in referral to art therapy, and the diagnoses of referred patients have extended over the whole spectrum of mental illness short of catatonia and severe agitation. Consequently the drawings are confined to neither those by patients in a particular diagnostic category, nor those by patients with a special aptitude for art. We maintain a climate such that resistance to graphic expression seldom outlasts the first session, and still more rarely persists into a third.

At intervals over the same period medical students, psychology interns, occupational therapy personnel, and psychiatric nurses-in-training were confronted with the same situation as were referred patients. Renderings of the mother-and-child theme made by four of these presumably normal persons are included in this study. While these trainees fall far short of supplying a control group, their pictures serve to indicate that the patients' drawings differ from those of others less than one might expect.

Before selections were made, each mother-and-child picture had been reproduced in a way that eliminated as far as possible the differences that were irrelevant for our purpose. All drawings were traced with a black, nylon-tipped pen, great care being taken, within the limits of this medium, to reproduce the character, although not the weight, of the original line. Thus, even the faintest lines would be clearly shown; otherwise a number of drawings too pale to register in a photograph would have had to be rejected regardless of the interest of their content. All but the smallest drawings were reduced when photographed so that *size* would not influence selection; the dimensions of the originals are shown next to the reproductions. In taking the liberty of altering the weight of the lines we do not mean to say that the strength or weakness of a line has no significance, for obviously it reflects the patient's self-confidence and capacity for making a definite statement. In this study, however, we are concentrating on the *content* of the patient's graphic expression as he responds to it. In our experience it is rarely that a patient is aware of, or reacts to, his own *style*.

Basis of Selection

Out of the drawings by forty-nine patients, twenty-five drawings by twenty-three patients were selected, solely on the basis of how much information was available about each in the written records, especially direct quotations from what the patients said during exploratory sessions. Records were of two kinds: comments or queries written directly on the drawing during the art-oriented interview; and clinical notes made afterward to assist the therapist's communication with the psychiatrist in charge. Notes were sometimes written on the drawing spontaneously by the patient, but more often were added by the therapist, who recorded the gist or the exact words of the patient's comments during the interview, with an occasional explanation of the part played by the therapist.

Basis for Sorting

The drawings were sorted according to the patient's success in recognizing the pathology of his relationship to his mother as it appears in the drawing, but with strong reservations about the validity of our estimation of pathology as revealed by pictures. Typically patients first react to apparent pathology by protesting that they "just can't draw." Bearing it in mind that, regardless of the graphic evidence, we do not *know* that the patient's relationship to his mother is as disturbed as the drawing seems to say, the therapist must proceed on the assumption that the patient is, so to speak, innocent until proved guilty. Nor is the metaphor inappropriate: strong feelings of guilt are inevitably associated with the discovery of previously unsuspected hostility toward one's mother.

Nevertheless, while the drawings were selected entirely on availability of records dealing with the *therapeutic* process, they contain material about which *diagnostic* inferences are almost automatic. One can scarcely glance at some of the drawings illustrated without immediately concluding that something was wrong with the person who made them, and there can be little doubt that at least a few reflect an extremely disturbed mother–child relationship. On the basis, then, of the patient's recorded response to this material, we have grouped the drawings under the following categories:

A: No recognition by the patient of the pathology apparent in his drawing.

B: Partial recognition.

C: Recognition of discrepancies between what was *intended*, and the result that *emerged*, producing emotional insight.

D: Reinforcement of previous insights by recognition of such discrepancies in a current drawing.

E: This group consists of five drawings made by four nursing students. Notes on these were very brief, since no attempt was made at exploration in any depth. Such information as did emerge was volunteered, and there was no effort to steer the discussion in a therapeutic direction.

Illustrative Examples

Sources of information will be distinguished below by certain typographical devices. Thus, notes spontaneously written on the drawing by the patient are capitalized, with quotes (e.g., "THIS IS MY MOTHER AND ME").

Direct quotations written by the therapist on the patient's drawing, or summaries of the gist of a patient's verbal responses, are capitalized without quotes. Where it is necessary to add explanatory material, this is placed within parentheses in lower case. Thus: SHE LOOKS STRANGE (Therapist: Why?) HER EYES (look) HARD.

Information derived from clinical notes or other records will resume normal typography. Names used are obviously fictional.

Supplementary comments will be prefaced by the word NOTE, in capitals. We suggest that the reader delay reading these comments until he has got his own firsthand impression by inspecting the drawing and reading the patient's response to it. Experienced art viewers will recognize how readily one may be influenced by reading *about* a work before actually seeing it.

Group A

Patients in this category got little or no benefit from their response to their drawings.

Albert (A-1)

This drawing was made in the presence of a group. Albert was one of ten chronic psychotic patients who had shown some response to drug therapy. He had had a prefrontal lobotomy some ten years before. He accepted the

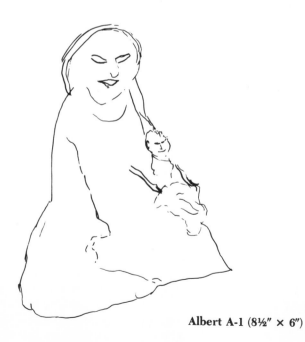

Albert A-1 (8½" × 6")

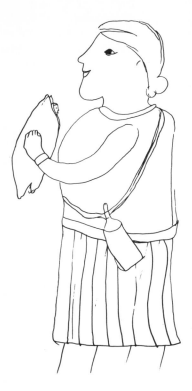

Alec A-2 (14″ × 7″)

therapist's assignment of a mother–child drawing, made after it became clear that he would not act on his own initiative. He was unable, however, to say anything about the resulting picture.

NOTE: the weak, detached arms of the mother, and the withdrawn attitude and expression of the child.

Alec (A-2)
"PRE-CHILDHOOD MEMORY, MAW, & I."
THE MOTHER IS GOING TO PUT THE BABY TO BED. (Therapist: What's the expression on her face?) CONTENT. (On the baby's face?) PEACE.

Over the years Alec had been referred several times by successive psychiatrists at times when he seemed to be on the verge of improving. His originally acute psychotic symptoms, slightly modified by a prefrontal lobotomy, were finally reduced by drug therapy; he became an infantile and ingratiating person with delusions of being female. An impression of therapeutic progress was created by recovery from relapses but he made no real gains. His subjects were usually hearts and flowers, rigidly conventional. The mother–child theme was assigned in the hope of exploring matters of greater emotional significance. The result was the woman holding a bundle. He added the baby's face only at the therapist's suggestion.

NOTE: patient's typical smile on mother's face!

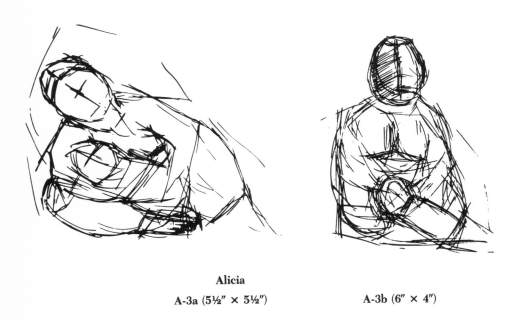

Alicia

A-3a (5½″ × 5½″)   **A-3b (6″ × 4″)**

Alicia (A-3a and 3b)
(Assignment: to show mother and child in two contrasting moods. Alicia decided to show the mother) LOVING (and) KILLING.

She was discharged on subsidence of overt symptoms a few months after admission. She made a poor response to art therapy, taking refuge in the kind of vague abstractions shown here.

NOTE: that neither love nor hate is allowed to emerge from these highly ambivalent drawings.

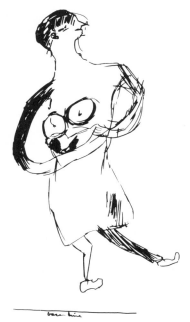

Andrew A-4 (8″ × 5″)

Andrew (A-4)
Andrew was a member of the same group as Albert. A lobotomized patient of long standing, he was still subject to cyclic expressions of rage. The mother–child subject was assigned. He made no response to art therapy.

NOTE: the insecurity of the pose, the strongly accentuated breasts, the perfunctory rendering.

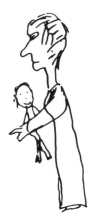

Anne A-5 (3½″ × 1½″)

Anne (A-5)
A KINDLY WOMAN—UNSMILING

Anne was quite blind to the insecure position of the baby in relation to the mother's arms. In this as in other sessions she did all she could to maintain intellectual control. Yet this drawing marks an advance over earlier drawings in which people were always rendered as stick figures. It was made a week after she had described three homosexual experiences. Two months later, in the course of a review of her accumulated drawings, she discovered a link between her homosexuality and her ambivalence toward her mother.

NOTE: the sternness of mother, the transparency of her upper arm and the insecurity of her stance; also, the smile and the withdrawn attitude of the child, both typically autistic.

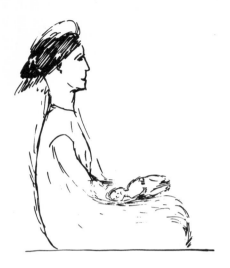

Arthur A-6 (5½″ × 4″)

Arthur (A-6)
(Referring to an early memory) I SORT OF ROUSED UP AND HEARD MOTHER SINGING ROCK-A-BYE BABY. (How old were you?) AGE ONE.

This drawing was made during a hopeful phase of Arthur's therapy. It emerged from discussion of a series of memory drawings. He derived few insights, however, regressing during the following months into conventional landscapes, ruled abstractions, and brief, abortive efforts to resume drawing childhood memories.

NOTE: mother's vanishing arms; the pathetic pose and insecurity of the baby.

Group B

This category consists of patients who were able to get partial glimpses through their drawings into their deeper feelings about mother.

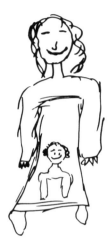

Barbara B-1 (4½″ × 2″)

Barbara (B-1)

"PHYSICAL AFFECTION—DOING THINGS TOGETHER. HAVE A WAY OF DISCIPLINE THAT YOUR CHILD UNDERSTANDS, NAMELY, SETTING A CHILD ON A CHAIR AND SETTING TIMER ON STOVE, WHEN IT RINGS CHILD IS ALLOWED TO GET DOWN."

EYES (of mother) SHOULDN'T BE LOOKING STRAIGHT AHEAD— SORT OF A NOTHING EXPRESSION. (Mother) SHOULD BE CUD-DLING THE CHILD—(her) ARMS JUST HANGING THERE. (The child has) NO ARMS—EYES DON'T SHOW MUCH EXPRESSION.

The mother–child subject was suggested after a discussion of Barbara's feelings about her mother. She was discharged a few weeks later, after some progress in art therapy, her symptoms having receded.

NOTE: that although Barbara saw a good deal of the apparent pathology, she failed to discover a striking feature: how, although she had tried to place the child securely in the mother's lap, she had achieved an effect of insulation and isolation from the mother.

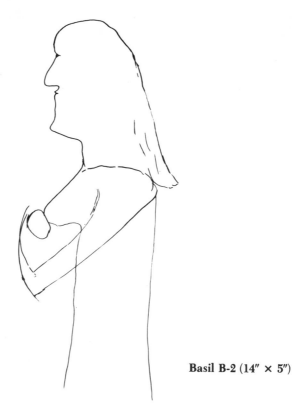

Basil B-2 (14″ × 5″)

Basil (B-2)

"IT IS IMPORTANT TO SEE THINGS AS THEY ARE. IT IS DIFFICULT TO IMAGINE THINGS AS THEY ARE NOT. WHAT IS THE SIMILARITY BETWEEN CONCENTRIC AND PARALLEL LINES? THE SIMILARITY IS TRULY OBVIOUS—WE MUST FIND IN THIS DRAWING THE OBVIOUS."

ARM SHAPED LIKE A SICKLE—A STRONG FACE—MASCULINE—MY MOTHER RUINED ME—SEX IS A DIRTY WORD WITH MOTHER.

This subject was suggested after Basil had discussed feelings about his mother at a somewhat superficial level. The contrast between his own written notes and the comments recorded on the drawing by the therapist reveal the conflict between his deeper feelings and his attempt at intellectual control.

NOTE: how the child is reduced to a cipher by an aggressive, threatening mother. The deeper message is clear in all its aspects, including the absence of the lower half of the body.

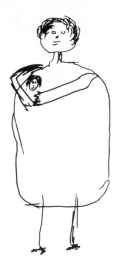

Beatrice B-3 (6″ × 2½″)

Beatrice (B-3)

MOTHER IS HUGGING THE BABY. (Her eyes are) VACANT (showing) NO INTEREST IN THE BABY.

Beatrice's drawing was formally assigned, the therapist instructing her to draw a mother and her baby to show in every possible way that they love each other. Direct assignments were made when it became apparent during two trial sessions that Beatrice lacked the confidence to decide on her own subject. Her comments on her drawing reveal some insight, but evidently she was frightened by what she saw. According to the clinical notes, "This patient is very sick. Her drawings and her completely inappropriate behavior to her daughter indicate more pathology than a severe neurosis." Two weeks later: "the patient says she is not getting anything from art therapy and this therapist is inclined to agree with her."

NOTE: the mother's fragile footing, and the floating, bodiless head of the child.

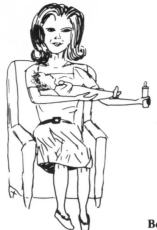

Belinda B-4 (6½″ × 4″)

Belinda (B-4)
(Therapist: Your intention?) THE WOMAN IS HAPPY BECAUSE BABY
HAS FINALLY GOTTEN TO SLEEP. (Therapist: The result?) BABY IS
ASLEEP—MOTHER IS PLEASED—MAYBE BABY'S LEGS ARE
STIFF—MOTHER IS PUTTING BOTTLE AWAY AND WATCHING TV.

The mother–child subject was suggested after a verbal exploration of
Belinda's family feelings. While noting the contradiction between the baby's
rigidity and its being asleep, Belinda was unable to see more deeply.
Superficial improvement soon led to Belinda's discharge, so that her capacity
for insight could not be put to any further test.

NOTE: the peculiar position of the bottle, as if being held away as far as
possible from the child.

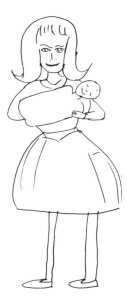

Bertha B-5 (7½″ × 3¼″)

Bertha (B-5)

(The drawing was assigned by the therapist: "Draw a mother loving her baby." When it was completed, he asked what feeling Bertha got from her drawing.) THE MOTHER HAS A HAPPY SMILE, BABY HAS A SMILE OF CONTENTMENT. (Would she make any criticism?) MOTHER'S ARM SHOULD BE IN FRONT OF THE BABY. THERE'S NOTHING TO HOLD IT THERE.

Bertha failed to notice the marked difference between the mother's and the baby's facial expressions. She achieved only partial recognition of the contradictions in the drawing and was unable to make any personal inferences.

NOTE: how the mother's arm appears to be *inside* the baby's covering, like a muff, and the mother's determined expression.

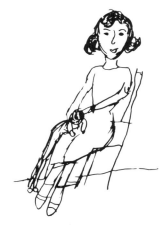

Bessie B-6 (4½″ × 2½″)

Bessie (B-6)
CRIED ON THE TABLE—I CANNOT REMEMBER CRYING ON MOTHER'S LAP.

This drawing emerged out of a series of childhood memories. Bessie recalled crying when she learned she was going to have an operation. She said that her "mother looks worried—the child is standing on the floor, burying her head in mother's lap. Mother is patting and comforting her." Bessie had several months of intensive art therapy both when she was hospitalized and as an outpatient. This drawing, in which she first glimpsed that her feelings about her mother were wishful rather than based on reality, was the starting point of substantial progress.

NOTE: the numerous ways in which Bessie's insecurity was expressed.

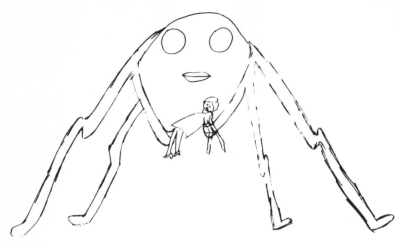

Brenda B-7 (12″ × 18″)

Brenda (B-7)

During a picture-centered group discussion of three prints (a Renoir and two Nativity paintings, all dealing with the relationship between mother and child) one patient, much given to banal sentiments, remarked, "What mother doesn't love her child?" Upon this, Brenda brought out drawing B-7 and pinned it up for the group to view. She declared that the mouth was too human, the spider-monster-mother wasn't vicious enough. When the group failed to share her feelings she was furious and tore up the drawing. In a subsequent group session she asserted that she had received *no* love as a child. In a series of drawings extending over several months of intensive art therapy she had been able, painfully, to sort out the various elements originally condensed in a single monstrous form that had haunted and frightened her to the point where she had a powerful compulsion to draw it; the spider-mother was one of these elements.

The drawing shown represents the high point in her therapy. Thereafter she began to deny earlier insights and her drawings regressed to stereotyped forms that she was unable or unwilling to interpret. Brenda had a long previous and subsequent history of discharges and readmissions, prefaced by a prefrontal lobotomy in 1948. The operation had no discernible effect on a pattern of loud-mouthed, aggressive attempts to cover up affectionate impulses from whose consequences she shied away the instant they were expressed.

NOTE: how eloquently the blank expression of the mother and the limp passivity of the little girl express the pathos of Brenda's unrequited childhood hunger for affection.

Group C
Patients in this category were able to gain significant insights through recognition of the discrepancies between what they had intended to show and what actually emerged in their drawings.

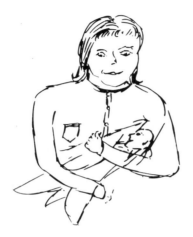

Carolyn C-1 (4″ × 3″)

Carolyn (C-1)
LOOKS LIKE A PUT-ON SMILE. (Mother is) LOOKING STRAIGHT AHEAD. (Intended to show) MOTHER CARRYING THE BABY CARE-FULLY AND GENTLY. THE BABY TO LOOK SECURE; (but in fact) ONE ARM IS GOING AROUND THE HEAD AND THE OTHER IS TOO FAR BACK. ACTUALLY IT (the baby) LOOKS UNCOMFORTABLE. TO SHOW LOVE THE MOTHER WOULD SIT AND ROCK OR HUG THE BABY. WHEN I WAS YOUNG I NEVER FELT MOTHER LOVED ME.

In this instance, as the therapist became aware of Carolyn's inability to express affection, the suggestion was made, among others, that she draw a mother and baby showing in every way possible that the mother *loves* her baby. This Carolyn rephrased as "draw a mother holding her baby to show the kind of a mother I would want."

Carolyn, then sixteen years old and with a fragile sense of her own identity, explored her childhood family relationships in some depth but could not link up past with present feelings. She is now nearly twenty and has been able to function outside the hospital only at brief, irregular intervals.

NOTE: how aggressively the mother is holding the baby, and the confusion of lines adjacent to the baby's head.

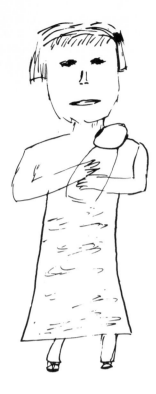

Charlie C-2 (10″ × 4″)

Charlie (C-2)
"ODD SHAPED SKIRT AND LEGS—NO EARS ON MOTHER—
COMMUNISM IS THE GROWN-UPS FAULT. CHILDREN MUST BE
PROTECTED."

(First response to therapist's invitation to Charlie to comment:) SHE
LOOKS HAPPY AND CONTENTED—SEEMS LIKE THE TYPE WHO
WOULD PROTECT THE BABY—SHE LOVES IT. (Later comment:) A
WEE BIT SAD (the mother), THE RIGHT KIND OF SADNESS. (Invited
to criticize the drawing:) BABY IS BETTER DRAWN THAN THE MOTH-
ER (her) MOUTH IS TOO WIDE—GIVES THE FACE A PLEASANT
LOOK—CLOSED EYES GIVE HER A CALM LOOK—BABY'S EARS
ARE DARKER THAN THE REST (they show more strongly in the original
drawing)—I KEEP HEARING THIS 60-CYCLE HUM.

This mother–child drawing was suggested by the therapist. During
exploration of it, Charlie recognized a struggle between the "happy,
contented" look he wanted to see in his drawing and his glimpses (e.g., "a
wee bit sad") of what he actually expressed. In later sessions he gained
substantial insight into his sexual ambivalence. Two months after this session

the clinical notes included: "has acquired considerable introspective ability, being already in better shape than many patients qualifying for discharge."

Charlie himself was discharged a few weeks later. Since his art-oriented interviews were the only psychotherapy he received during his hospital stay, there is good reason to believe that art therapy contributed substantially to his recovery.

NOTE: the transparency of the mother's arms.

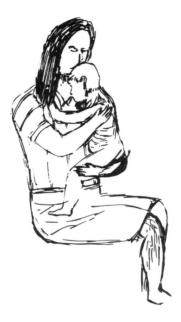

Conrad C-3 (7¼" × 3½")

Conrad (C-3)

(Intentions:) TO SHOW BABY AND MOTHER HOLDING OUT ARMS TO EACH OTHER—IF IT WAS NURSING OR HELD CLOSELY IT WOULD NOT SHOW THAT THEY *BOTH* LOVE EACH OTHER. (Results:) I COULDN'T GET THIS THE WAY I WANTED IT. I WANTED THE MOTHER'S HAND SUPPORTING THE WEIGHT. I WANTED THE MOTHER TO BE SMILING—(she) SEEMS SAD AND WISTFUL.

The subject was assigned. In further explorations Conrad discovered how wide a discrepancy there was between his intentions and the results: the ambivalence of the child, at once reaching for and pushing away the mother, and the concern about the mother's supporting arm which is drawn and redrawn, suggesting to the viewer an anxiety associated with the child's genital area. Conrad's craving for and rejection of female domination led later to recognition of his own sexual confusion, which was amply illustrated in subsequent drawings.

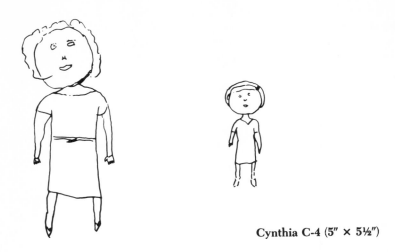

Cynthia C-4 (5″ × 5½″)

Cynthia (C-4)
(Reaction to mother:) SHE DOESN'T LOOK TOO TIDY—SEEMS TO BE
HAPPY—ONE LEG IS SHORTER—HEAD IS LOPSIDED. (Reaction to
daughter:) I HADN'T THOUGHT BEFORE, BUT SHE DOESN'T LOOK
VERY HAPPY—SHE'S SUPPOSED TO HAVE FRIENDS.

The words "I hadn't thought before" express the surprise of discovery that
is typical of significant insights. This drawing emerged from a series of
childhood memories and was followed by further highly fruitful sessions.

NOTE: how Cynthia tries to close the *spatial* gap (standing for an
emotional one) by imitating her mother's stance and expression.

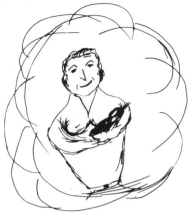

Cyril C-5 (6″ × 5½″)

Cyril (C-5)
(Intentions:) I GOT THE FEELING I WANTED—WARM, COMFORT-
ABLE, SECURE, BEING HELD—SOMETHING I REALLY GO FOR.
(Later reaction:) THE WHOLE THING IS PHONY. MOTHER'S NOSE IS
TOO POINTED—I LIKE THE SMILE—THE HAIR IS SCRAGGLY—NO
HANDS OR ARMS ON BABY—JUST A COUPLE OF O's.

Cyril, who was twenty-two years old, habitually drew his personal
symbol, a tramp, whom he described as a "sad sack." The concept of the
baby as two zeros amply confirms his feeling of worthlessness and his
pessimism about making his way in the world. Later this patient made
substantial progress.[2] The drawing shown here emerged out of a discussion
of Cyril's feelings about his mother.

2. For a reproduction of the "sad sack," see *ibid*.

Group D

Recognition of similar discrepancies between intentions and results on the part of patients in this category served to strengthen and confirm insights they had arrived at earlier.

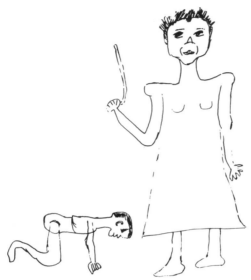

Dennis D-1 (9″ × 7½″)

Dennis (D-1)

THIS (referring to mother) COULD BE A MAN FROM MARS. (Referring to face:) IT'S A SKELETON.

This drawing was made after Dennis had begun to deal verbally with his feelings about his parents. When the therapist suggested that he draw his mother he objected, but agreed to draw "an attractive woman." The child was added during the next session, after Dennis offered some resistance, quoting the biblical dictum, "Honor thy father and mother." The therapist approved this sentiment but pointed out that Dennis was exploring childhood feelings which might not necessarily be those he now had. According to a clinical note, this drawing expressed "the very real problems of Dennis's early childhood when both his parents (his father a war cripple fiercely resentful of his helplessness) took out their frustrations on him, laying a foundation for his 'dislike' of women, and recurrent hostility to males."

As a patient he seemed to relate to staff and others *only* through outbursts of abuse, as if anger were the only social bridge he knew. Between such outbursts he became autistic. Well aware of his angry feelings toward his parents, Dennis was able to express them in too limited a way to benefit from their ventilation.

NOTE: the difficulty Dennis had in connecting the mother's anger with the child, who is facing the punishment of the strap head-on.

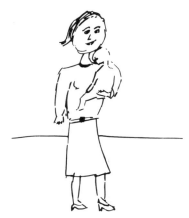

Desmond D-2 (4½″ × 1¼″)

Desmond (D-2)
(Asked to criticize his drawing:) HAIR LIKE A MOP—NECK LIKE ON OSTRICH—JAW LIKE A BRICKLAYER—SHOULDERS LIKE A FULL-BACK. (Asked to describe the feelings he saw in the drawing:) MOTHER HAS A HAPPY FACE—A WIDE-EYED SMILE—LOOKING OUT-WARDS. BABY HASN'T MUCH EXPRESSION—LITTLE ORPHAN ANNIE STYLE—MOTHER IS JUST HOLDING THE BABY—BABY'S HAND IS JUST HANGING—NOT AROUND THE MOTHER'S NECK.

Before making this drawing, Desmond had begun to explore childhood memories, but nothing significant had emerged. At the start of this session the therapist found him staring at the blank paper. He discussed the "nothing" he saw there. He said he was "in a fog" and expected to be all his life. To break the therapeutic impasse the therapist suggested that he draw a mother and child. At first he thought the negative aspects of his drawing were accidental, but later he decided that they did express feelings about his mother who was "a stubborn person—strong willed" who overorganized his life. Yet Desmond could not accept the evidence of his drawing that his present feelings about his mother had so early an origin. In later sessions he was able to trace back his feelings of sexual inadequacy to the relationship between his mother and father where the former played the male role. These insights were amply reinforced when he reviewed this drawing, and helped to promote the breakthrough that came when discharge was imminent.

NOTE: the vagueness ("nothingness") of the baby's head.

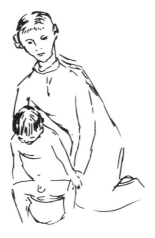

Donald D-3 (4″ × 2½″)

Donald (D-3)

Donald, who had graduated brilliantly into his chosen profession, was subject to periodic emotional storms which made relations with his wife impossible. Attempts to establish himself in his profession invariably failed, because of his inability to tolerate male authority figures, and his repeated emotional entanglements with overprotective females who were prone to anxiety attacks which invariably "infected" him and brought on new storms. Children complicated the situation, with tragic results for one of them.

Donald made many competent drawings expressive of the full range of his inner and outer life, rarely breaking through the intellectual control he was able to maintain between incapacitating attacks of anxiety.

In this drawing he illustrated his mother's distaste for toilet training. Discussing it, he clearly recalled the turbulence of his own experience, his mother's coldness and his father's fury when he deliberately withheld his feces. His therapy was characterized by sessions in which he could coolly analyze his problems alternating with others in which he went into acute panic reactions and, more rarely, burst into a rage. Later he was treated in another hospital and left his profession. A more stable pattern has developed, although he is still subject to attacks of anxiety. Donald is one of those acutely intelligent people whose intellectual insights have been used to head off significant emotional confrontations.

NOTE: that what appear to be conspicuous ears actually represent coils of hair which the mother wore over her ears, perhaps suggesting that she rarely listened to him.

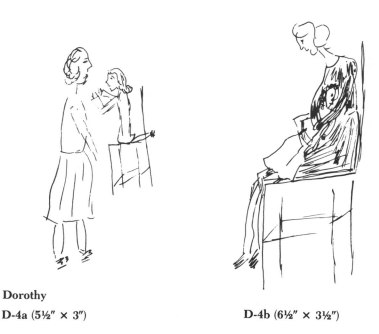

Dorothy

D-4a (5½″ × 3″)   **D-4b (6½″ × 3½″)**

Dorothy (D-4a and 4b)
(Spontaneous explanation:) I PUT A CHAIR IN BECAUSE I USED TO KISS HER GOOD-BYE ALWAYS—THAT'S WHY I PUT IN THE CHAIR. (A later comment:) SHE COULD HAVE BENT DOWN. I SHOULDN'T NEED A CHAIR. (Still later, withdrawing the implied criticism:) I COULD HAVE DRAWN IT THE OTHER WAY.

The first drawing was one of a series of childhood memories. Her second drawing was an attempt to show mother and child "the other way."

(Comments on second drawing:) I'M THE BABY—IT SEEMS SHE'S GOING TO SLIP OUT AT ANY MOMENT—SHE COULD SLIDE OFF

ON THE FLOOR. (Recognizing discrepancies:) NOW IT DOESN'T LOOK SO NICE TO ME ANYMORE—MOTHER IS LOOKING AWAY FROM THE CHILD—SHE DOESN'T SEEM TO BE INTERESTED IN THE BABY. (Reversing her judgment:) MOTHER WAS IN A HURRY. SHE COULD HAVE BEEN PREGNANT. (Becoming critical again:) THE BABY COULD HAVE SAT SO IT FILLED IN THE CORNER (referring to the angle made by the mother's lap). THAT PART OF THE BODY (the genital zone) SHE DOESN'T WANT ANYONE CLOSE TO. (Why?) SHE DOESN'T LIKE IT.

Dorothy was well aware of her insecurity both as a child and as an unmarried woman in her late twenties. She also realized how sexually inhibited she was. She undertook drawings of childhood feelings to test their relationship to current ones. They proved to be the prelude to a series of expressions of her current feelings, and these prompted dreams which were in turn explored graphically. Finally, significant insights into the reasons for her sexual inadequacy emerged.

NOTE: the swings, typical of Dorothy's emotional confusion, between confession and recantation, as her defenses alternately softened and hardened.

Douglas (D-5)

"WEAPON OR SACRIFICE?—THE CHILD IS PIPESTEM STIFF AS SHE (the mother) BRANDISHES HIM OVER THE FATHER FURNACE."

Douglas had received wide recognition for his creative achievements when he entered the hospital in a state of extreme thought disorder. Following a course of chemotherapy, he was referred to art therapy in a more rational state. He had already come to realize that his parents were prone to use him as a weapon in their quarrels, and he had acquired insight into long-standing sexual problems.

His drawings served to confirm earlier insights and to bring them together in a less piecemeal fashion. A majority of his pictures were concerned with sex and death, with women appearing in various monstrous forms. Here he was able for the first time to show his mother as human. In a part of the same drawing not here shown, his father is symbolized as a mass of red scribbling, interspersed with heavy black blobs to represent the "fuel" that kept the "father-furnace" burning.

Through exploring these drawings he achieved a new integration of his feelings, and after discharge he resumed his creative work, with no further serious breakdown over the past six years.

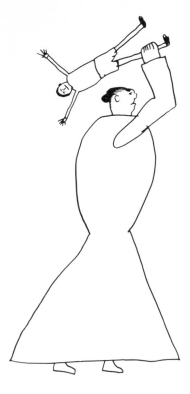

Douglas D-5 (11″ × 5″)

Group E

These five drawings were made by psychiatric nurses-in-training during a short course designed to give them some insight into the usefulness of graphic and plastic expression as a therapeutic medium. In the first session each nurse was confronted with the same situation as that faced by a patient in his first art therapy session: drawing materials, and the instruction to "Draw anything you feel like drawing—anything that comes to mind." In the second session the nurses were asked to "Draw a mother and her baby, showing in every possible way that they love each other." These five drawings were selected from the work of the trainee group on the same basis as the patients' work, namely, they are the ones about which the most information had been recorded.

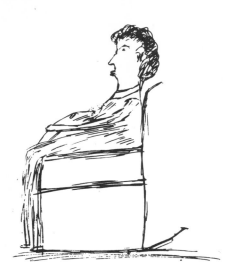

Edith E-1 (5½″ × 3½″)

Edith (E-1)

In conversations with Edith, the therapist learned that she was unmarried, in her early fifties, and was a member of an ethnic minority of European origin, so that her mastery of English was limited. She had undertaken to become a psychiatric nurse to increase her financial contributions to her widowed mother and two stay-at-home adult siblings. Being in training was acutely uncomfortable for her, and she constantly feared failure.

NOTE: the peculiar lips of the mother (suggesting displaced sexuality) and the extreme vagueness of the baby.

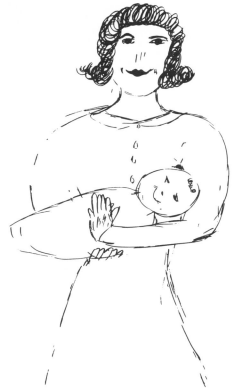

Estelle E-2 (12″ × 6″)

Estelle (E-2)

Each nurse, before her exploratory session with the therapist, was told that she need not comment aloud on her reactions to her drawing, but could merely make mental notes of them. Estelle, however, was the only one to say nothing about her drawing. Her silence, in view of the apparent pathology, is understandable.

NOTE: the mother's hand that seems both to hold and reject the baby, and the mother's eyes staring beyond her child as if at a viewer. The baby appears to be smugly happy although it is so bundled up that it can make no gesture with hands or arms toward the mother.

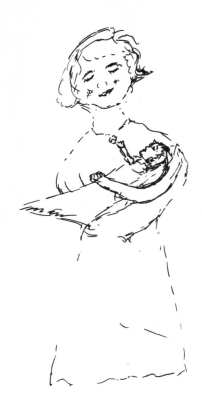

Ethel E-3 (9″ × 4″)

Ethel (E-3)
THE MOTHER AND BABY HAVEN'T ANY FEET—THE MOTHER IS
VERY HAPPY—THE CHILD IS TRYING TO REACH FOR THE
MOTHER—THE BABY'S FACE IS TOO OLD, MORE LIKE HER LATE
TEENS.

Ethel's comments and criticisms were made without any prompting from
the therapist. In her personal and professional relationships there was every
indication that Ethel was a healthy, productive person.

NOTE: the contrast between the mature-looking outreaching child and
the mother, who is vaguely rendered in a way that suggests uncertainty.

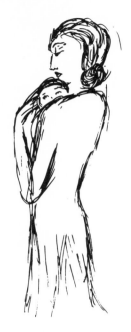

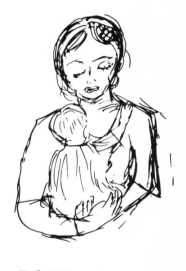

E-4b (6½″ × 4″)

Evelyn
E-4a (8½″ × 3½″)

Evelyn (E-4a and 4b)
Evelyn felt that she had evaded the problem by showing a rear view of the mother and only a bare glimpse of the child. She made the second drawing on her own initiative.

NOTE: the physical closeness achieved in both drawings.

Discussion

There were three kinds of motivation that prompted the twenty-five drawings made by twenty-three patients. For eight patients the mother–child subject was *assigned*, that is, the patient was directed to undertake the drawing of it. For seven others, the subject was *suggested*, it being made very clear that alternatives, whether initiated by the patient or offered by the therapist, were equally acceptable. Thus if the mother–child subject was elected, the choice was free even though prompted. The remaining eight patients spontaneously chose this subject, the choice arising out of either a series of childhood memories or from a discussion of parental relationships. This group includes what we call semispontaneous drawings, those made in response to indirect suggestions. For example, when Arthur recalled his mother singing him to sleep, the therapist asked, "Could you draw that?" and he responded enthusiastically, the wish to make the drawing evidently having already been present.

Responses to Assignment of Subject

Of the eight patients to whom the mother–child subject was assigned, *Albert, Alec, Alicia,* and *Andrew* were chronic psychotics with little capacity for self-exploration and unlikely ever to have undertaken such a drawing on their own initiative. Their drawings are revealing, but only to the viewer. *Beatrice* and *Bertha* caught a glimpse of what may be termed their graphic ambivalence. Beatrice was too ill to make any constructive use of this momentary insight. Bertha had great difficulty in recognizing her own feelings and was assigned the mother–child subject in the hope that some emotion might be stirred up by the drawing. So it seems to have been, but Bertha was too little able to recognize what she had expressed for her to get any real benefit from exploring the strange content of this drawing. Although *Anne* got little out of exploring her drawing at the time, the insights she gained from reexamining it two months later were substantial. In *Conrad's* case the therapist sensed that he was ready for a breakthrough and deliberately assigned the mother–child subject as a means of focusing on his sexual ambivalence which, as had already become apparent, was a major area of concern for him. The results confirmed the correctness of the therapist's decision.

Responses to Suggestion of Subject

The mother–child subject was suggested to seven of the patients whose drawings are illustrated, and it should be mentioned that patients to whom choices including this subject were offered chose others quite frequently. Early in therapy, in a search for the approach that would be most rewarding for the patient, he might be offered choices ranging from fantasy and recollected dreams to drawings of current, actual situations. Appropriate *specific* subjects, on the other hand, are more likely to be suggested when a therapeutic impasse has been reached.

All seven of the patients who chose the alternative of drawing a mother and child from among a number of suggestions had undergone some advance preparation: *Barbara, Basil, Carolyn,* and *Desmond* had discussed and drawn family relationships, and *Belinda* and *Dennis* had also explored feelings about their families but only in words. *Charlie's* drawing grew out of discussion of a drawing he had made in the previous session which represented "a sexually divided person." In Belinda's drawing the extraordinary contrast between the rigid body of the child and the pleasant, relaxed mother (who nevertheless holds the bottle away from her very masculine-looking baby) tempts one to diagnostic inferences. Belinda was referred for art therapy so close to the time of her discharge that family relationships were brought up promptly in the hope that a quick breakthrough might be achieved with this relatively intact person. This hope was not realized. The drawing nevertheless illustrates the kind of graphic response that under more favorable circumstances might have led to substantial gains.

Charlie's drawing was a means of exploring the origins of his sexual ambivalence. As noted earlier, the tentative insights gained in immediate exploration of this drawing were reinforced in later sessions. A striking advantage of the graphic approach is the opportunity to review and explore in greater depth a drawing that the patient was unable to understand fully at an earlier stage of therapy.

Although Carolyn's sense of identity was exceedingly fragile, her overt symptoms always became so mild after a few days in hospital that she was frequently discharged and readmitted, and therefore could not receive any consistent treatment.

Desmond recognized the negative aspects of his feelings about his mother that appeared in his drawing, but resisted the implications as to their childhood origin until his discovery in later sessions that her dominant role in the family was at the root of his sexual inadequacy.

Although Dennis achieved a substantial exploration of childhood memories, these were so consistently negative that a picture of his parents emerged in which it seemed that affection was utterly absent, and open hostility the rule. His adult behavior, too, suggested that the only emotion he knew was anger, as if growing up in a totally hostile environment his only security was associated with direct expression of rage. His drawings could reinforce angry feelings toward his parents he had long been aware of, but he could find nothing positive in any of his graphic explorations.

Results of Spontaneous Choice of Subject

All of the eight patients whose drawings of mother and child emerged spontaneously or semispontaneously achieved some therapeutic progress.

With *Brenda, Arthur,* and *Donald,* this progress was limited. Brenda's therapeutic peak was reached with the illustrated drawing. Almost as soon as she recognized the spider figure as her mother her drawings became less expressive. It seems that the depth of her hostility frightened her. She was never able to recognize the sexual conflicts that were clearly expressed in a concurrent series of drawings. Arthur tackled childhood memories with some vigor, but somewhere along the line therapy failed him, and he regressed to making sterile abstractions. Donald explored a wide range of childhood memories and recurrent and current dreams, reinforcing insights he had gained unaided through his superb intelligence and his capacity for detachment. But his drawings were almost entirely confined to his periods of intellectual control, and even in a panic his drawings were more a means of recovering control than graphic releases of feeling. In the course of eight years his symptoms subsided, but it seems doubtful whether he profited therapeutically from his art sessions.

The remaining five made substantial progress. *Dorothy* derived from art therapy at least a foundation for the gradual improvement she was able to achieve. This followed on her taking part in a form of positive reinforcement group treatment, with a less intensive kind of art therapy as a continuing adjunct.

In *Bessie's* case, the apparent lack of any substantial gain from exploration of her mother–child drawing was deceptive. Returning to this drawing later in her therapy, she recognized it as the starting point of insights she achieved later. Her response had been deeper than it seemed at the time.

In his creative work *Douglas* had already acquired and expressed insights at a symbolic level. In the drawing shown he was able to depict his mother in a direct rather than a symbolic style, but he did not reach this level in representations of his father. Evidence since his discharge suggests that he has become more productive and has been able to cope more successfully with continuing symptoms. *Cynthia* and *Cyril* both followed up their successful mother–child explorations with steady progress.

Some Comparisons

Table I provides too small a sample for statistical analysis so that the pattern it presents of increasingly therapeutic responses to increasingly spontaneous choice of the subject may be deceptively clear. Yet the table also indicates that it is worthwhile to suggest and even to assign the mother–child drawing, in view of the long-term gains achieved by Anne, Conrad, Charlie, and Desmond.

The main point of including the drawings by four nurses who were not in treatment, and for all of whom the subject was assigned, is to illustrate how apparent pathology may emerge from among the drawings of persons who are *not* patients: women who had successfully practiced an exacting profession and were now being trained as specialists in a difficult area. Two of the five drawings present features which, if they appeared in the drawing of a mental patient, might be used as evidence of his pathology. Such evidence, unless reinforced by the patient's own exploration of his drawing under the aegis of a competent psychotherapist, may be grossly misleading.

Edith voiced some of her insecurity but did not relate it to her drawing which, however, provides supporting evidence. *Estelle's* silence on looking at her drawing suggests some apprehension, and the ambivalence and detachment seen in the picture suggest that her concern may have been justified. Yet there was no further reason to suspect any pathology. *Ethel's* drawing is perhaps the most interesting of the group. One may speculate

	SUBJECT ASSIGNED BY THERAPIST	SUBJECT SUGGESTED AMONG ALTERNATIVES	SUBJECT CHOSEN SPONTANEOUSLY BY PATIENT	TOTALS
NO THERAPEUTIC RESULTS	A-1, Albert A-2, Alec A-3, Alicia (a&b) A-4, Andrew 4	0	0	4
LIMITED THERAPEUTIC PROGRESS	B-3, Beatrice B-5, Bertha 2	B-1, Barbara B-2, Basil B-4, Belinda C-1, Carolyn D-1, Dennis 5	A-6, Arthur B-7, Brenda D-3, Donald 3	10
SUBSTANTIAL LONG-TERM THERAPEUTIC GAINS	A-5, Anne C-3, Conrad 2	C-2, Charlie D-2, Desmond 2	B-6, Bessie C-4, Cynthia C-5, Cyril D-4, Dorothy (a&b) D-5, Douglas 5	9
TOTALS	8	7	8	23

Table 1: Therapeutic Results Related to Degree of Spontaneity

about the meaning of a mature and well-defined little person in the arms of an affectionate but weakly rendered and rather vague mother figure. *Evelyn's* two drawings look the healthiest.

Ethel's drawing invites speculation about what might have emerged had she drawn *father* and child. Obviously this is the logical sequel to the mother-and-child drawing. Drawing this subject becomes especially desirable when the father is absent from a series of childhood memories. Frequently, in such instances, the therapist encounters powerful resistance, confirming the significance of the omission.

Yet it is impossible to generalize about the direction in which therapy should move as a sequel to explorations of a mother–child drawing. Nor do we wish to suggest the use of this subject itself as a routine. Rather it exemplifies one of many doors that may be opened occasionally or more often in the course of verbal therapy as well as in art therapy.

The strong reservations we have always felt about the diagnostic use of such drawings remain. Even in so seemingly obvious a case as Edith's we must note that she has succeeded in filling a useful role in society and in coping with the insecurity that threatened her while she was in training. She obtained her certificate and is now working in a hospital where her native language is used. Among patients' drawings it is instructive to study D-3 and D-5, first impressions of which might lead to a completely mistaken diagnostic comparison.

In assisting patients to explore such drawings, facile diagnostic inferences, subtly conveyed by the therapist to the patient, can destroy the usefulness of the work. Yet the temptation is always present and must be dealt with, perhaps by saying to oneself as one sits down beside the patient who has made a seemingly pathological drawing, "This looks really sick. I wonder what we'll *actually* find?" As one learns from experience how frequently such diagnostic judgments are personal projections, this attitude becomes more and more natural.

Conclusion

Drawings of significant subjects appear to be almost equally useful whether they emerge spontaneously or are deliberately assigned. It is our hope that, by presenting the concrete example of responses to a single subject, we may reach psychotherapists who have hitherto shied away from using such procedures merely out of their unfamiliarity with art.

People in the field of art and the obscure discipline of esthetics associated with it are indeed sometimes characterized by preciousness or even arrogance to a degree which naturally makes the uninitiated feel excluded. Yet when one looks at these mother–child drawings there is no esthetic or artistic wall between them and the viewer. If there is any complexity it is that of feelings with which we are all familiar: the relationship between a mother and her child. Experience in encouraging patients to explore their drawings certainly makes the therapist better able to promote maximum therapeutic use of the procedure, but this requires a training no more esoteric—possibly less so—than do purely verbal techniques of psychotherapy. Indeed, all the therapist learns about the drawing is taught him by the patient; beyond that lie mere surmise and conjecture. It is even possible that an individual with no artistic background or inclinations might be better able to help a patient explore his graphic production than another person whose preconceptions, developed out of long familiarity with art, could prove to be a handicap.

In short, although there may be a few patients who cannot, for various reasons, enter this therapeutic door, there are surely no psychotherapists— whatever technique they may rely on primarily—who cannot show their patients that there is such a door, and at least occasionally encourage them to open it and make a brief exploratory excursion within.

An Experiment Dealing with Color and Emotion

Rebecca R. Crane

Much has been written about the possible emotional impact of color on the individual. Rorschach color theory, which has been prominent in this discussion, derives from Rorschach's discoveries that percepts motivated by color alone correlate with inability to control primitive impulses while percepts motivated primarily by form coincide with controlled emotion.

Attempts to verify these conclusions by direct experimentation with the Rorschach test have been rather inconclusive because of the extreme difficulty in controlling all possible variables which might influence results. A number of investigators of basic theory[1] have reached the conclusion that people reacting primarily to the color on the blot are reflecting a lack of detachment in their emotional experience as well as considerable passivity. They found that those who have greater organizing energy tend to emphasize form over color in their imagery.

Outside of research with the Rorschach, others have experimented with color-sorting tests and geometric designs. One very interesting study by Oeser[2] combined the two, along with Rorschach evaluation of the personality of the subjects. Oeser showed subjects a standard which consisted of a red triangle. This was projected briefly on a screen. He then showed them a group of colored forms arranged in a circle. One of these was a green triangle and opposite it was a red square. The other forms were non-red and non-triangle. After a brief exposure he asked the subjects to locate the standard. Two groups of people resulted, one drawn to the form pole and the other to the color pole. Subsequent testing by the Rorschach showed that the form-dominated gave no color responses, or very few, while the

1. David Shapiro, "Color-Response and Perceptual Passivity," *Journal of Progressive Technology*, Vol. 20, 1956, pp. 52–69.
2. O. A. Oeser, "Some Experiments on the Abstraction of Form and Color," Parts I and II, *British Journal of Psychology*, Vol. 22, 1932, pp. 200–215, 287–323.

color-dominated gave many color responses, the form of which bore scant resemblance to the actual blot. The personality structure of the two groups also differed markedly. The form-dominated were more precise and specific, more inhibited and controlled. The color-dominated were more spontaneous, more expansive and extroverted.

Choice of color has been another aspect for investigation. Working with children of different ages, Alschuler and Hattwick[3] clearly demonstrated that the colors used by children in painting shifted with age as the personality developed, and that color preference was related to the personality.

Wexner[4] attempted to show a relationship between color and mood by associating color with words that have emotional significance. Her results are expressed as frequencies of choice in a rather abstract experimental situation, and no attempt was made to scale the emotional value of the colors.

Since reaction to colors appears to have significance for the way in which a personality functions, and since research has by no means solved the place of color in personality theory, the present experiment was undertaken to study the association between colors and specific emotional situations. The experiment was carried out at a university with 134 undergraduate students in psychology courses as the subjects. There were 72 men and 62 women.

Eight questions having emotional implications were selected. Two implied a strong-pleasant emotional experience; two implied pleasant emotional experience that was mild in nature; two portrayed strong-unpleasant emotional experience; and, finally, two denoted emotional experiences that were unpleasant but relatively mild. To illustrate, one question was: "Which man has just won a hotly contested election?" (strong-pleasant). Another was: "Which man has just bumped his knee on the door?" (mild-unpleasant). It was planned to associate each of these situations with the colors: violet, blue, green, yellow, orange, and red.

To bring out the emotional content and ensure an emotional context for the response, the colors appeared on cards in the silhouette shape of men, identical in every respect except for the color. Since the study was not concerned primarily with the physical properties of color, but with the phenomenology of color, it seemed best to use those which are generally accepted as red, yellow, etc., instead of trying to equalize brightness and saturation. After studying samples carefully, the investigators selected poster paints in spectrum colors because they are easily applied and give a clear, flat, and even surface.

3. R. H. Alschuler and L. A. Hattwick, "Easel Painting as an Index of Personality in Preschool Children," *American Journal of Orthopsychiatry*, Vol. 13, 1943, pp. 616–625.

4. Lois Wexner, "The Degree to Which Colors (Hues) Are Associated with Mood-Tones," *Journal of Applied Psychology*, Vol. 38, No. 6, 1954, pp. 432–435.

The cards with the colored male figures were placed in pairs, one pair at a time, on the chalk ledge of the blackboard in a classroom. The one to the left was under a large letter A, and the one to the right was under a large letter B. The subjects were asked to choose between them in response to the question asked. Altogether, the 134 subjects made 2,010 choices for each question, with a grand total of 16,080 choices for all eight. Then, some rather intricate statistical procedures were needed to obtain values for each of the colors in relation to each specific emotional situation which had been presented. These values could then be placed along scale intervals on a graph so that the results could be visualized.

The results were impressive and clear. All of the colors were distributed rather nicely along the scales instead of being bunched at either end. On the color scales related to questions which had been judged to be pleasant, yellow and orange have the highest values while violet has the lowest. These scale positions are almost entirely reversed for the unpleasant questions. Violet has the highest value for the two strongly unpleasant questions with yellow and orange the lowest. There is some variation when the mildly unpleasant questions are considered but the pattern can be clearly seen. Red has the highest value here, but violet is next to it. The light colors, in terms of brightness, are evidently important for pleasantness while the reverse is true for unpleasantness where violet and red are emphasized with blue a close second.

If the results are examined in more detail, some very interesting facts emerge. Both of the strongly unpleasant questions are concerned with death and they have exactly the same scale positions for the colors from top to bottom with violet the highest, blue next, then red. In the two mildly unpleasant questions, which are concerned with minor frustrations, the red is at the top, then violet, then orange. It is interesting to note that when annoyance is involved rather than grief and despair, red moves up on the scale and displaces violet. This conforms to the popular notion that one sees red when he is angry.

Another variation is seen in the scales for the pleasant questions which seems to have significance. Here the scale for one that was judged strongly pleasant is more like one that was judged mildly pleasant than either is like the other one in its own category. On studying these two questions it is observed that they are very similar in nature. Both are concerned with pleasurable anticipation. In one, the man is anticipating an adventurous voyage around the world; in the other, he is about to go fishing. The judges decided that the emotional experience was stronger in anticipating the voyage than the fishing trip, but the scales are almost identical. The only difference is the reversal of the blue and green positions which are very close together on both scales and exactly in the middle, with two colors above and two below them.

Obviously, the kind of emotional experience is an important factor in determining scale positions of colors, and it seems to be of greater significance than the strength of the emotion involved. The emotional meaning of each association is important but more experimentation is needed to determine the specific implication of each of the colors for personality.

Another point that has not been approached in this study is the relation of cause and effect. While the results obtained support the theory that certain colors are associated with specific emotional situations, the experiment made no effort to determine what brought about this relationship. Was it the result of cultural influences, an organic or neurological predisposition, or a combination of several such factors? There is need for much more research into the associations found between colors and emotional experience.

Contributors

Suzanne Israel Black holds an M.A. in art therapy from The George Washington University in Washington, D.C. Now devoting her time to raising her child, she worked earlier with abused and neglected children temporarily placed at the Children's Shelter of Essex County in Belleville, New Jersey.

Walter Carter is a student in the Master of Arts degree program in art therapy at The George Washington University in Washington, D.C., and is teaching art in a public school in Arlington, Virginia. Formerly an art instructor at Bloomsburg State College in Bloomsburg, Pennsylvania, he was greatly influenced by his correspondence with Margaret Naumburg.

Susan Castelluccio—see Susan Castelluccio-Michal.

Susan Castelluccio-Michal, ATR, is an art teacher in the Interrelated Arts Program of the Montgomery County, Maryland, public schools. A graduate of the Master of Arts degree program in art therapy at The George Washington University, Ms. Michal has worked with children with a variety of handicapping conditions.

Drew Conger earned her M.A. in the Master of Arts degree program in art therapy at The George Washington University and is an art therapist at the Geriatric Day Care Center of the Downtown Cluster in Washington, D.C. She works with both physically and mentally disabled adults.

Rebecca R. Crane, now retired, was a research assistant in clinical psychology at Georgetown University in Washington, D.C., at the time this article was written.

Henriette de Knegt is employed as an art therapist at a county hospital. She works with both mentally retarded and schizophrenic adults.

Irene W. Dewdney, ATR, has had extensive experience as an art therapist at various treatment centers in southwestern Ontario, Canada, where she and her husband, Selwyn Dewdney, pioneered the picture-centered group session. At present she serves as a consultant with the Western Ontario Therapeutic Community Hostel and conducts an art therapy training program, as well as a private practice.

Selwyn Dewdney developed various art therapy approaches in several mental health facilities in southwestern Ontario, Canada, between 1947 and 1972. Later he lectured on Amerindian art in Canada at the Ontario College of Art in Toronto, and was associated with the Royal Ontario Museum's Department of New World Archaeology.

Judith Finer, ATR, is assistant professor of art therapy at Salem College and art therapist at the Mandala Center, a private psychiatric hospital, both in Winston-Salem, North Carolina. She received her M.A. in art therapy from The George Washington University in Washington, D.C.

Sondra Kitt Geller, currently a candidate for an M.A. in art therapy at The George Washington University in Washington, D.C., is a former teacher of French. She serves as editor of the Newsletter of the Potomac Art Therapy Association in the Washington, D.C., area.

Lena L. Gitter received training in Europe in the Montessori method of educating children. For many years a teacher in Montessori schools, she now serves as a Montessori consultant and lecturer. A staunch advocate of preschool education for the poor and of day care centers, Ms. Gitter was awarded a medallion for her services by the International Montessori Commemorative Committee.

Susan E. Gonick-Barris, ATR, is director of art therapy studies in the Fine Arts Department at Montclair State College, New Jersey, and a doctoral candidate at Columbia University in New

York City. Ms. Gonick-Barris studied with Dr. Laura Perls and has a master's degree in art therapy from Pratt Institute. Her award-winning paintings have been widely exhibited.

Brian Halsey, a full-time painter and printmaker whose works have been exhibited throughout the United States and in France and Switzerland, earned a B.A. in art from Wheaton College in Wheaton, Illinois, an M.A. in church history and the creative arts from Trinity Divinity School in Deerfield, Illinois, and a Ph.D. in humanities from Florida State University in Tallahassee.

Margaret C. Howard, ATR, now retired, worked as director of art therapy at Children's Medical Center in Tulsa, Oklahoma. She has also lectured extensively on art therapy at several educational and clinical settings in the Midwest. Her training in art therapy included study with Margaret Naumburg at New York University in New York City.

Suzanne Israel—see Suzanne Israel Black.

Norman Jones is currently director of Early Childhood Services of the CATCH Community Mental Health/Mental Retardation Center in Philadelphia. A past-president of the Delaware Valley chapter of the Association of Black Psychologists, Mr. Jones is a contributor to *Mental Health: A Challenge to the Black Community,* published in 1978.

Carolyn Refsnes Kniazzeh, ATR, a graduate of Wellesley College who received art therapy training from Margaret Naumburg, is a doctoral candidate at New York University. An art therapist in private practice, Ms. Kniazzeh is also an exhibiting painter.

Edith Kramer, ATR, HLM, painter, sculptor, and author of three books and numerous articles on art therapy with children, teaches in the Master of Arts degree programs in art therapy at The George Washington University in Washington, D.C., and New York University in New York City. She also serves as assistant professor of child psychiatry at Albert Einstein College of Medicine, Bronx, New York.

Hanna Yaxa Kwiatkowska, ATR, HLM, is an associate professor of art therapy at The George Washington University, Washington, D.C., and a visiting professor at the Catholic University of Rio de Janeiro, Brazil. Known for her writings, research, and pioneering clinical work in family art therapy, she introduced the art therapy program at the National Institute of Mental Health and directed it for twelve years. Her sculpture has been exhibited in the United States, Europe, and Brazil. She is the author of *Family Therapy and Evaluation Through Art.*

Mildred Lachman—see Mildred Lachman-Chapin.

Mildred Lachman-Chapin, ATR, director of activity services at the Barclay Hospital in Chicago, Illinois, earned a master's degree from the American University in Washington, D.C., and trained in art therapy at the Washington School of Psychiatry. She has taught art therapy at the university level, given workshops and demonstrations throughout the country, served as a consultant, and maintained a private practice.

Bernard I. Levy, Ph.D., FAPA, ATR, HLM, holds his doctorate in psychology from the University of Rochester, New York. He is currently professor of psychology at The George Washington University in Washington, D.C., where he also directs the Master of Arts degree program in art therapy. A watercolor painter and teacher of the art, Dr. Levy is also the author of many research articles concerning art therapy.

Claire A. Levy was trained as an English teacher in New York University. She has served the *American Journal of Art Therapy* as editorial assistant for eighteen years and as book editor for seven.

Saul Lishinsky, ATR, a practicing artist who trained at the Art Students League in New York City and with Hans Hoffmann in Provincetown, Massachusetts, works as an art therapist in a community mental health center in New York City. He is also the founder and director of Bronx Community Murals, Inc., which creates and promotes a public form of fine art.

Lee B. Macht, M.D., is professor and chairman, Department of Psychiatry, Harvard Medical School, and chief of psychiatry, the Cambridge Hospital.

Hilde Meyerhoff, ATR, earned a B.A. in psychology and art at the University of California at Los Angeles. Since moving to Israel in 1965, she has held several institutional art therapy positions and is at present in private practice. She lectures widely on art therapy and art psychotherapy, and has published a number of articles in the field.

Susan C. Michal—see Susan Castellucio-Michal.

Margaret Naumburg, ATR, HLM, is recognized internationally as a pioneer in the field of art therapy and has published many books and articles on the subject. A certified psychologist and a psychotherapist specializing in analytically oriented art therapy. Ms. Naumburg was the founder and first director of the progressive Walden School in New York City.

Geraldine A. Nestingen studied art therapy at The George Washington University in Washington, D.C. At present she serves as a part-time art therapist at Georgetown Hospital in Washington, D.C., and as a staff assistant in the Washington office of Congressman John M. Murphy.

Carolyn Refsnes—see Carolyn Refsnes Kniazzeh.

Janie Rhyne, Ph.D., ATR, earned her doctorate in psychology from the University of California at Santa Cruz in 1979. Author of *The Gestalt Art Experience*, Dr. Rhyne is currently assistant professor at the Institute of the Expressive Therapies at the University of Louisville in Kentucky, teaching and conducting research linking personal constructs with expressive form in visual communication.

Edna Salant, ATR, has served since 1969 as consultant in art therapy at the National Child Research Center, a large, private preschool in Washington, D.C. Her discussion paper for the International Year of the Child on "Play and Art Therapy with the Very Young Child" has been translated into French and Spanish, and will be made available around the world.

Stewart R. Smith, M.D., was formerly an instructor in psychiatry at the Harvard Medical School. He is now in the private practice of psychiatry and psychoanalysis in Boston, Massachusetts.

Linda St. Germain earned an M.A. in art therapy at The George Washington University. Formerly a professional graphic artist, she has also worked as a crisis counselor and publications director for the Rape Crisis Center in Washington, D.C.

Elizabeth Cohn Stuntz was a psychiatric social worker at the Woodburn Center for Community Mental Health in Fairfax, Virginia, and has done volunteer work in a variety of community organizations. She holds a master's degree from Smith College School for Social Work.

Lauri Tanner studied art therapy in the Master of Arts degree program at The George Washington University, Washington, D.C.

Jane Teller, ATR, is a professional artist whose wood sculptures have been widely exhibited. Ms. Teller prepared for art therapy by studying with Margaret Naumburg and with E. S. Weber, M.D., a psychiatrist on the staff of Princeton Hospital, New Jersey. She works as an art therapist at the Carrier Clinic in Belle Meade, New Jersey, and at the New Jersey Neuropsychiatric Institute.

Elinor Ulman, ATR, HLM, is an associate professor and coordinator of training in the Master of Arts degree program in art therapy of The George Washington University, Washington, D.C. In 1961 she founded the *Bulletin of Art Therapy* which, as the *American Journal of Art Therapy,* she continues to edit and publish. She has done clinical work in a variety of settings and contributed numerous articles in the field, some of which are included in two books, *Art Therapy in Theory and Practice* and *Art Therapy Viewpoints,* of both of which she was the senior editor.

Anna Wagner serves as art therapist at the Olomana School, a public alternative high school on Windward Oahu, and in the Expressive Arts Program of the Human Services Department of Castle Hospital in Kailua, Hawaii. In the past she has taught introductory courses in art therapy at Hawaii Loa College and Chaminade College in Hawaii.

Katherine J. Williams, ATR, teaches in the Master of Arts degree program in art therapy at The George Washington University in Washington, D.C., where she earned her M.A. in art therapy, and Vermont College of Norwich University in Montpelier, Vermont. She serves as consultant in art therapy at Walter Reed Army Medical Center in Washington, D.C., and also maintains a private practice.

Laurie Wilson, Ph.D., ATR, is director of the graduate training program in art therapy at New York University, and art therapist at the Jewish Board of Family and Child Services, both in New York City. She collaborated with Edith Kramer on *Childhood and Art Therapy: Notes on Theory and Application.*

Betty L. Zeiger, ATR, holds master's degrees in painting from American University and in art therapy from The George Washington University, both in Washington, D.C. She is supervising art therapist at the Hebrew Home of Greater Washington in Rockville, Maryland, and has served as a visiting consultant in art therapy at the Jerusalem Mental Health Center in Israel. Her paintings have been widely exhibited.

Index

Acrylic paints, 267, 268
Aged and art therapy, 187–94
Aggression
  and control, 17–26
  and constructive energy, 14, 26, 31
  in human relationships, 14
  nature of, 14
  venting of, 15–17
Alphabet learning and the mentally retarded, 234–35
Alschuler and Hattwick study, 359
American Art Therapy Association, 34
American Journal of Art Therapy, 4, 188
Analysis of drawings
  by mentally retarded patients, 55–65
  of mother-child relationship, 351–57
  by psychiatric patients, 70–80, 83–84, 111–13
Angry drum, 235–38
Anti-art, 4
Art
  anti-, 4
  definition of, 4
  and the demands of the artistic process, 40–41
  Freud on, 85–95
  function of, 41
  importance of quality in, 36
  integrative character of, 41
  and maturation, 40–41
  nature of, and mental health, 174
  pseudo-, 43
  rehabilitative use of, 174–86
  and the value of symbolizing, 34
Art as Therapy in a Group Setting: The Stories of Batja and Rina, 214–31
Art education
  activities for, 42–44
  and alphabet learning, 234–35
  distinction from art therapy, 39
  for the emotionally disturbed, 38–46
  goal of, 41
  history of, 45–46
  and learning problems of minimal brain dysfunction, 199–200

teaching requirements for, 41–42, 44–45
Art Education for the Emotionally Disturbed, 38–46
Art for Children with Minimal Brain Dysfunction, 197–213
Art in a Class for Mentally Retarded Children, 232–45
An Art Therapist Looks at Her Professional History, 102–05
Art therapists
  basic task of, 6
  and the bicameral mind, 34–37
  in community mental health center, 174–86
  description of patient-therapist relationship, 106–18
  for the elderly, 176, 177, 187–94, 249–52
  Gestalt, 8
  and judging psychopathology from paintings, 316–20
  Jungian, 8
  and the mentally retarded, 48–49
  and minimal brain dysfunction, 197–213
  and the parent-child relationship, 69–81
  and psychiatric illness, 153–73
  and the use of slides, 138–52
Art therapy
  and aggression, 14–31
  for alcoholics, 268
  and basic task of art therapist, 6
  and the bicameral mind, 32–37
—*for children:* aggressive child, 15–31; focus of art therapy with, 10–11; handicapped, 103–04; in hospital setting, 214–31; mentally retarded, 49–53; with minimal brain dysfunction, 197–213; as psychiatric patients, 105; of separated parents, 282–93
—*color in:* and the bicameral mind, 33, coloring-in of scribble, 308; and communication, 268; and emotion, 358–61; meaning of sharp contrasts, 180–81; and the mentally retarded, 57, 62; and minimal brain dysfunction, 206; and rehabilitation